Imaging of the Spine

A TEACHING FILE

Imaging of the Spine

A TEACHING FILE

MAURICIO CASTILLO, M.D.

Professor of Radiology
Chief of Neuroradiology
The University of North Carolina School of Medicine
Chapel Hill, North Carolina

JOHN H. HARRIS, JR., M.D., D.SC., F.A.C.R.

Professor and Chief, Emergency Radiology
John S. Dunn Distinguished Chair in Radiology
Professor, Emergency Medicine
The University of Texas Houston Medical School
Houston, Texas

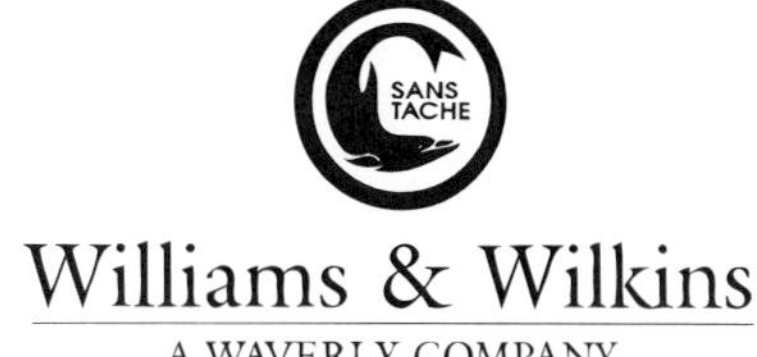

Williams & Wilkins
A WAVERLY COMPANY

BALTIMORE • PHILADELPHIA • LONDON • PARIS • BANGKOK
BUENOS AIRES • HONG KONG • MUNICH • SYDNEY • TOKYO • WROCLAW

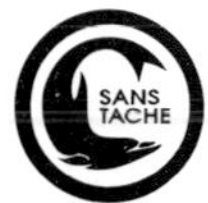

Editor: Charles W. Mitchell
Managing Editor: Marjorie Kidd Keating
Production Coordinator: Raymond E. Reter
Project Editor: Kathleen Gilbert
Design Coordinator: Mario Fernandez
Illustration Planner: Maryland Composition Co., Inc.
Typesetter/Digitized Illustrations: Maryland Composition Co., Inc.
Printer/Binder: RR Donnelley & Sons Company

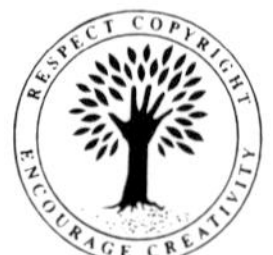

Library of Congress Cataloging-in-Publication Data

Castillo, Mauricio.
    Imaging of the spine : a teaching file / Mauricio Castillo, John H. Harris, Jr.
      p.   cm.
    Includes bibliographical references and index.
    ISBN 0-683-30244-2
    1. Spine—Imaging—Case studies.   I. Harris, John H., 1925– .
  II. Title
    [DNLM: 1. Spinal Diseases—radiography—case studies. 2. Spinal Injuries—
radiography—case studies.   WE 725 C352i 1998]
    RD768.C38   1998
    617.5′607572—dc21
    DNLM/DLC
    for Library of Congress   97-44168
                                               CIP

Con cariño para mi madre. A pesar de la distancia que nos separa, nuestros corazones permanecen juntos.

M.C.

To my grandchildren—Emily, C.J., Ben, and Chelsea—with love.

J.H.H., Jr.

Teaching Files are one of the hallmarks of education in Diagnostic Radiology. There has long been a need for a comprehensive series of books, using the Teaching File format, that would provide the kind of personal "consultation with the experts" normally found only in the setting of a teaching hospital. Williams & Wilkins is proud to have created such a series. Our goal is to provide the resident and practicing radiologist with a useful resource that answers this need.

Actual cases have been culled from extensive teaching files in major medical centers. The discussions presented mimic those performed on a daily basis between residents and faculty members in all radiology departments.

The format of the books is designed so that each case can be studied as an unknown, if desired. A consistent format is used to present each case. A brief clinical history is given, followed by several images. Then, relevant findings, differential diagnosis, and final diagnosis are given, followed by a discussion of the case. The authors thereby guide the reader through the interpretation of each case.

We hope that this series will become a valuable and trusted teaching tool for radiologists at any stage of training or practice, and that it will also be a benefit to clinicians whose patients undergo these imaging studies.

The Publisher
Williams & Wilkins

PREFACE

The purpose of this book is to illustrate and descibe both common and unusual disorders involving the spine. We have used cases from our personal collections as well as from the teaching archives at both of our institutions. The illustrations used here were chosen because they demonstrate the most common imaging features of the disorders discussed. We hope that the material chosen will reflect real-life cases, hopefully similar to those found at the view box every day.

The format for this book is simple. The reader may use it as an "unknown" casebook or for a review. Each case begins with a short description of the entity presented and then addresses the imaging findings. For each entity, examples from one or more cases were used. We have tried to label the most important findings in each figure without giving the case away, thereby preserving the ability to use this book for a self-examination. Differential diagnoses are discussed only when pertinent. In some cases, the imaging tends to be pathognomonic of the pathology, and there should be only one diagnosis. Each discussion is short but provides the reader with a basic understanding of the disorder shown.

The cases are grouped into seven chapters, making it easy to review specific areas of spinal imaging according to the reader's interest. The illustrations for all of the cases reflect what is now considered state of the art in spinal imaging. Therefore, the section on trauma is heavily weighted toward radiographs and computed tomography (CT), while the remaining sections use mostly CT and magnetic resonance imaging.

It is our desire that readers find this book fun. We have tried to acknowledge all of those persons who provided us with some of the cases. Any omission is unintended and we apologize for it.

Mauricio Castillo, M.D.
John H. Harris, Jr., M.D.

CONTENTS

chapter 1

DEGENERATIVE SPINE DISORDERS

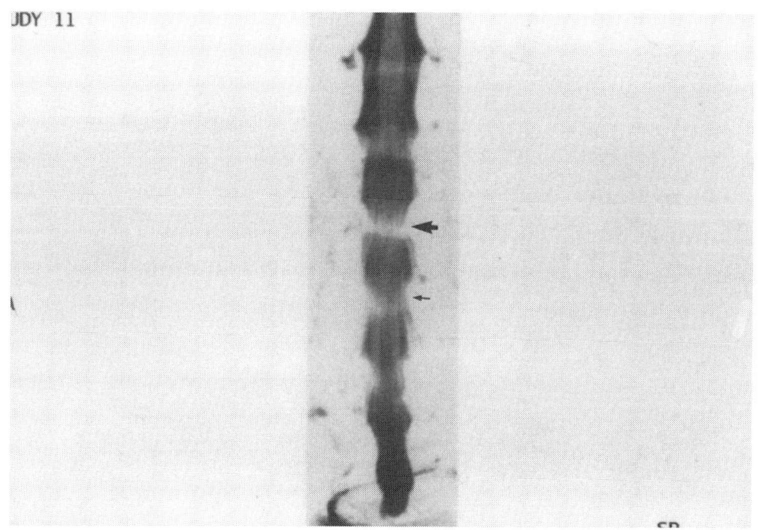

CASE 1

Clinical History: 55-year-old female with bilateral lower extremity pain and a mild weakness that worsens after walking more than two blocks.

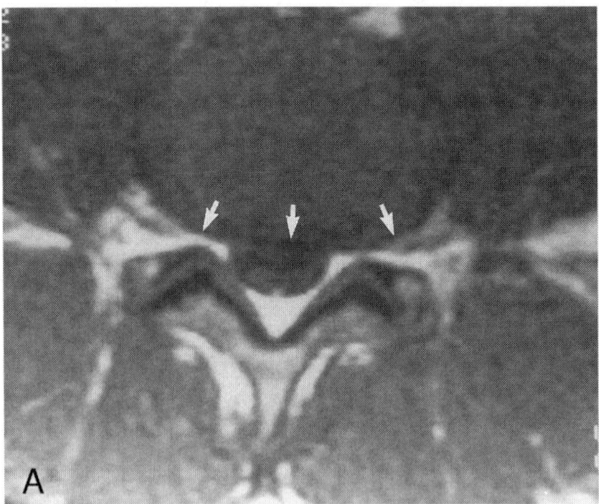

Figure 1.1 A

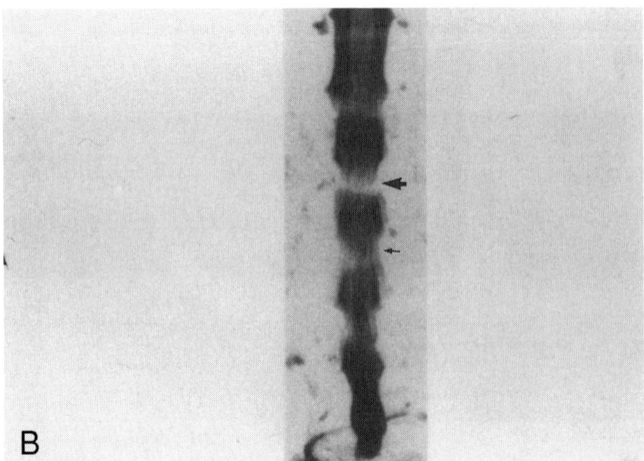

Figure 1.1 B

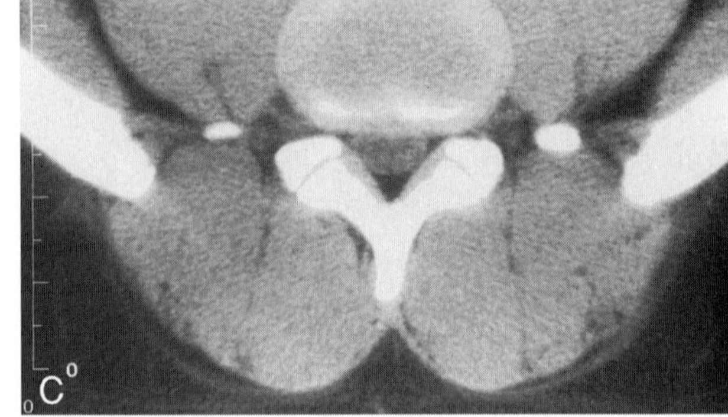

Figure 1.1 C

Findings: Axial MR T1-weighted image (Fig. A) shows central lumbar stenosis at the level of L3-L4. The thecal sac is narrowed in its anteroposterior diameter by a disk bulge (arrows) and mild degeneration of facet joints. MR myelogram shows constriction of the thecal sac at L3-L4 (larger arrow) and a similar, but less severe abnormality, at L4-L5 (smaller arrow) (Fig. B). Axial CT (Fig. C) at same level as Fig. A shows the diffuse disk bulge equally well.

Diagnosis: Acquired central spinal canal stenosis.

Discussion: The patient exhibits the classical clinical features of neurologic claudication. Neurologic claudication generally improves in a recumbent position and, unlike vascular claudication, it may increase with the patient standing still.

Acquired central spinal canal stenosis generally occurs in the lumbar region and is multifactorial. Degenerative changes result in bulging or herniated disks, which in combination with a thickened ligamentum flavum (actually buckling as ligaments do not undergo hypertrophy) and overgrowth of the facet joints, leads to compression of the spinal canal. Classically the thecal sac assumes a triangular configuration in axial imaging in cases of central stenosis. Surgery involves unroofing of the spinal canal by removal of the posterior elements, and if the facet joint hypertrophy has narrowed the lateral recesses, partial facetectomies may be indicated.

Unlike acquired spinal stenosis, congenital stenosis occurs secondary to bone dysplasias, Morquio disease, and achondroplasia. In these patients, the pedicles are short.

CASE 2

Clinical History: The following three patients all present with chronic low back pain.

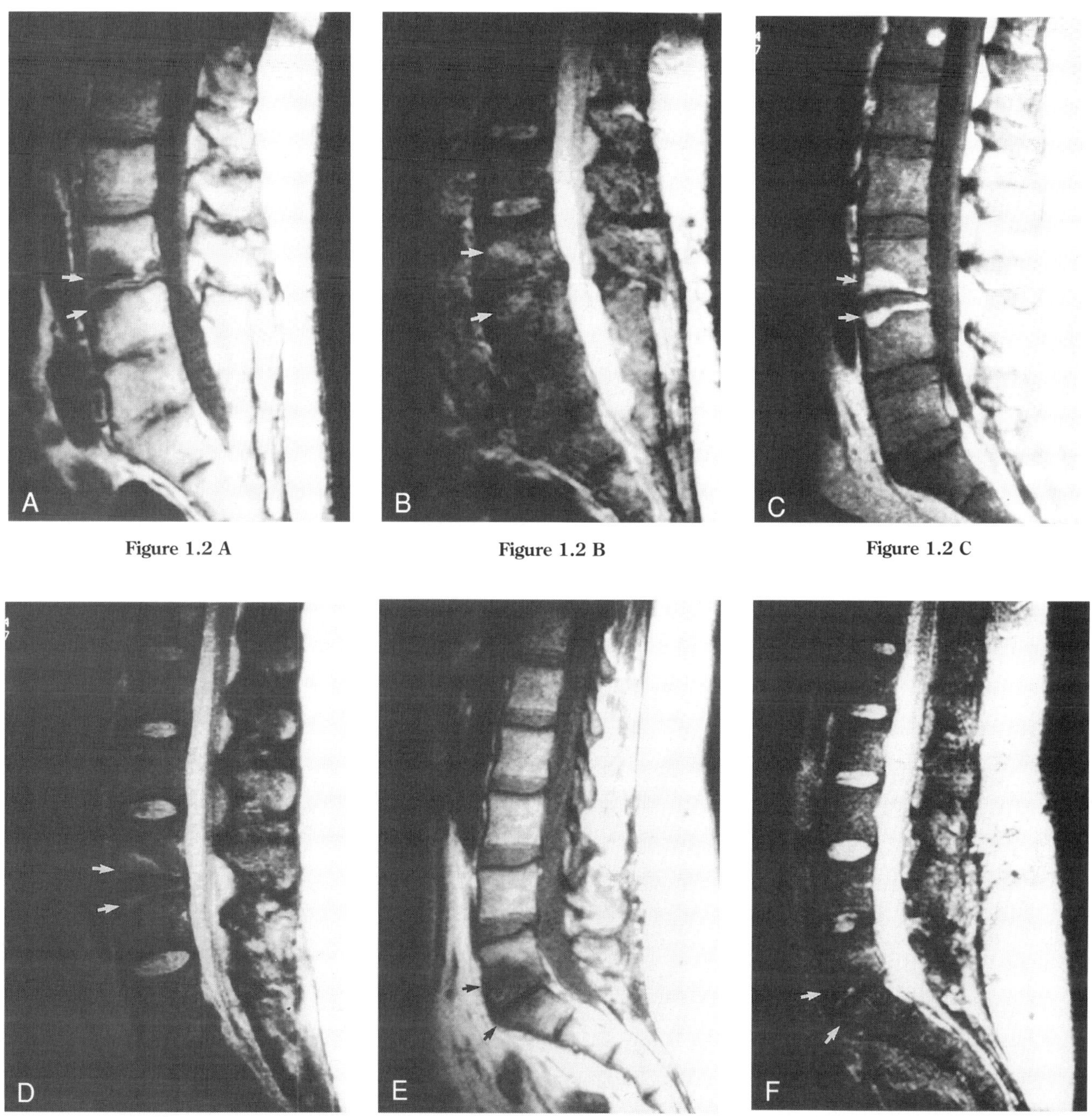

Figure 1.2 A   Figure 1.2 B   Figure 1.2 C

Figure 1.2 D   Figure 1.2 E   Figure 1.2 F

Findings: Midsagittal MR T1-weighted image (Fig. A) in the first patient shows decreased height of the L3-L4 disk. There is low signal intensity (arrows) in the anterior aspect of the inferior end-plate of L3 and the superior end-plate of L4. Corresponding T2-weighted image shows the end-plate abnormalities (arrows) to be bright (Fig. B). Midsagittal MR T1-weighted image (Fig. C) in patient #2 shows high signal intensity in the end-plates (arrows) abutting the L3-L4 disk. On a corresponding T2-weighted image (Fig. D) these changes (arrows) are of low signal intensity. The L3-L4 disk is hypointense. In the third patient, midsagittal MR T1-weighted image (Fig. E) shows low signal intensity from the end-plates (arrows) abutting the L5-S1 disk. On a corresponding T2-weighted image (Fig. F) the end-plates (arrows) remain hypointense.

(continued)

Diagnosis: Vertebral end-plate changes secondary to degenerative disease.

Discussion: The clinical significance of degenerative changes in the vertebral end-plates is uncertain. Some patients may have a nonspecific low back pain while others are asymptomatic. By MR imaging, changes in the end-plates may be divided according to the Modic classification. Early on, the end-plates are infiltrated by water (edema) and as such are of low T1 signal intensity and of high T2 signal intensity. This appearance is similar to that of early infectious diskitis. These type 1 changes may progress and the end-plates become infiltrated by fat. As such, they are of high T1 signal intensity and of low T2 signal intensity (particularly using conventional spin echo). These type 2 changes may also progress and the end-plates become infiltrated by fibrous tissues and new bone formation. This is reflected by low T1 and T2 signal intensity. Type 3 changes are seen on radiographs as end-plate sclerosis. In all of these changes, the corresponding disk tends to be hypointense on T2-weighted images.

CASE 3

Clinical History: 45-year-old male with low back pain and mild lower extremity weakness.

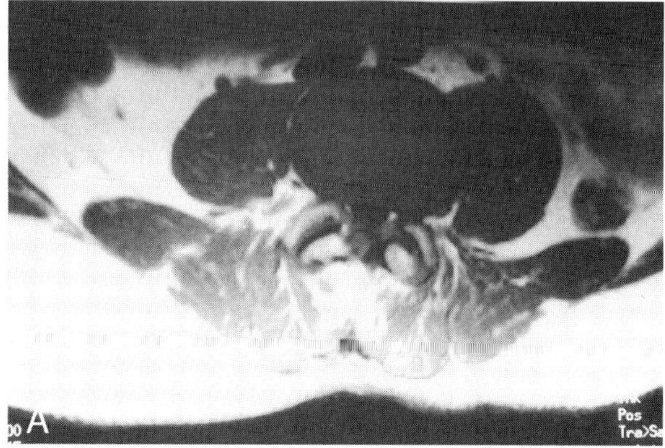

Figure 1.3 A

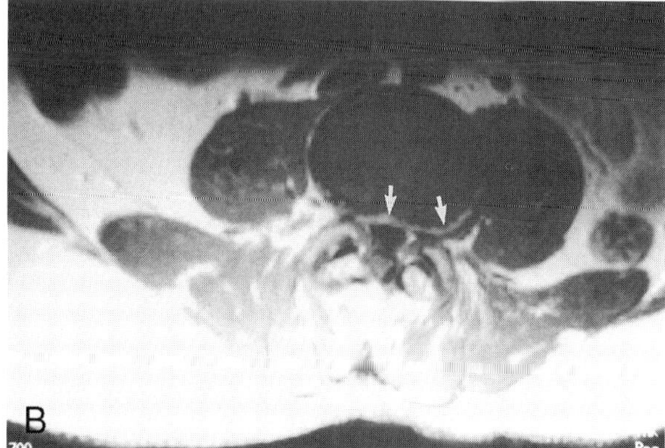

Figure 1.3 B

Findings: Axial precontrast MR T1-weighted image (Fig. A) at L4-L5 shows a diffuse bulging disk, mild thickening of the ligamentum flavum, and facet joint hypertrophy resulting in central stenosis. Corresponding postcontrast image (Fig. B) shows peripheral and curvilinear enhancement (arrows) of the posterior disk margin.

Diagnosis: Acquired central spinal canal stenosis with an enhancing radial annular tear.

Discussion: Bulging disks occur secondary to a generalized relaxation of the annulus fibrosus. As such, they are diffuse and are not focal defects. A bulging disk may be defined as one that extends at least 3 mm beyond the margins of the corresponding vertebral end plates. Many of them are associated with radial (circumferential) tears of the annulus fibrosus. T2-weighted images have a sensitivity close to 70% (when compared with microtome sections) in the detection of annular tears. These appear as focal areas of increased T2 signal intensity in the posterior annulus. In an attempt to repair the tear, there is proliferation of granulation tissue that grows into the tear. The relative hypervascularity of this granulation tissue leads to enhancement after gadolinium administration.

Clinical History: 40-year-old male with sudden onset of low back pain and bilateral S1 radiculopathy.

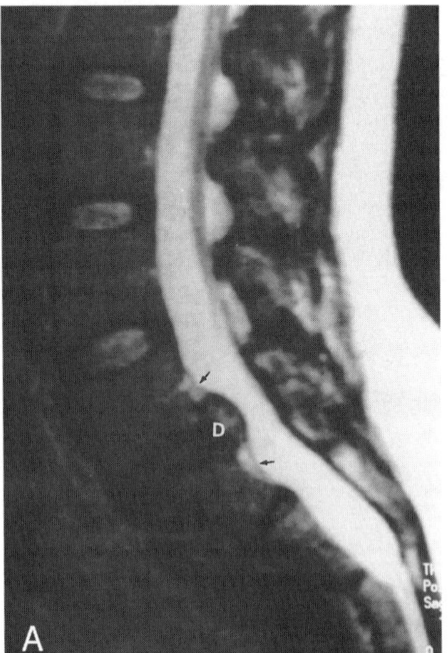

Figure 1.4 A

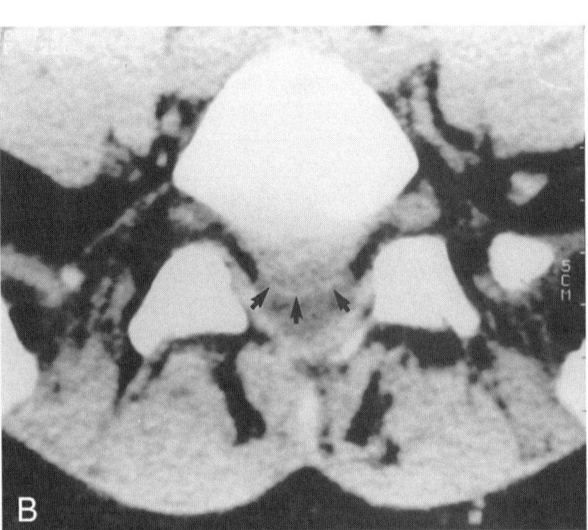

Figure 1.4 B

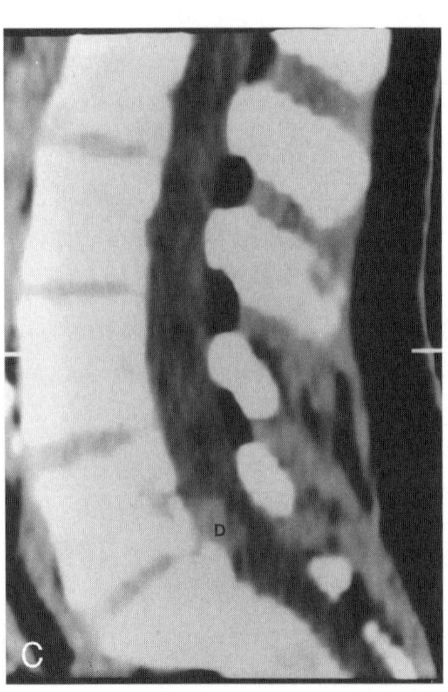

Figure 1.4 C

Findings: Midsagittal MR T2-weighted image (Fig. A) shows a central herniated disk (D) at the L5-S1 level. Note that the herniated fragment is slightly hyperintense to the parent disk. The posterior longitudinal ligament (arrows) is elevated, implying that this herniated disk is subligamentous. CT 3-mm thick axial section (Fig. B) in the same patient also clearly shows the central disk herniation (arrows). Midsagittal CT reformation nicely shows the disk herniation (d) (Fig. C) and loss of height of the parent disk.

(continued)

Diagnosis: Central disk herniation at L5-S1.

Discussion: Herniated disks represent extrusion of the nucleus pulposus through a transverse tear in the annulus fibrosus. In the lumbar region, they are more common at the L4-L5, L5-S1, and L3-L4 levels. They usually compress the nerve roots one level below them. If the posterior longitudinal ligament is intact, they are considered to be subligamentous. Subligamentous herniated disks may be central or eccentric. Eccentricity may be secondary to the presence of a dense fibrous septum, which attaches the posterior longitudinal ligament to the midline of the vertebrae and the annuli. Herniated disks may migrate inferiorly or superiorly with equal frequency. High T2 signal intensity is not uncommon in herniated disk fragments. Its etiology is uncertain, but may be related to increased water content. Some investigators recommend initial screening of the patient with low back pain using only sagittal and axial fast spin echo T2-weighted images of the spine. This may allow for a lesser fee and increased utilization of an MR unit. However, if abnormalities are identified, a complete set of images is indicated.

CASE 5

Clinical History: 35-year-old male with a sudden onset of low back pain and a right S1 radiculopathy following weight lifting.

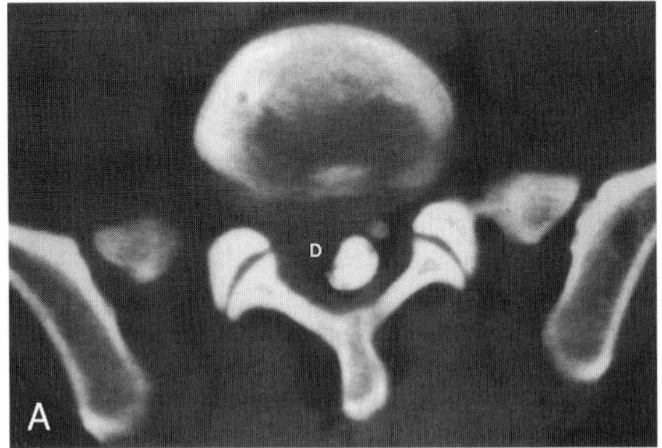

Figure 1.5 A

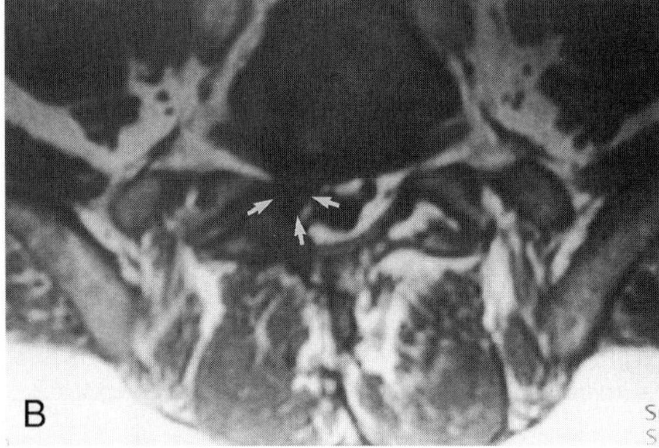

Figure 1.5 B

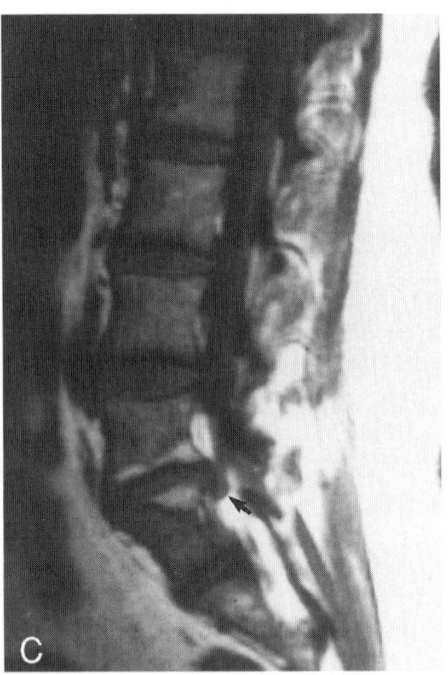

Figure 1.5 C

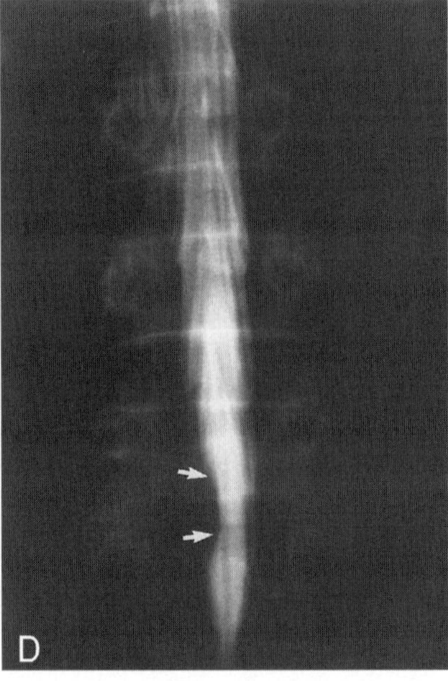

Figure 1.5 D

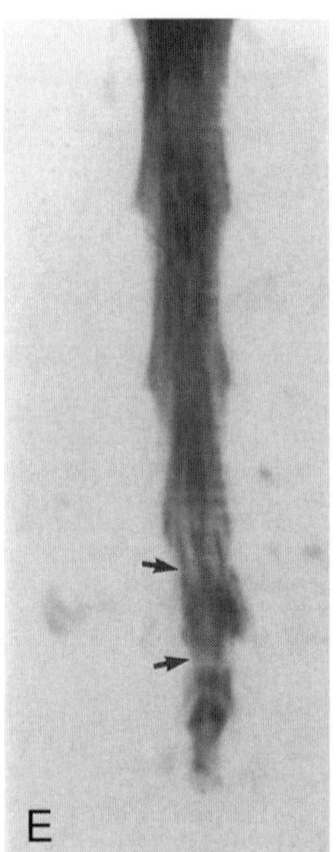

Figure 1.5 E

Findings: Postmyelogram axial 3-mm thick CT section (Fig. A) shows a right lateral disk herniation (D) with compression of the right S1 nerve root sleeve and compression of the adjacent ventrolateral thecal sac. Axial MR T1-weighted image (Fig. B) in the same patient shows the herniated disk (arrows). Right parasagittal MR T1-weighted image (Fig. C) shows the disk herniation (arrow) and also fatty infiltration of the vertebral end-plates (Modic type 2 changes, see Case 2). Frontal view from the conventional myelogram (Fig. D) in the same patient shows compression (arrows) of the right lateral aspect of the thecal sac by the herniated disk. Frontal view from the MR myelogram (Fig. E) shows compression of the thecal sac (arrows) similar to Fig. D.

(continued)

Diagnosis: Right parasagittal L5-S1 disk herniation.

Discussion: Trauma is a relatively frequent cause of disk herniations. Lateral disk herniations are more common than central ones. This is caused by the presence of a midline septum in the anterior epidural space (attaching the posterior longitudinal ligament to the periosteum of the dorsal surface of the vertebrae) and a relative decrease in the thickness of the off midline annulus fibrosus. They are similar to central disk herniations and usually compress the nerve root exiting below the level of herniation. Only approximately 10% of patients with acute low back pain show abnormalities at imaging. Conversely, approximately 50% of patients with chronic low back pain have imaging abnormalities that may be related to the symptoms. Of the patients who present with an acute onset of isolated radiculopathies, 72% show a herniated disk by MR imaging. However, in 80–90% of patients with radiculopathy/low back pain, the symptoms resolve after 8–10 weeks of conservative treatment. Therefore, imaging may be indicated only in patients who do not respond to conservative management and those with atypical symptoms, such as muscle function impairment or suspected lesions in the cauda equina and/or conus medullaris.

CASE 6

Clinical History: 28-year-old male with sudden onset of a left C6 radiculopathy and interscapular pain.

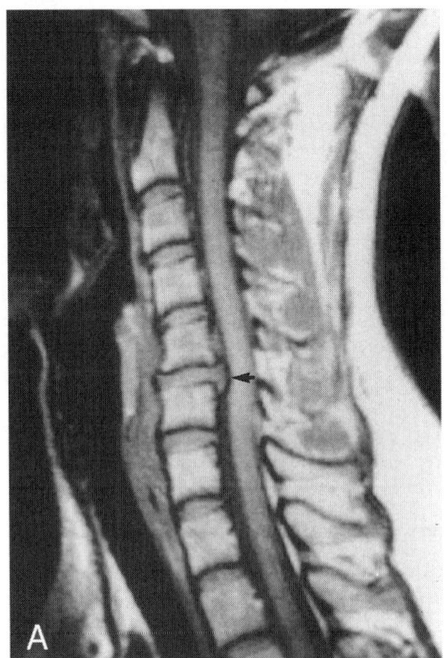

Figure 1.6 A

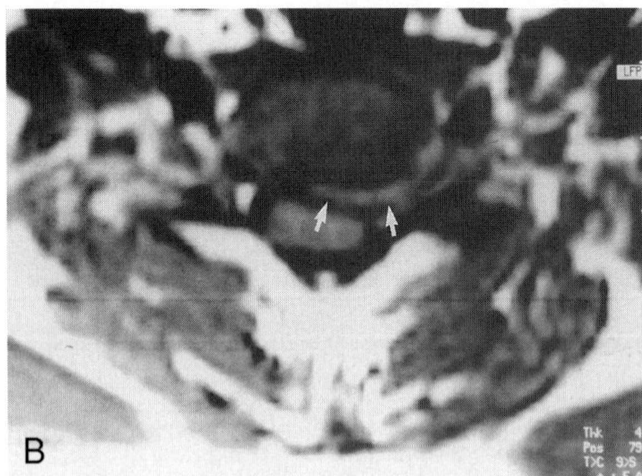

Figure 1.6 B

Findings: Midsagittal MR T1-weighted image (Fig. A) shows a disk herniation (arrow) at the C5-C6 level. There is compression of the ventral subarachnoid space and ventral surface of the spinal cord. The signal intensity from the spinal cord was normal on T2-weighted images (not shown). An axial T1-weighted image (Fig. B) shows that the herniated disk (arrows) is central and leftward explaining the patient's symptoms. Note the compression of the spinal cord.

Diagnosis: Central and leftward C5-C6 disk herniation.

Discussion: Cervical disk herniations are generally encountered in patients 20–40 years of age. Unlike lumbar disk herniations, they are generally not associated with trauma. There are eight cervical nerve roots, each pair exiting through the neural foramina *above* the corresponding level. Therefore, a herniated disk at C5-C6 results in compression of the C6 nerve root. Most herniated disks in the cervical spine occur at the C6-C7 (60%) and C5-C6 (30%). Gadolinium administration is not routinely needed for the evaluation of degenerative disease of the cervical region. However, contrast administration is helpful by increasing the signal intensity of the epidural space and highlighting extradural abnormalities. Gradient echo imaging is routinely done in an attempt to obtain an adequate "myelographic effect," particularly on the axial plane. Gradient echo images do, however, overestimate the degree of foraminal stenoses. Axial imaging of the cervical spine requires sections that are no more than 3 mm thick (for both MR imaging and CT).

CASE 7

Clinical History: The first patient (Figs. A and B) is a 35-year-old male with progressive T7 sensory loss and lower extremity spasticity. The second patient (Fig. C) is a young female with lower thoracic back pain.

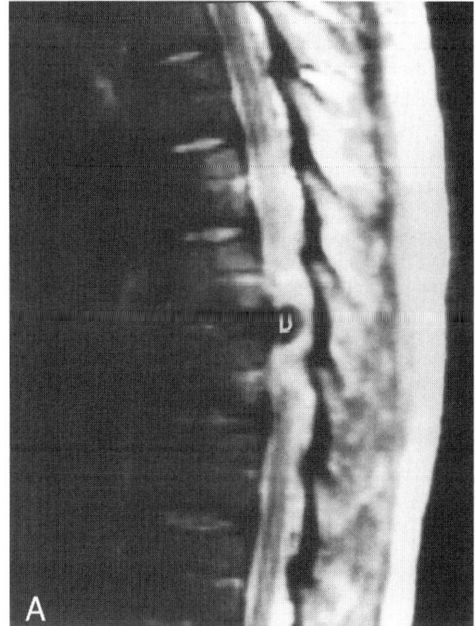

Figure 1.7 A

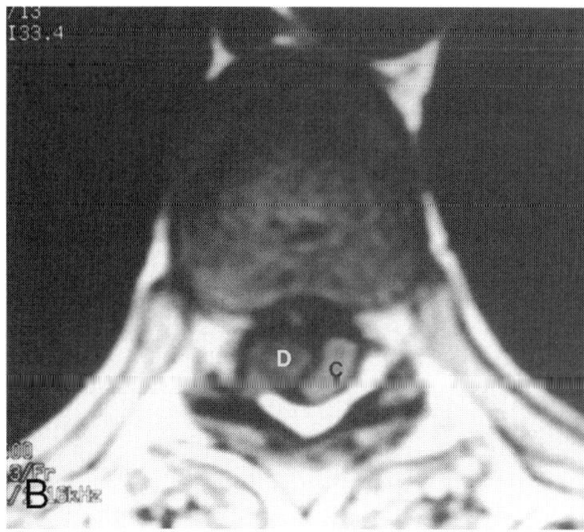

Figure 1.7 B

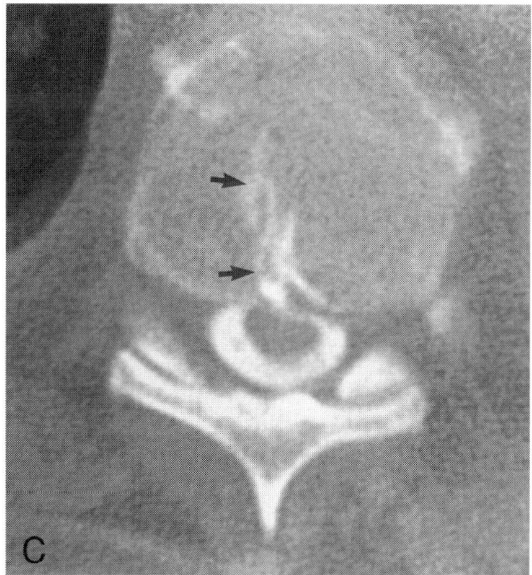

Figure 1.7 C

Findings: Midsagittal MR T2-weighted image (Fig. A) shows a hypointense herniated disk (D) at T7-T8. Axial MR T1-weighted image (Fig. B) at that level shows the herniated disk (D) to be in the right lateral region and to result in significant compression of the spinal cord (C). In the second case, axial postmyelogram CT section (Fig. C) at the T10-T11 level shows a small, mostly central disk herniation with an area of bone sclerosis (arrows) in the superior end plate of T11.

Diagnosis: Thoracic herniated disks.

Discussion: Thoracic disk herniations are less common than lumbar and cervical ones. Most thoracic disk herniations occur in the mid- to lower regions. Most small thoracic disk herniations are asymptomatic, whereas larger ones result in myelopathic symptoms such as sensory loss, paresthesias, paresis, and spasticity. Many of them do, however, present with nonspecific and often confusing clinical findings. The correct clinical diagnosis may be made in only 50% of patients. MR imaging is the method of choice for the evaluation of suspected thoracic disk herniations, but small ones may be difficult to see when pulsation artifacts (from the heart and great vessels) are present. Thoracic disk herniations may have very low signal intensity on both T1- and T2-weighted sequences. By CT, an area of bone sclerosis in the vertebral end plates which tracts into the herniated disk is often seen. This has been termed a nuclear "tail" or "trail," and when present, one should rule out the presence of disk herniation.

CASE 8

Clinical History: 45-year-old male with right S1-S2 radiculopathy.

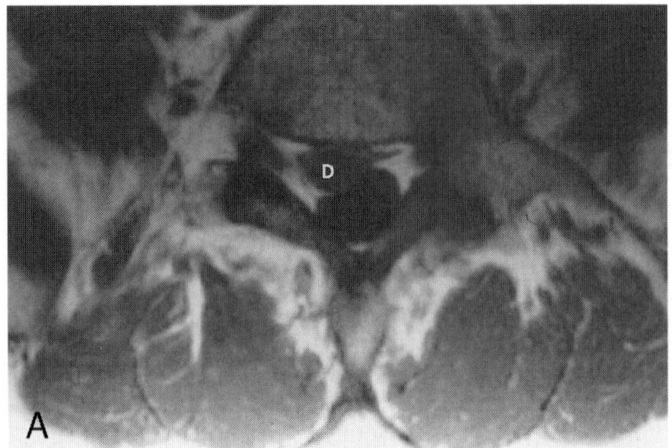

Figure 1.8 A

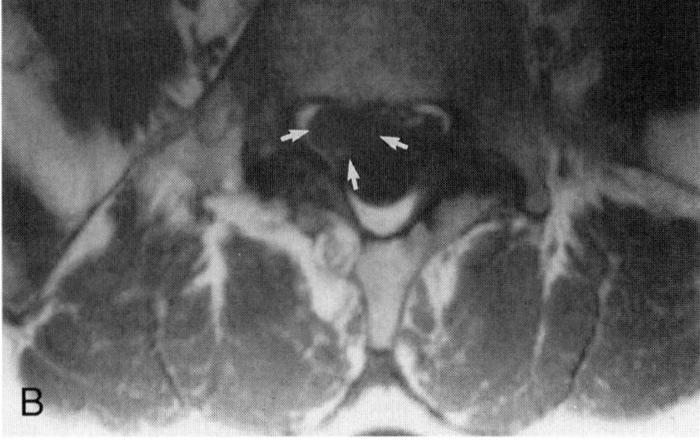

Figure 1.8 B

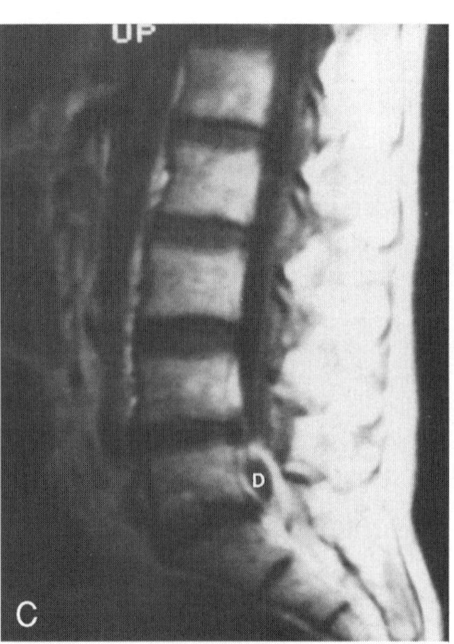

Figure 1.8 C

Findings: Axial MR noncontrast T1-weighted image (Fig. A) at the midlevel of a transitional L5 vertebra shows a fragment of herniated disk (D) in the ventral epidural space compressing the thecal sac. MR T1-weighted image (Fig. B) obtained slightly below Fig. A shows the disk fragment (arrows) sequestered within the lateral recess. Midsagittal MR T1-weighted image (Fig. C) shows the free fragment of herniated disk (D) sequestered in the ventral epidural space at L5 level. Determining the parent disk in this case is not possible.

(continued)

Differential Diagnosis: Epidural abscess, extradural tumors (neurofibroma, lymphoma, metastasis), synovial and ganglion cysts, free herniated disk fragment.

Diagnosis: Free herniated disk fragment (sequestered disk).

Discussion: A free herniated disk fragment has become detached from its parent disk and is no longer contained by the posterior longitudinal ligament. It commonly migrates superiorly or inferiorly along the ventral epidural space. It may become lodged (sequestered) in the lateral recesses or in the posterior epidural space. On rare occasions, it may burrow into the thecal sac and become intradural. Intradural free disk fragments are more commonly found in the lumbar region. Most free fragments are eccentric in location. When they become sequestered within a lateral recess they may erode the bone. Epidural abscesses are generally the result of diskitis and therefore are easily differentiated from a free disk fragment. However, differentiating an epidural abscess of hematogenous origin (without bone or disk abnormalities) from a free disk fragment may be difficult. Extradural tumors demonstrate enhancement and are easily differentiated from free disk fragments which do not enhance. Synovial and ganglion cysts occur in the dorsolateral epidural space always adjacent to a degenerated facet joint.

Clinical History: Patient shown in Fig. A presents with acute onset of a right L3 radiculopathy. Patient shown in Fig. B presents with a right L4 radiculopathy, and the patient shown in Fig. C presents with an acute left C7 radiculopathy.

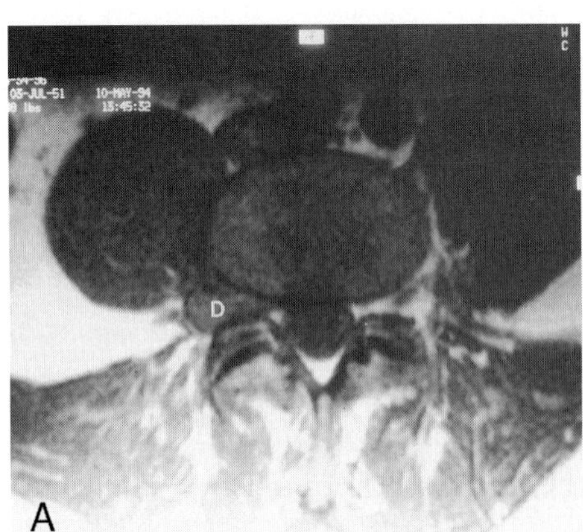

Figure 1.9 A

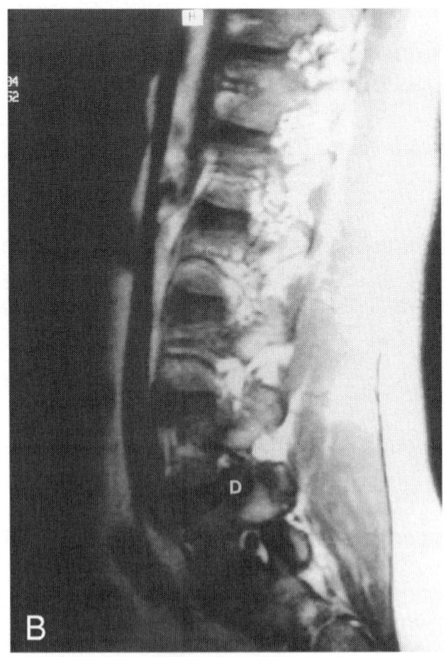

Figure 1.9 B

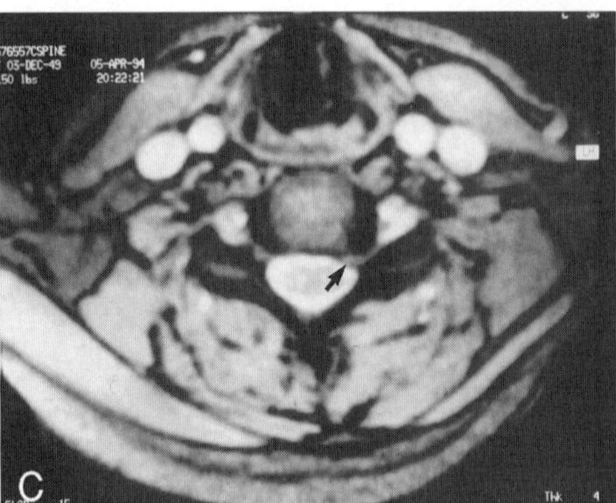

Figure 1.9 C

Findings: Axial noncontrast MR T1-weighted image (Fig. A) shows a large disk herniation (D) in the right neural foramen at the L3-L4 level. Note complete effacement of the normal fat in that foramen. Fig. B is a right parasagittal T1-weighted image showing a disk herniation (D) in the neural foramen at the L4-L5 level. In Fig. C, there is a disk herniation (arrow) in the left neural foramen at the C6-C7 level. Note the moderate stenosis of the ipsilateral neural foramen as a consequence of overgrowth of uncovertebral joint.

(continued)

Differential Diagnosis: Neurofibroma, schwannoma, metastasis, lymphoma, conjoined nerve roots, perineurial cysts, foraminal (far lateral) disk herniations.

Diagnosis: Foraminal (far lateral) disk herniations in the lumbar and cervical spine.

Discussion: Lateral disk herniations may be foraminal or even extraforaminal. They generally compress the nerve root exiting at that level rather than the one below. The central and paracentral disk herniations tend to compress the level below. They are easily seen in the lumbar spine as they efface the normal fat within the neural foramina. In the cervical region, they are more difficult to identify because of the normal absence (or very little amounts) of fat in the epidural space. Lateral disk herniations account for approximately 10% of all disk herniations in the lumbar region. They are more common in older individuals, particularly males. Most are found at L2-L3 and L3-L4, therefore slightly higher than central and paracentral disk herniations. They may produce bone erosion. Most tumors arising in the neural foramina enhance and therefore may be distinguished from lateral disk herniations. Conjoined nerve roots occur mostly at the L5 and S1 levels. Perineurial cysts are fluid-filled and tend to follow the signal intensity of CSF in all sequences and do not enhance.

CASE 10

Clinical History: Patient shown in Fig. A presents with acute onset of bilateral lower extremity pain and weakness. Fig. B is from a patient with left S1 and S2 radiculopathies.

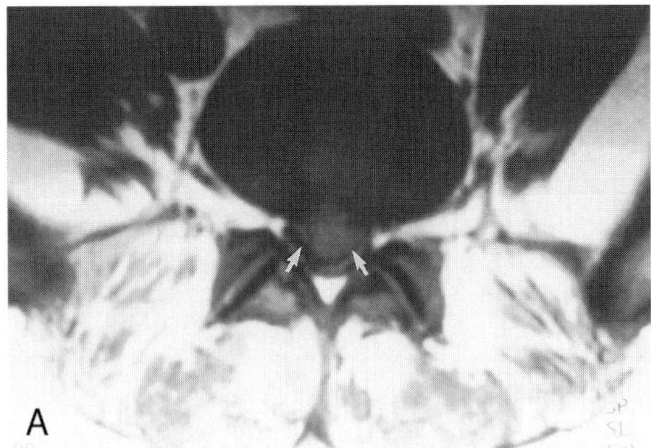

Figure 1.10 A

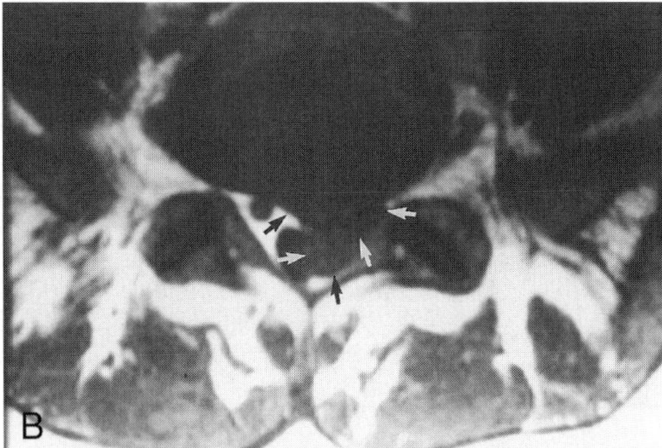

Figure 1.10 B

Findings: Axial noncontrast MR T1-weighted image (Fig. A) shows a very large central disk herniation (arrows) at the L4-L5 level. Note slight hyperintensity of disk herniation and almost complete obliteration of the thecal sac. In a different patient, a noncontrast MR T1-weighed image (Fig. B) shows a large right paracentral disk herniation (arrows) with effacement of the left S2 nerve root sleeve and compression of the thecal sac.

Diagnosis: "Giant" disk herniations.

Discussion: Giant disk herniations differ from the more common disk herniations only in their size. Because of their volume, resolution of symptoms after conservative management is uncommon in these patients. Giant disk herniations are more common in younger patients, particularly children. Most occur at the L4-L5 and L5-S1 levels and result in sciatica. Common sciatica refers to pain at the distribution point of the L5 and S1 nerve roots. Paresthesia is common, and the patient generally assumes a "flexed" position that relieves the pain. The pain is aggravated in the standing or sitting positions. The pain extends from one or both buttocks down the posterior mid- to inner-thigh and calf and to the dorsal and lateral foot (or feet). It is possible that many giant disk herniations represent a combination of nucleus pulposus and epidural hematoma (see Case #12).

CASE 11

Clinical History: 50-year-old male presenting with a left L3 radiculopathy.

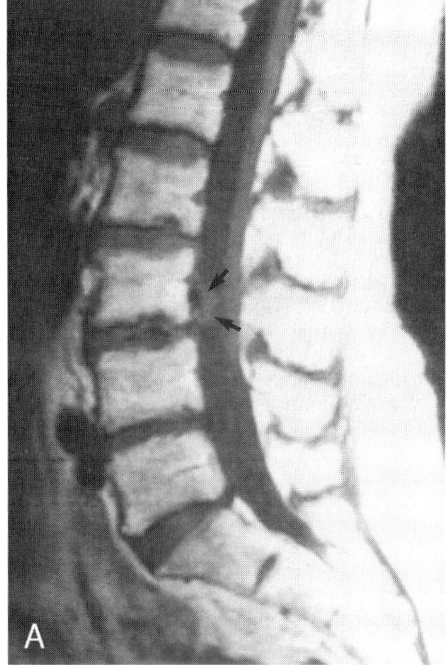

Figure 1.11 A

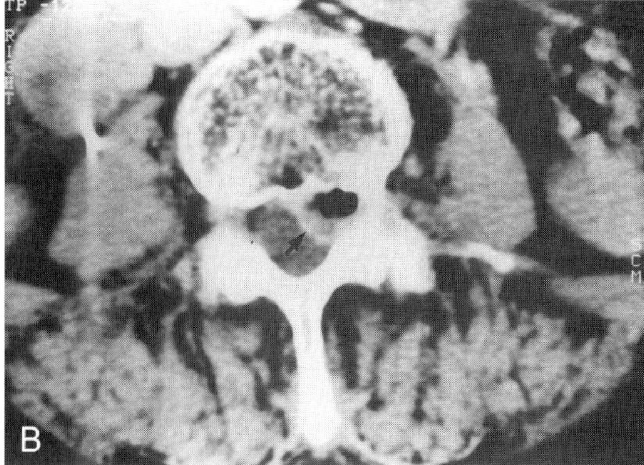

Figure 1.11 B

Findings: Midsagittal MR T1-weighted image (Fig. A) shows a herniated disk fragment (arrows) in the ventral epidural space at L3. This disk fragment contains very low signal intensity centrally. Low signal intensity also at the L3-L4 intervertebral disk is related to the presence of gas (vacuum phenomenon). Axial 3 mm CT section (Fig. B) in the same patient shows the herniated disk (arrow) in the left ventral epidural space at L3. Note gas in the herniated disk fragment.

Differential Diagnosis: Synovial cyst, gas in herniated disk fragment.

Diagnosis: Gas in herniated disk fragment.

Discussion: Intradiscal gas or vacuum phenomenon generally occurs secondary to disk degeneration. This gas is mostly nitrogen. CT is a more sensitive method to detect intradiscal gas than is MR imaging or radiographs. Intradiscal gas has no significance by itself. Diskitis almost never results in accumulation of gas in the disk. However, intradiscal gas may be seen in cases of trauma or may be associated with compression fractures caused by metastatic vertebral involvement. Gas-containing masses located in the epidural space include disk herniations and synovial cysts. When a synovial cyst contains gas, the corresponding facet joint also almost always contains gas.

CASE 12

Clinical History: 48-year-old male with acute onset of low back pain and bilateral lower extremity weakness and pain.

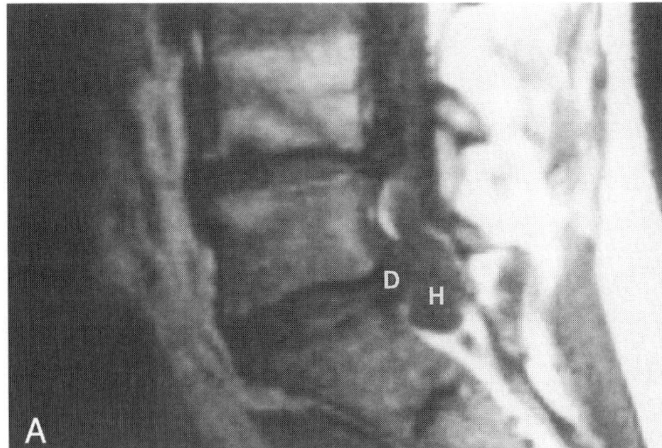

Figure 1.12 A

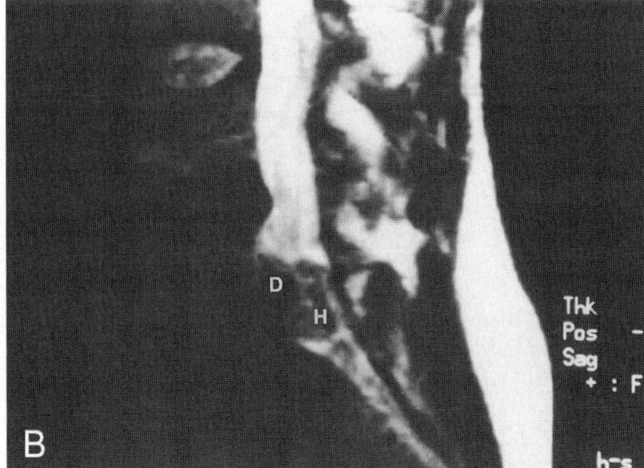

Figure 1.12 B

Findings: Midsagittal MR T1-weighted image (Fig. A) shows a disk herniation (D) at the L5-S1 level. There is a large component (H) of intermediate signal intensity posterior to the herniated disk. On a midsagittal MR T2*-weighted image (Fig. B), this large component (H) is clearly separable from the disk herniation (D) and is of very low signal intensity. The herniated disk is well seen. At surgery, a disk herniation and an epidural hematoma were found.

Diagnosis: Spontaneous epidural hematoma associated with lumbar disk herniation.

Discussion: Most spontaneous epidural hematomas are found in the cervical and thoracic regions. Most are located in the dorsal and lateral epidural compartments. Spontaneous epidural hematomas in the lumbar region may be isolated or in combination with disk herniations. Most so-called giant disk herniations are probably a combination of nucleus pulposus and hematoma. Lumbar ventral epidural hematomas may account for some of the disk herniations that rapidly resolve with conservative management. Epidural hematomas probably result from rupture or tearing of the fragile epidural veins located adjacent to a bulging annulus or herniated disk. By MR imaging, these epidural hematomas are of intermediate signal intensity on T1-weighted sequences and are bright on T2-weighted images. Gradient echo imaging suggests the presence of epidural hematomas when the lesions are of very low signal intensity. Lumbar spontaneous epidural hematomas tend to extend superiorly or inferiorly in the ventral epidural space and tend to be larger at the mid-vertebral body level.

CASE 13

Clinical History: 32-year-old male presenting with bilateral C6 radiculopathies and low neck pain.

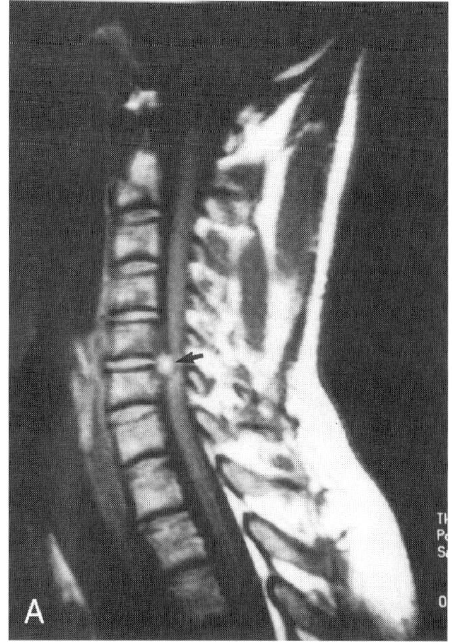

Figure 1.13 A

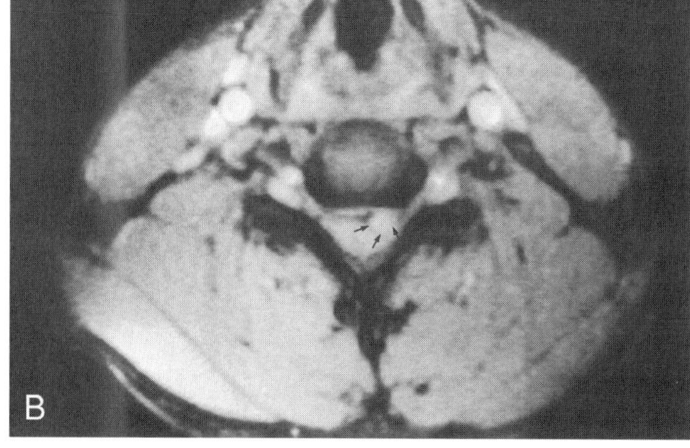

Figure 1.13 B

Findings: Midsagittal MR T1-weighted image (Fig. A) shows a bright abnormality (arrow) in the ventral epidural space. This abnormality is contiguous with the C5-C6 intervertebral disk. On an axial T2*-weighted image (Fig. B), the abnormality (arrows) is also of high signal intensity.

Differential Diagnosis: Spontaneous epidural hematoma (see Case #12), bright disk herniation.

Diagnosis: Bright disk herniation.

Discussion: High signal intensity on MR T1-weighted images may be present in the intervertebral disk or in herniated disks. Intervertebral disk hyperintensity is believed to be related to the presence of calcifications. Intradiscal calcifications are generally not significant but in adults may be related to metabolic disorders, such as ochronosis or chondrocalcinosis. In children, disk calcifications may be transient after trauma or even possibly inflammatory. Intradiscal high T1 signal intensity after trauma may reflect hemorrhage (methemoglobin). The T1 and T2 hyperintensity in herniated disk fragments may be related to hemorrhage or hydrated calcifications. These hyperintense disk herniations may be indistinguishable from ventral epidural hematomas by MR imaging. However, bright disk herniations tend to be more focal than hematomas.

CASE 14

Clinical History: Figs. A and B correspond to a patient with chronic mid-thoracic back pain. Fig. C is from a 57-year-old patient with chronic low back pain.

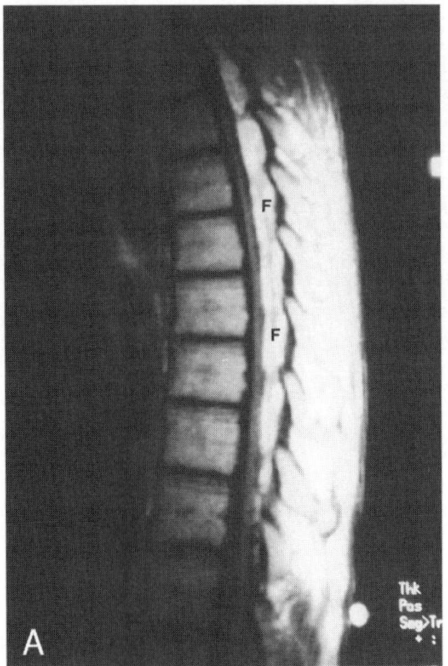

Figure 1.14 A

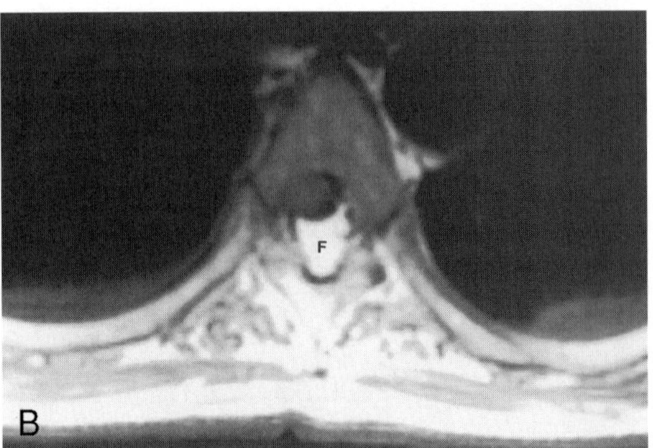

Figure 1.14 B

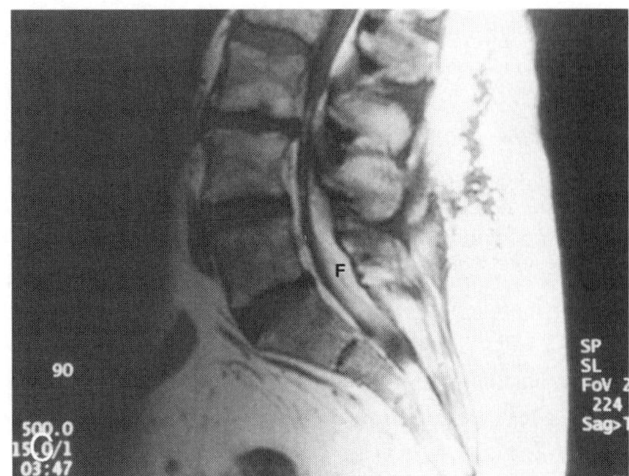

Figure 1.14 C

Findings: Midsagittal MR T1-weighted image (Fig. A) shows hypertrophy of the fat (F) in the dorsal epidural space. Note the diffuse narrowing of the spinal canal and compression of the spinal cord, which appears thin. Axial mid-thoracic MR T1-weighted image (Fig. B) in the same patient shows the large amount of fat (F) displacing the spinal cord anteriorly and to the right. In a different patient, midsagittal MR T1-weighted image (Fig. C) shows increased epidural fat (F) (dorsal greater than ventral) in the lower lumbar spine. Note markedly reduced diameter of thecal sac.

(continued)

Differential Diagnosis: Epidural hematoma, intraspinal lipoma, epidural angiolipoma, epidural lipomatosis.

Diagnosis: Epidural lipomatosis.

Discussion: Hypertrophy of the epidural fat may be idiopathic and may be related to exogenous steroid administration, Cushing disease, or obesity. In most cases, epidural lipomatosis involves the thoracic region. The lumbar region is less commonly affected. In the thoracic spine, the hypertrophy of the fat tends to involve the dorsal epidural space, whereas in the lumbar spine, it tends to be concentric. Patients with thoracic epidural lipomatosis present with myelopathy and pain. In the lumbar region, affected patients present with radiculopathies, neurologic claudication, and pain. Histologically, the fat is not encapsulated and is normal. Epidural hematomas generally present acutely and involve the upper thoracic region more commonly. Unlike lipomatosis, their signal intensity is not nulled by using fat suppression techniques. Intraspinal lipomas are focal masses and may be associated with dysraphism or cutaneous abnormalities, such as dermal sinus tracts. Angiolipomas are unusual tumors composed of fat and vascular elements. They are found in the posterior epidural space in the thoracic and lumbar regions. Angiolipomas are focal masses averaging 2–5 vertebral bodies in length. They generally show some enhancement after contrast administration and may demonstrate serpiginous defects within them, probably related to the presence of vessels.

CASE 15

Clinical History: 55-year-old female with an isolated left C6 radiculopathy.

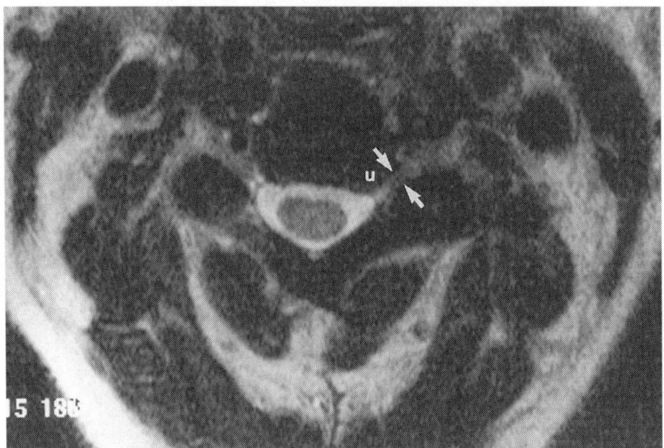

Figure 1.15

Findings: Axial T2*-weighted image at the C5-C6 level shows narrowing of the left neural foramen (arrows). This is secondary (mostly) to hypertrophy of the uncinate process (u) of the corresponding uncovertebral joint.

Diagnosis: Narrowing of the left C5-C6 neural foramen secondary to degenerative joint disease.

Discussion: The uncinate processes are short bridges of bone arising from the posterolateral and superior aspect of the vertebral bodies of C3 through C7. They articulate with a notch in the inferior end-plate of the vertebral body above. Together they form the so-called uncovertebral joints or joints of Luschka. The uncinate processes form the anterior border of the cervical neural foramina. In the cervical region, the neural foramina are obliquely oriented (45° in the coronal plane). Their margins are the inferior pedicle superiorly, the superior pedicle inferiorly, the facet joint posteriorly, and the uncinate process anteriorly. The normal neural foramina measure approximately 4–5 mm in diameter. Degenerative changes involving the uncovertebral and facet joints are generally responsible for narrowing of these foramina. Narrowing of the cervical neural foramina is better visualized by CT. MR imaging using gradient echo sequences tends to slightly overestimate the degree of narrowing.

CASE 16

Clinical History: Two cases of young patients with chronic low back pain.

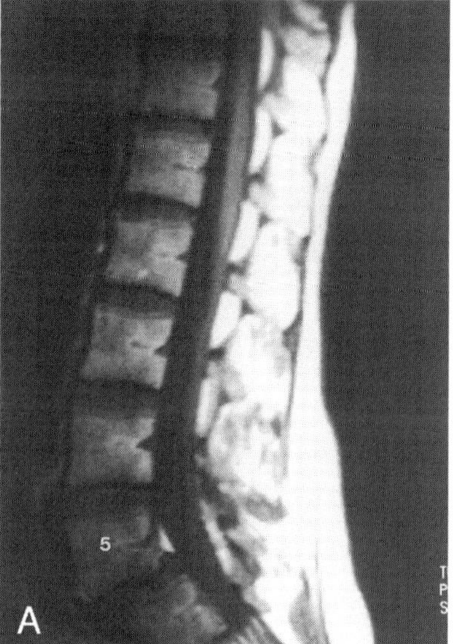

Figure 1.16 A

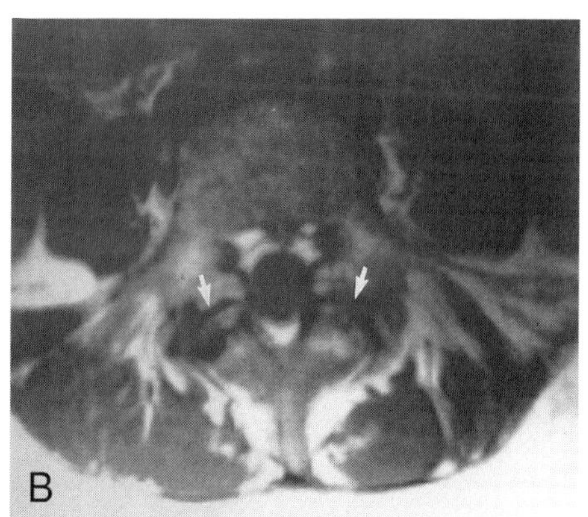

Figure 1.16 B

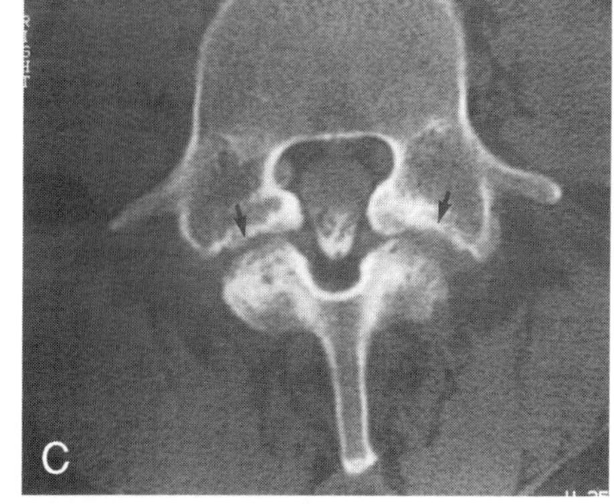

Figure 1.16 C

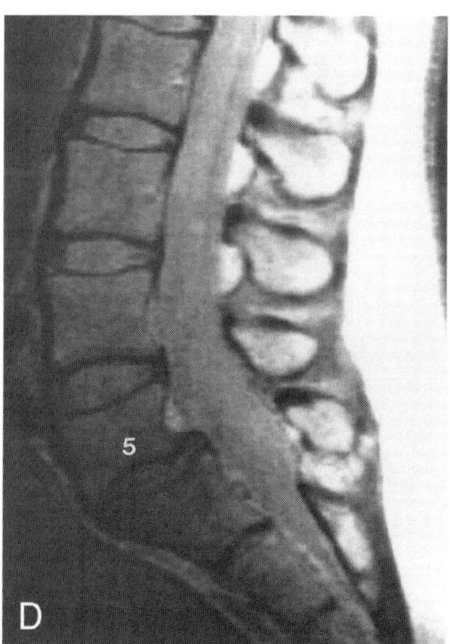

Figure 1.16 D

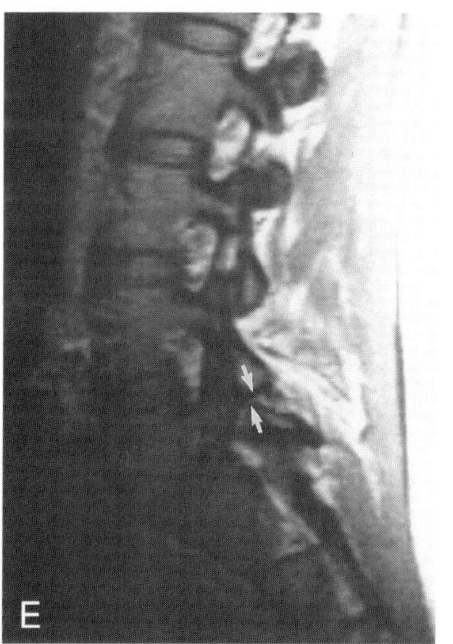

Figure 1.16 E

(continued)

Findings: In the first patient, a midsagittal MR T1-weighted image (Fig. A) shows mild (grade 1) anterior displacement of L5 (5) on S1. Axial MR T1-weighted image (Fig. B) shows defects (arrows) in both pars interarticularis at L5. In the same patient, CT axial section (Fig. C) at same location reveals clefts (arrows) in both pars interarticularis. In the second patient, a midsagittal proton density image (Fig. D) shows mid-anterior displacement of L5 (5) over S1. Note widening of the spinal canal at this level. Parasagittal T1 weighted image (Fig. E) shows a pars defect (arrows) at L5. Similar findings were present on the opposite side (not shown).

Diagnosis: Bilateral spondylolysis of L5 and grade 1 anterior spondylolisthesis of L5.

Discussion: Spondylolysis refers to a cleft involving the posterior vertebral arch at the level of the pars interarticularis. This abnormality is also known as an "isthmic" or "open arch" defect. It is probably the result of repeated microtrauma. The clefts are bridged by fibrous tissues. They are most commonly bilateral and at the L4 and L5 levels. Uncommonly, they are found in the cervical spine. They occur in approximately 1–5% of the population. Patients generally present with low back pain and/or radiculopathies.

Spondylolisthesis refers to the displacement of one vertebra in relation to the adjacent ones. Displacement is more commonly anterior, but posterior displacement may also occur. The degree of displacement may be graded by dividing the underlying normal vertebra into three segments and determining the position of the posterior border of the displaced vertebra in relation to these segments. Spondylolisthesis may be secondary to spondylolysis or to relaxation of the facet joints ("closed" type) caused by degeneration. On midsagittal MR images, widening of the spinal canal at the level of a spondylolisthesis most likely indicates underlying spondylolysis.

Plain radiographs continue to be one of the most reliable and easiest ways to diagnose spondylolysis. The pars defects may be difficult to appreciate on axial images because they may be confused with the facet joints.

CASE 17

Clinical History: 40-year-old male status post right-sided L5 microdiscectomy for a previous herniated disk presents with persistent pain and a right S1 radiculopathy.

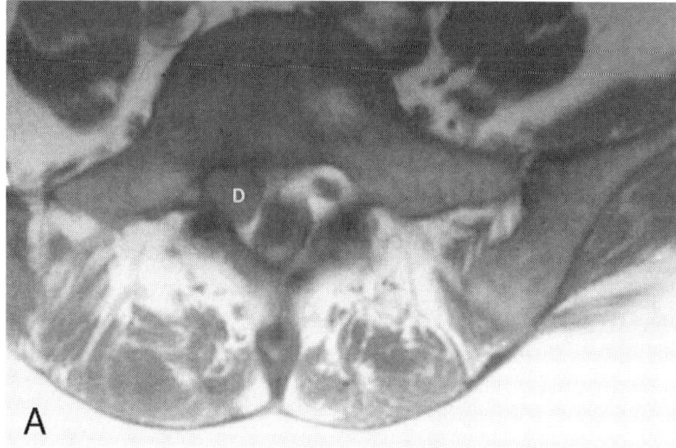

Figure 1.17 A

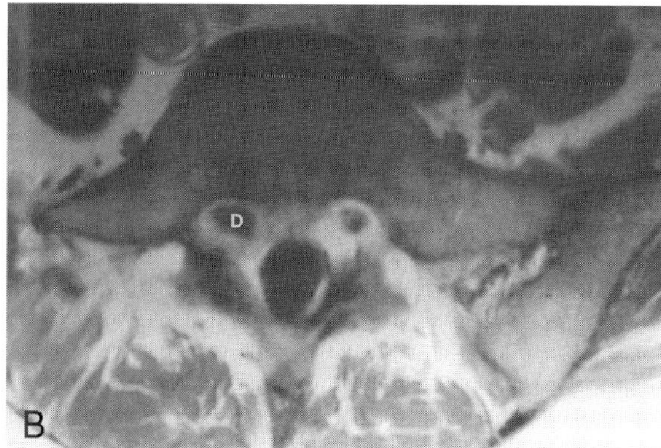

Figure 1.17 B

Findings: Axial precontrast MR T1-weighted image (Fig. A) shows a mass (D) of intermediate signal intensity in the right lateral recess compressing the corresponding nerve root and also the thecal sac. Postcontrast MR T1-weighted image (Fig. B) shows only peripheral enhancement of the abnormality (D).

Diagnosis: Recurrent/residual disk herniation.

Discussion: Recurrent or residual pain occurs in 10–40% of patients after lumbar surgery for disk disease. One of the most common reasons for this is the presence of a recurrent or residual disk herniation. Disk herniations are responsible for 12–16% of failed back syndrome cases. More than 50% of these disks are located laterally, particularly in the lateral recesses. They tend to be polypoid and of low T2 signal intensity. Because the disk is avascular, it does not enhance after contrast administration. Peripheral enhancement secondary to presence of granulation tissues is common. However, on delayed (greater than 20 minutes) postcontrast MR images, a recurrent/residual disk herniation may enhance due to ingrowth of granulation tissue. MR imaging with contrast has a greater than 96% accuracy in the differentiation of recurrent/residual disk herniation versus epidural scar.

CASE 18

Clinical History: 35-year-old female with low back pain 6 months after surgery for a leftward disk herniation at L5-S1.

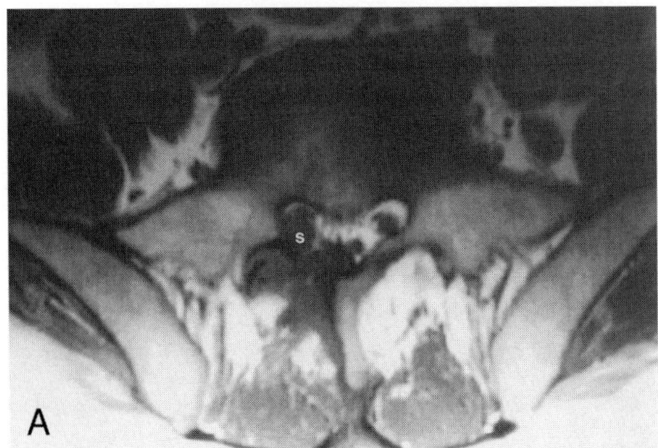

Figure 1.18 A

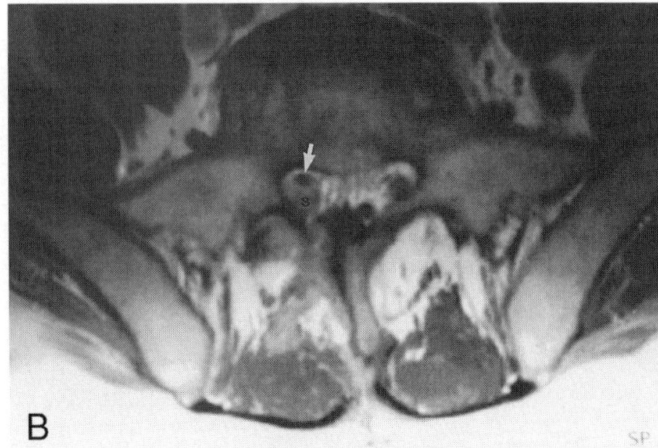

Figure 1.18 B

Findings: Precontrast axial MR T1-weighted image shows a zone abnormal intermediate signal intensity (s) in the right lateral recess of S1 (Fig. A). Note postsurgical changes involving the corresponding lamina and paraspinal fat. Axial MR T1-weighted (Fig. B) immediately after gadolinium administration shows enhancement of the abnormality (s) clearly differentiating it from the corresponding nerve root sleeve (arrow), which is mildly compressed.

Diagnosis: Postsurgical epidural fibrosis (scar).

Discussion: The causes of the failed back syndrome include: recurrent/residual disk herniation, epidural scar, arachnoiditis, unrecognized and untreated stenoses of lateral recesses, instability, nerve injury, and surgery at the wrong level. Epidural scar is responsible for 6–8% of failed back syndrome cases. It is hypointense to isointense to muscle on T1-weighted images and bright on T2-weighted sequences. It generally produces retraction of the thecal sac but may also result in mass effect with compression of the thecal sac and the nerve root sleeves. It is richly vascular and enhances immediately after gadolinium administration (herniated disks do not enhance immediately after contrast administration). If MR imaging is done less than 3 weeks after surgery, 38% of patients show findings that are very similar to their presurgical study regardless of their clinical status.

CASE 19

Clinical History: This patient underwent an L4-L5 diskectomy 1 month before this study and now presents with nonspecific mild low back pain.

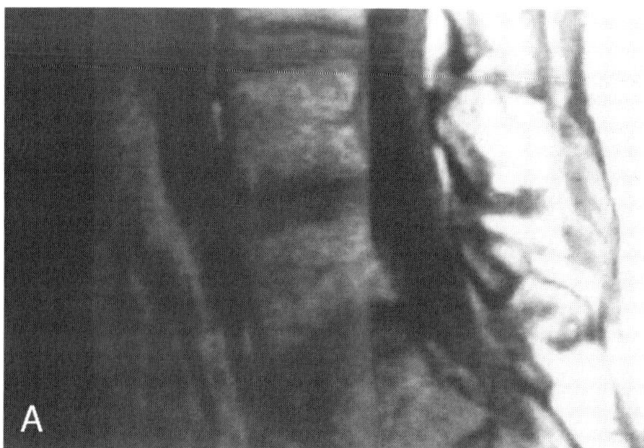

Figure 1.19 A

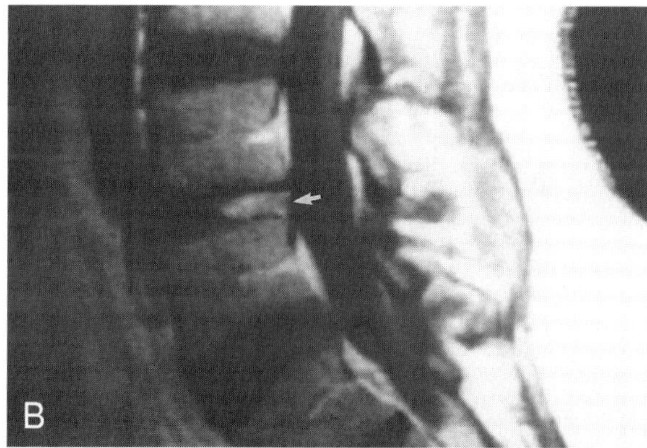

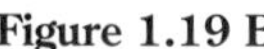

Figure 1.19 B

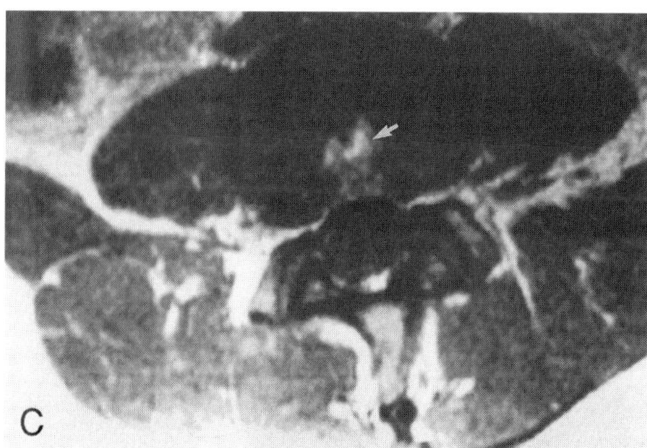

Figure 1.19 C

Findings: Precontrast midsagittal MR T1-weighted image (Fig. A) shows no abnormality. Postcontrast midsagittal MR T1-weighted image (Fig. B) shows enhancement (arrow) in the posterior aspect of the L4-L5 intervertebral disk. Axial postcontrast MR T1-weighted image (Fig. C) also shows the enhancement (arrow). Note lesser signal-to-noise in Fig. A when compared with Fig. B. Fig. A was obtained with only one signal average.

Diagnosis: Enhancement along curretaged region of a previously herniated disk.

Discussion: Postsurgical diskitis and osteomyelitis occur in less than 1–3% of all patients. The absence of vertebral endplate abnormalities and epidural abnormalities make the diagnosis of infection less likely in this case. In addition, this patient was afebrile. This patient has no evidence of recurrent/residual disk herniation; therefore, the cause of the back pain is undetermined. The area of enhancement reflects the presence of vascularized granulation tissue where the herniated disk material was resected.

CASE 20

Clinical History: The patient shown in Figs. A and B underwent epidural anesthesia with incorrect placement of the needle. Fig. C shows a patient who had a laminectomy at L4 for disk herniation. A different patient who had undergone repeat myelography for degenerative disease is shown in Figs. D and E. All patients had low back pain at the time of these studies.

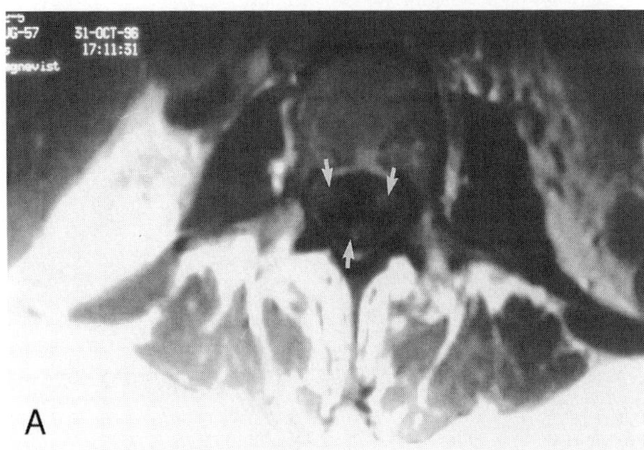

Figure 1.20 A

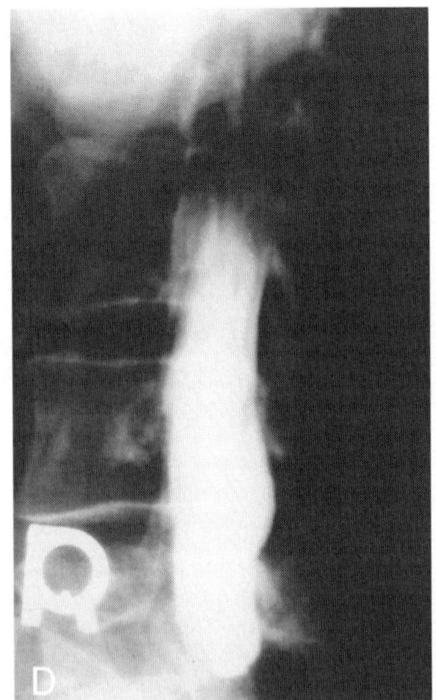

Figure 1.20 D

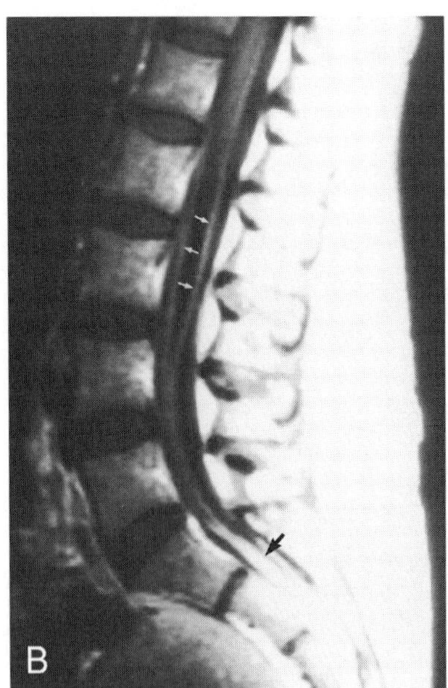

Figure 1.20 B

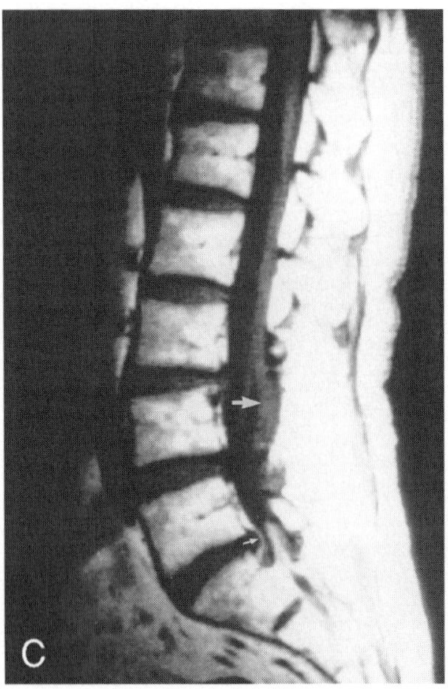

Figure 1.20 C

Findings: Figs. A and B show clumping of the lumbar nerve root (white arrows) compatible with arachnoiditis. The black arrow in Fig. B points to an incidental lipoma of the distal filum terminale. The patient in Fig. C shows slight posterior protrusion of the thecal sac at L4 secondary to a laminectomy. The nerve roots (larger arrow) of the cauda equina and matted and adherent to the surgical site. Note enhancement of the posterior annulus (smaller arrow) at the L5-S1 intervertebral disk from an incidentally found annular tear. Fig. D is an oblique view from a myelogram showing a "featureless" thecal sac. There is no filling of the nerve root sleeves due to arachnoiditis. In the same patient, Fig. E shows clumping of nerve roots (arrows).

Diagnosis: Arachnoiditis (see Case #25, Chapter 2).

(continued)

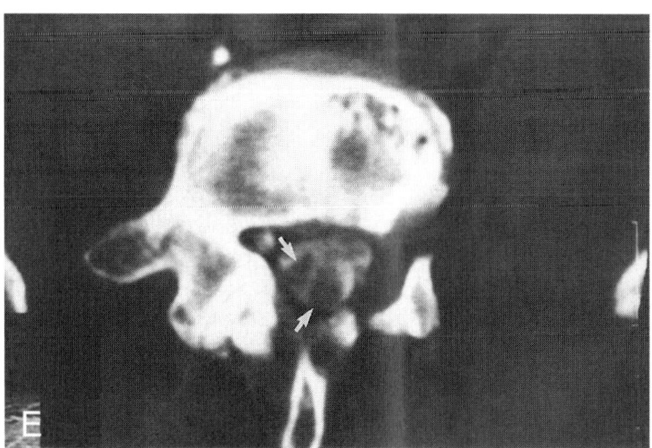

Figure 1.20 E

Discussion: Arachnoiditis is a misnomer because the process involves the dura, arachnoid, and pia matter. It is a relatively common cause of the failed back syndrome, accounting for 6–16% of these patients. Other causes for arachnoiditis are prior myelography, intrathecal administration of steroids and anesthetics, trauma, prior subarachnoid hemorrhage, and radiation. The most common symptoms of arachnoiditis are chronic pain radiating to both lower extremities, hyperthesias, and occasionally paraparesis. Pain is probably the result of traction of the nerve roots by adhesions. Arachnoiditis surrounding the spinal cord may result in the formation of syringohydromyelia. Arachnoiditis may be asymptomatic.

By conventional myelography, arachnoiditis may be divided according to its severity. Initially there may be a featureless sac. The thecal sac may appear empty secondary to adhesion of the nerve roots to the dura. More severe changes include clumping of the nerve roots and enhancement of them by MR imaging. Tumefactive arachnoiditis refers to a mass-like lesion composed of adhesions and nerve roots. By MR imaging, tumefactive arachnoiditis is usually of low T2 signal intensity. Occasionally, arachnoiditis calcifies and receives the name of arachnoiditis ossificans. These calcifications tend to occur in the dura. MR imaging is less sensitive than myelography and postmyelography CT in the identification of mild arachnoiditis.

Clinical History: Patient with mild low back pain who had spinal procedure many years before the present study.

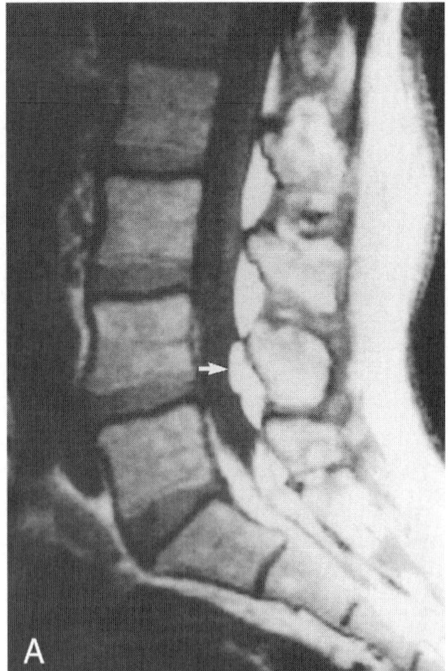

Figure 1.21 A

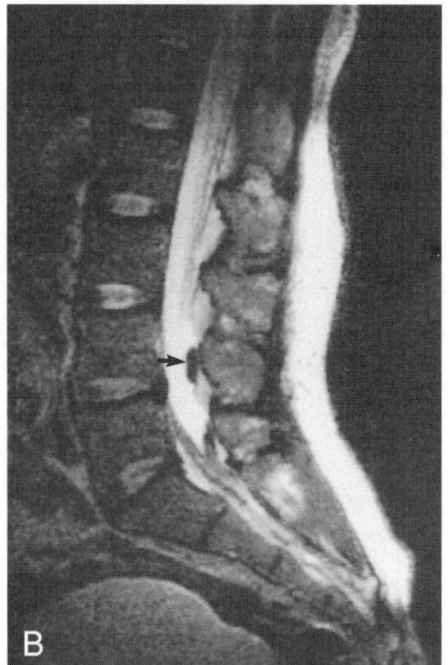

Figure 1.21 B

Findings: Midsagittal MR T1-weighted image (Fig. A) shows a small, very bright focal abnormality (arrow) abutting the posterior epidural space at the L4-L5 level. On a corresponding MR T2-weighted image (Fig. B), the abnormality (arrow) is very hypointense (lower than the signal intensity of fat).

Differential Diagnosis: Intraspinal lipoma, residual pantopaque in the spinal canal.

Diagnosis: Residual pantopaque in the spinal canal.

Discussion: Pantopaque was introduced as a radiographic contrast medium in the early 1940s and was later supplanted by the water-soluble metrizamide, which was introduced in the late 1960s and early 1970s. The relatively hyposmolar and nonionic contrast media have been employed for myelography since the mid-1980s. Pantopaque is composed of ethylesters of iodophenylundecylic acids bound to iodine. It is fat-soluble and is resorbed from the subarachnoid space at a rate of approximately 1 mL per year. In the United States, an attempt was made to remove all pantopaque after myelography; in some European countries the contrast was left in place. Pantopaque may result in inflammation and subsequent arachnoiditis. Pantopaque has typical MR imaging characteristics. It has a short T1 relaxation time and a short T2 relaxation time at long repetition times (TR). It is bright with respect to CSF at TRs less than 1000 msec. It is isointense to CSF at TRs 1000–2000 msec, and hypointense to CSF at TR greater then 4000 msec. Therefore, its signal characteristics are markedly different from those of fat when imaged with long TE/TR, and this should allow for easy differentiation from a spinal lipoma.

CASE 22

Clinical History: Patient with a right S1 radiculopathy.

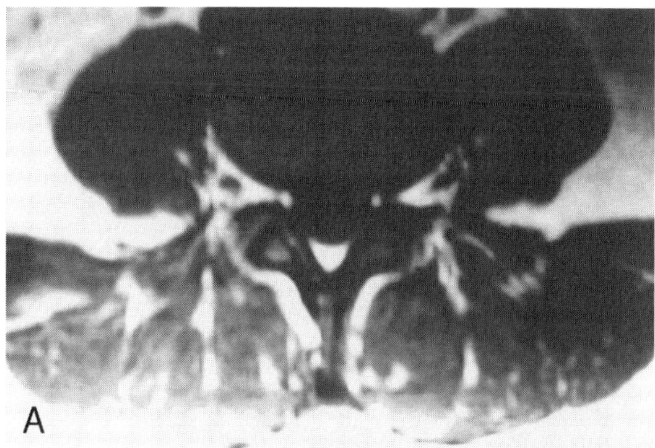

Figure 1.22 A

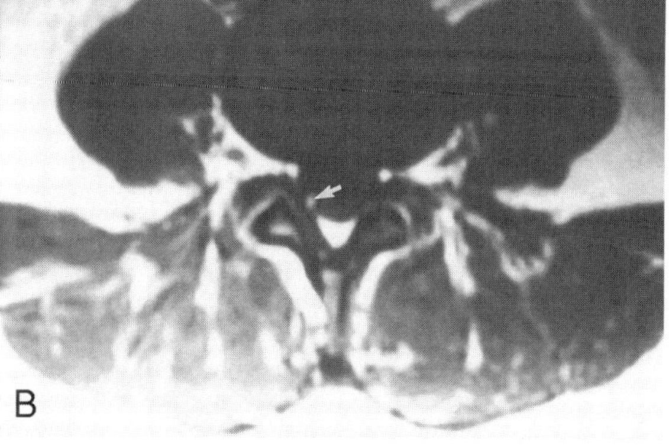

Figure 1.22 B

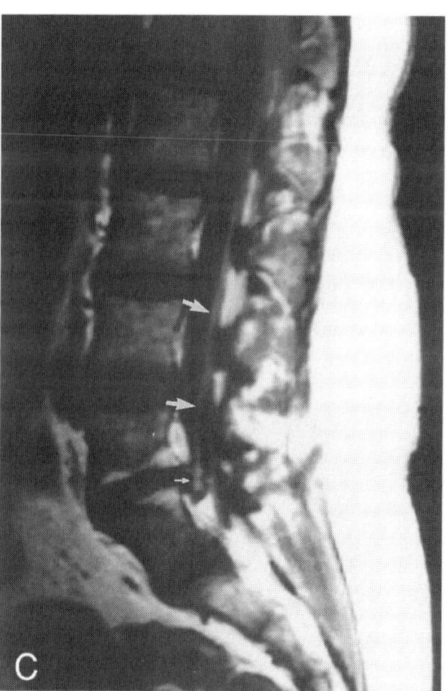

Figure 1.22 C

Findings: Precontrast axial MR T1-weighted image (Fig. A) at the L4-L5 level shows only a mildly bulging disk. Postcontrast image (Fig. B) at the same level shows enhancement of one (arrow) nerve root. Right parasagittal MR T1-weighted image (Fig. C) shows a long segment of enhancement (arrows) involving the right S1 nerve root. Note a small lateral herniated disk (tiny arrow) at the L5-S1 level directly compressing the enhancing nerve root.

(continued)

Differential Diagnosis: Enhancing lumbar radicular vein, arachnoiditis, leptomeningeal spread of tumor, enhancing nerve root secondary to irritation by a herniated disk.

Diagnosis: Enhancing nerve root secondary to irritation by a herniated disk.

Discussion: Contrast enhancement of nerve roots may be seen with herniated disks, spinal stenosis, and previous laminectomies. Careful observation reveals some degree of contrast enhancement in nerve roots in approximately 50% of all enhanced MR imaging studies of the lumbar spine. Pathologic enhancement is, however, more prominent. Enhancing nerve roots are seen in 21% of patients of focal lumbar disk protrusions. Nerve root enhancement is also dose-dependent and is seen more commonly after triple-dose than after single-dose examinations. Nerve root enhancement extends from the level of compression to the conus medullaris. Histologically, these abnormal nerve roots demonstrate Wallerian degeneration and inflammation and disruption of the endothelium of the capillaries leading to breakdown of the nerve-blood barrier. Enhancement of a nerve root has been considered as a marker for active neural disease.

Enhancement of the major lumbar radicular vein(s) may be easily mistaken for an enhancing nerve root. If no disk protrusions are associated, an enhancing vein should be considered. Arachnoiditis usually involves more than one nerve root (same observation applies for Guillain Barré and cytomegalovirus radiculitis). In addition, other signs of arachnoiditis are usually identified (see Case #20). In subarachnoid (leptomeningeal) dissemination of tumor, there are multiple areas of involvement and these tend to be nodular, unlike the thin enhancement of a compressed nerve root.

CASE 23

Clinical History: You are shown images in two different patients. Fig. A is from a patient presenting with low back pain and right L5 and S1 radiculopathies. Figs. B and C are from a patient with a similar history but on the left side.

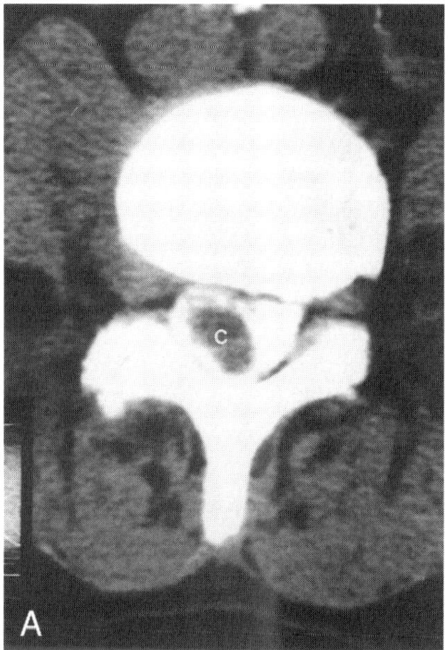

Figure 1.23 A

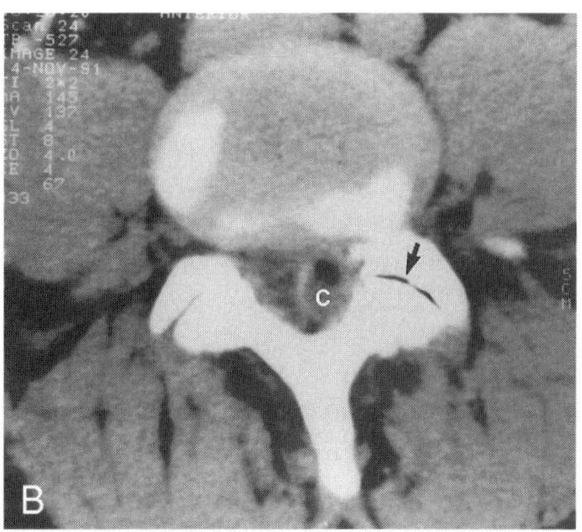

Figure 1.23 B

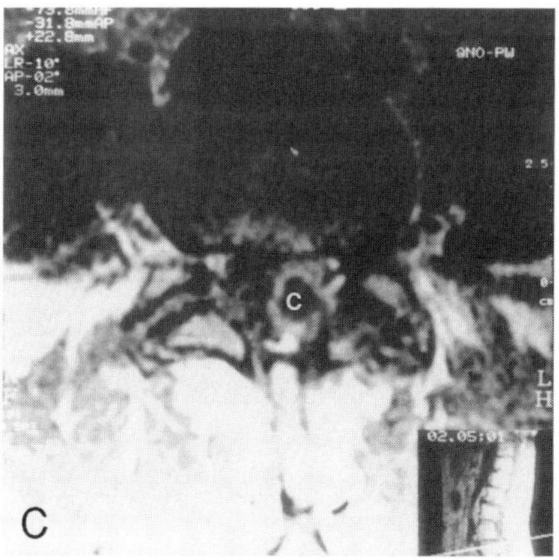

Figure 1.23 C

Findings: A postmyelogram CT axial image (Fig. A) shows a mass (C) in the right posterior epidural space displacing the opacified thecal sac towards the left. Note the center of low density and the calcified surrounding rim. The adjacent facet joint is degenerated. Fig. B is an axial CT image showing a mass (C) in the left posterior epidural space compressing the thecal sac. Note the gas in the mass and in the adjacent facet joint (arrow). Postcontrast MR T1-weighted image (Fig. C) in the same patient shows peripheral enhancement of the mass (C).

(continued)

Differential Diagnosis: Sequestered disk fragment, arachnoid cysts, epidural hematoma, ganglion cysts, synovial cysts.

Diagnosis: Synovial cysts.

Discussion: Juxta articular synovial cysts are uncommon extradural lesions usually occurring in the lumbar region, particularly at L4-L5, L3-L4, and L5-S1. However, they may also occur in the cervical spine, particularly the lower region. Synovial cysts arising at the C1-C2 levels are generally seen in association with rheumatoid arthritis. They arise adjacent to highly mobile facet joints secondary to proliferation of articular tissues. True synovial cysts are lined with synovium; ganglion cysts are not. In addition, ganglion cysts are filled with a myxoid material and are not connected to the facet joint. This differentiation is mostly academic; they are difficult to tell apart by imaging and basically require the same treatment. It is possible for a synovial cyst to differentiate into a ganglion cyst. Synovial cysts generally present with radiculopathy and/or intermittent pain. They commonly decompress spontaneously. In the cervical region they may result in a myelopathy.

Synovial cysts are always adjacent to a degenerated facet joint. By CT, their capsule may be calcified or of high density, probably related to hemorrhage. They may contain gas that may be tracked into the corresponding facet joint. They opacify with contrast if the facet joint is injected. On T1-weighted images they are hypointense to slightly hyperintense to CSF (unless filled with blood). If they are filled with blood, differentiation from a small posterior epidural hematoma may be difficult. On T2-weighted images, they are bright and surrounded by a capsule of low signal intensity. The capsule may enhance after gadolinium administration.

Clinical History: A 34-year-old Japanese male with neck stiffness and hyperreflexia in all extremities.

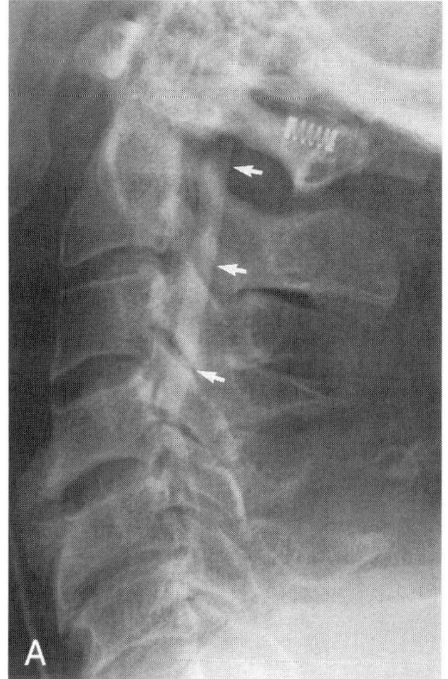

Figure 1.24 A

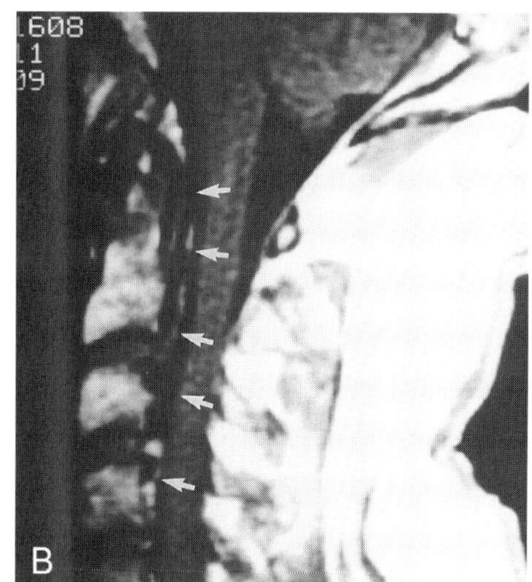

Figure 1.24 B

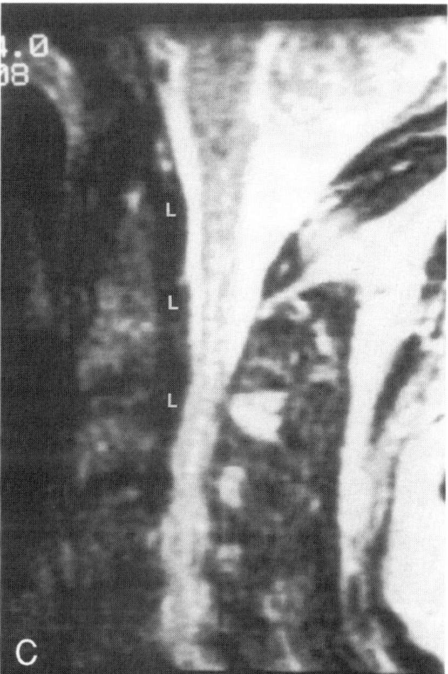

Figure 1.24 C

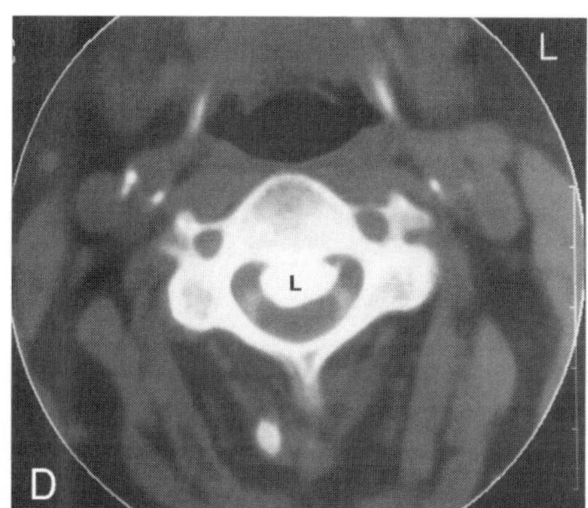

Figure 1.24 D

(continued)

Findings: Lateral radiograph (Fig. A) of the cervical spine shows a bar of bone (arrows) in the spinal canal abutting the posterior margins of the C2-C4 vertebrae. Note coarse anterior osteophytes C4-C6 in this patient who also had diffuse idiopathic skeletal hyperostosis. Midsagittal MR T1-weighted image (Fig. B) shows the bar of bone as an area of low signal intensity (arrows) containing some linear regions of hyperintensity. Note that the posterior aspect of this abnormality is indistinguishable from ventral subarachnoid space. Midsagittal MR T2*-weighted image (Fig. C) shows the abnormality (L) to be hypointense. Postmyelogram axial CT section (Fig. D) confirms that the abnormality (L) is heavily calcified.

Differential Diagnosis: Meningioma (particularly of the "en plaque" type), siderosis, osteophytosis (especially in the segmental type of OPLL), ossification of the posterior longitudinal ligament (OPLL), continuous type.

Diagnosis: Ossification of the posterior longitudinal ligament (OPLL), continuous type.

Discussion: OPLL is endemic to Japan where it is found in 2–3% of the population. However, it occurs in a worldwide distribution. In southeast Asia, ossification of the ligamentum flavum may be more common than OPLL (see Case #25). In the United States, most cases of OPLL occur in the setting of diffuse idiopathic skeletal hyperostosis (DISH, see Case #26). Approximately 50% of patients with DISH have evidence of OPLL. Initially, there is proliferation of small vessels in the ligament, which later ossifies. The ossified ligament may contain areas of bone marrow (including fat). Bone marrow is found in 56% of patients with continuous OPLL and in less than 10% with segmental type. Most patients present with a myelopathy. Myelopathy occurs when the anteroposterior diameter of the canal is less than 10 mm. Posterior decompression of the spinal canal is a common treatment.

By imaging, OPLL may be segmental, continuous, or mixed. The segmental type is commonly associated with disk degeneration. Continuous involvement is typical of OPLL. The most common sites of involvement are C3-C5 and T4-T8. OPLL may be difficult to identify by MR imaging, particularly in the absence of marrow. On T1-weighted images it may be indistinguishable from the ventral CSF. An ossified ligament greater than 3 mm thick is readily seen on sagittal T2-weighted images. MR imaging is, however, ideal to visualize the degree of spinal cord compression by OPLL. Increased T2 signal intensity in a compressed spinal cord may be indicative of edema and/or myelomalacia. Spinal cord abnormalities are seen on 35% of patients with continuous OPLL and in 16% of those with segmental OPLL. OPLL is, however, easily seen on lateral radiographs of the spine or by CT.

Clinical History: 45-year-old patient presenting with cervical myelopathy.

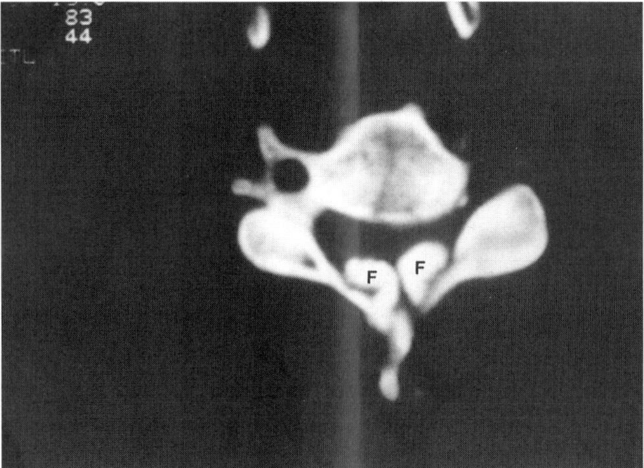

Figure 1.25

Findings: Axial CT section shows ossification in the region of the ligamentum flavum (F) bilaterally.

Differential Diagnosis: Osteophytes, osteochondiomas, calcified synovial cysts, ossification of the ligamentum flavum.

Diagnosis: Ossification of the ligamentum flavum.

Discussion: Ossification of the ligamentum flavum (OLF) is considered by some as a variant of ossification of the posterior longitudinal ligament (OPLL) (See Case #24). It is more common in southeast Asia but is found worldwide. It is said to occur to some degree in 20% of Asians older than 65 years of age. OLF is the most common cause of compression of the dorsal aspect of the spinal cord. OLF and OPLL may occur together. Some patients may also have ossification of the nuchal ligament. OLF is most commonly found in the thoracic region followed by the cervical and lumbar spine. Most patients present with myelopathy and radiculopathies. OLF may occur in patients with calcium pyrophosphate dihydrate crystal deposition. Treatment involves laminectomy with facetectomy and en-bloc resection of abnormal ligament.

OLF is better seen on CT images. When segmental and in the lumbar spine it may be confused with osteophytes arising from the facet joints or synovial cysts. Formation of bone marrow within OLF is very rare. Ossification of this ligament involves both its capsular and interlaminar portions. OLF is usually bilateral and is separable from the underlying lamina. MR imaging is unable to differentiate OLF from the more common hypertrophy (buckling) of the ligamentum flavum.

CASE 26

Clinical History: 55-year-old male with neck and diffuse joint pain and mild dysphagia.

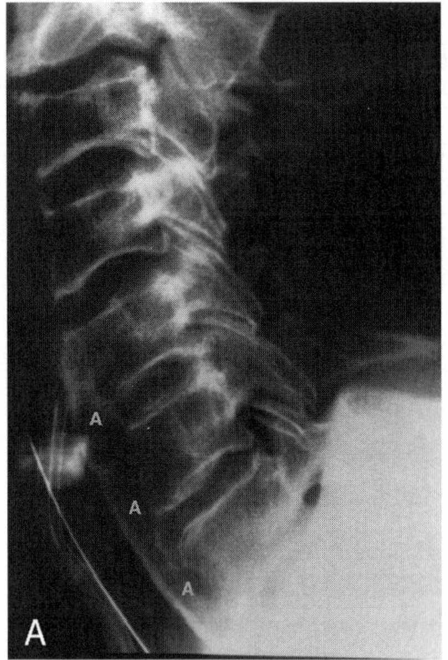

Figure 1.26 A

Figure 1.26 B

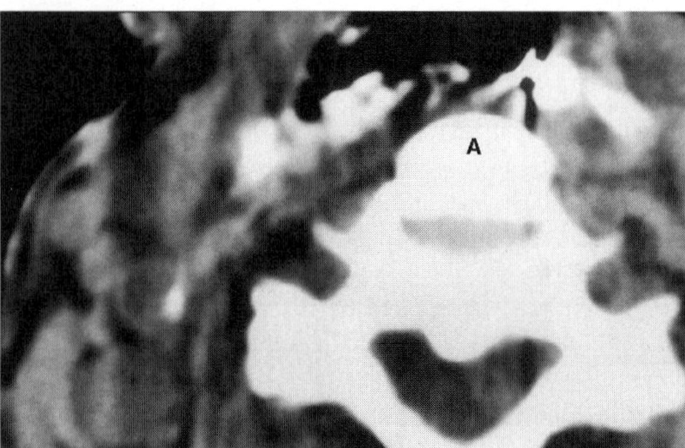

Figure 1.26 C

Findings: Lateral radiograph of the neck (Fig. A) shows a bar-like ossification (A) of the anterior longitudinal ligament. Lateral view of the thoracic spine (Fig. B) shows significant and coarse anterior osteophytes. Axial CT section (Fig. C) in same patient shows significant calcification (A) anterior to C6. Midsagittal MR T1-weighted image (Fig. D) shows that the calcified anterior longitudinal (A) ligament is bright probably secondary to infiltration by bone marrow. Frontal radiograph (Fig. E) of the lumbar spine shows bridging syndesmophytes.

Diagnosis: Diffuse idiopathic skeletal hyperostosis (DISH).

(continued)

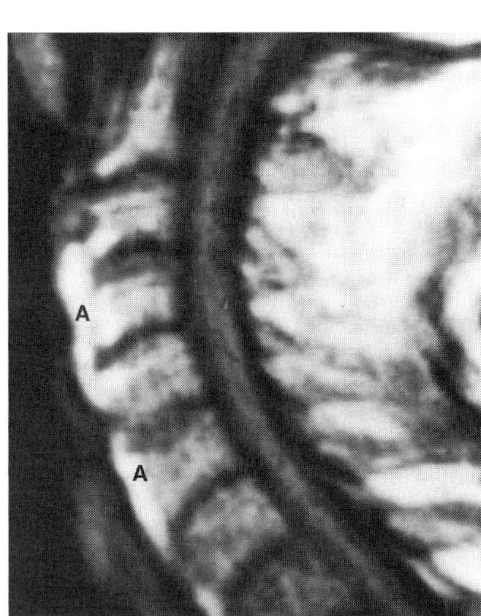

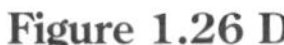

Figure 1.26 D

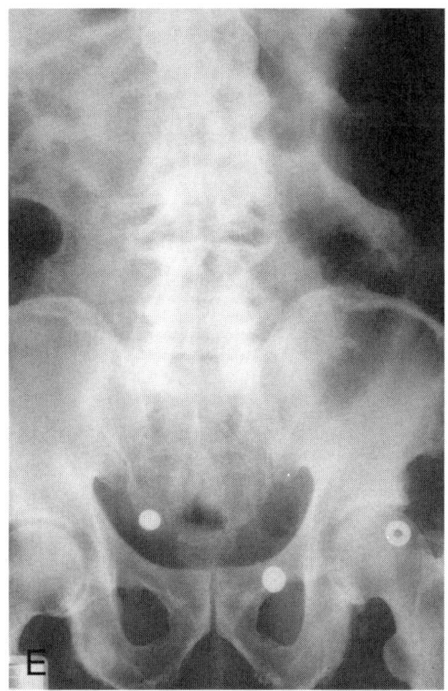

Figure 1.26 E

Discussion: DISH is also known as Forestier disease. It is an idiopathic disorder that affects predominantly elderly individuals. In the United States, approximately 20% of individuals over 70 years of age show radiographic changes compatible with DISH. Radiographic criteria for DISH include calcification/ossification of the anterior longitudinal ligament for at least four continuous vertebrae, normal intervertebral disk height, absence of apophyseal joint ankylosis, and evidence of sacroiliac joint inflammatory disease. The main differential diagnosis is spondylosis deformans.

The thoracic region (mostly lower) is most commonly affected, followed by the cervical and lumbar spine. Anterior cervical disease may result in dysphagia, and ossification of the posterior longitudinal ligament may produce a myelopathy (see Case #24). Extra spinal manifestations of DISH include whiskering at the insertion of ligaments in bone (entheses).

Clinical History: 40-year-old male with chronic bilateral sciatica and gluteal pain.

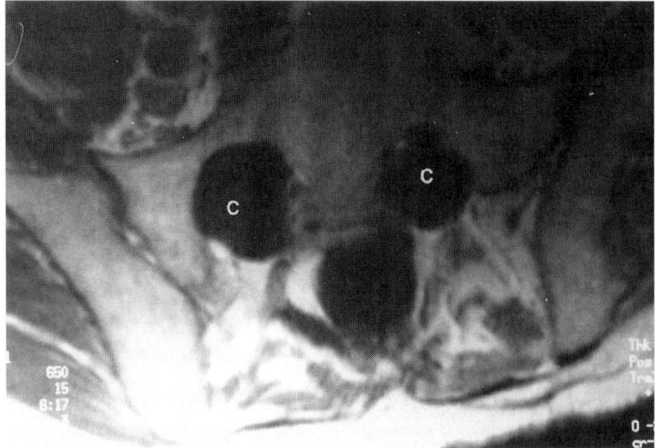

Figure 1.27

Findings: Axial MR T1-weighted image shows cystic structures (C) in the region of the sacral foramina and smooth erosion of the sacral foramina. Note also a prominent spinal canal.

Differential Diagnosis: Intrasacral meningocele, dural ectasia (neurofibromatosis, Marfan, Ehlers-Danlos), cystic schwannomas, Tarlov (perineurial) cysts.

Diagnosis: Tarlov (perineurial) cysts.

Discussion: Tarlov cysts arise in the potential space between the perineurium and the endoneurium generally at the junction of a nerve root with its dorsal ganglion. They occur in up to 15% of the population. Although commonly asymptomatic, they may result in pain and radiculopathies. This is probably the result of compression of the nerve roots against bone by the cysts and/or necrosis of the dorsal ganglion. These cysts have variable communication with remaining subarachnoid space. Some may even harbor a valve-ball type of communication that allows CSF to enter the cyst and remain there. This mechanism may be responsible for the growth of some cysts. When the cysts are symptomatic, treatment may be indicated. Image-guided aspiration resulting in resolution of the symptoms may be used to forecast the outcome of surgery. Surgical unroofing to establish a communication with the thecal sac is at times indicated.

By imaging, Tarlov cysts are commonly multiple and bilateral but asymmetric. They produce smooth bone remodeling. The margins of the affected neural foramina may be sclerotic. The cysts do not enhance after contrast administration. After myelography, they may fill (generally in an asymmetrical fashion) with contrast or remain unopacified. They tend to parallel the signal intensity of CSF on all MR imaging sequences. Because in some cysts the fluid is relatively stagnant, differences in protein concentrations and pulsatility may result in signal intensities that are different from those of normal CSF.

chapter 2

INFECTIOUS AND INFLAMMATORY PROCESSES

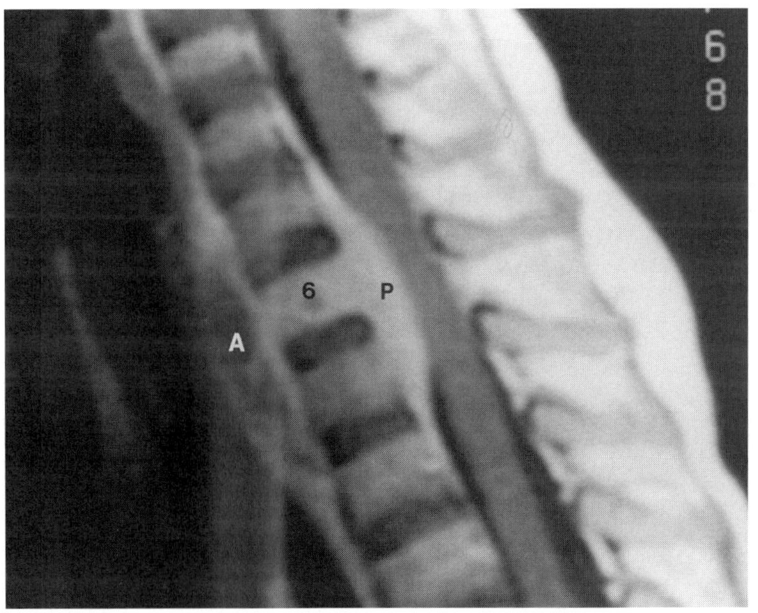

CASE 1

Clinical History: 40-year-old female with a 3-week history of low back pain and fever.

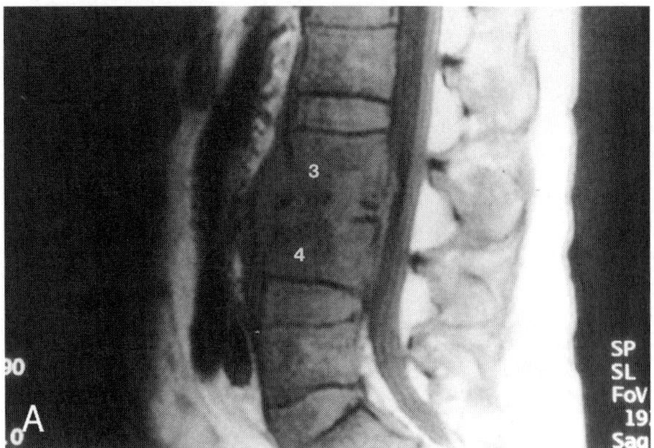

Figure 2.1 A

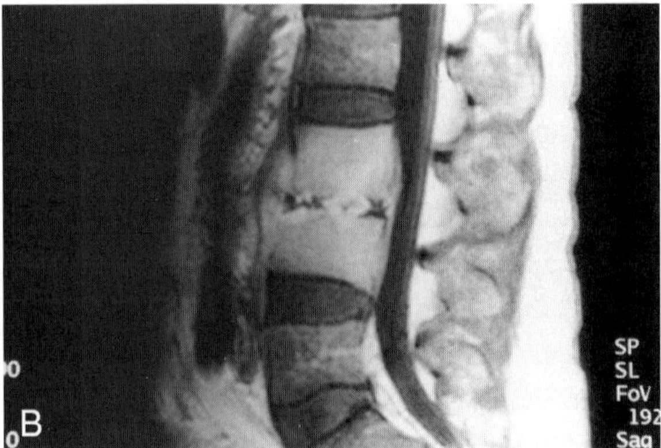

Figure 2.1 B

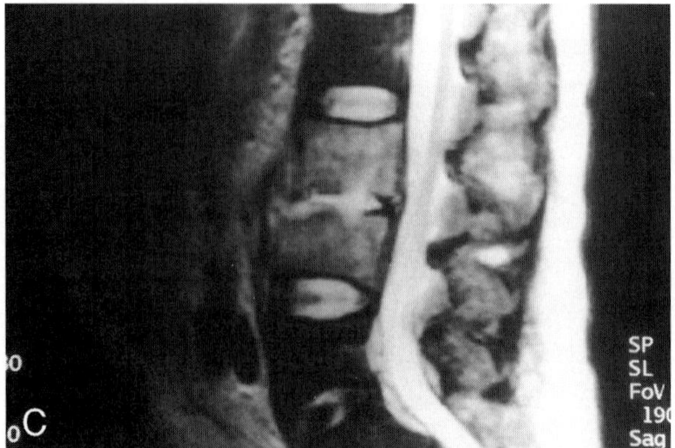

Figure 2.1 C

Findings: Noncontrast midsagittal MR T1-weighted image (Fig. A) shows low signal intensity from the L3 (3) and L4 (4) vertebral bodies. The inferior end-plate of L3 and superior end-plate of L4 are indistinct. The height of the L3-L4 disk is decreased. Under the anterior longitudinal ligament there is abnormal signal intensity at L3 and L4. Corresponding postcontrast image (Fig. B) shows significant enhancement of L3 and L4, the disk, and of the anterior and posterior phlegmons (not absence of necrosis). Corresponding T2-weighted image (Fig. C) shows increased signal intensity in the L3 and L4 vertebral bodies and the disk.

(continued)

Diagnosis: Diskitis and osteomyelitis at L3 and L4. Phlegmons under the anterior longitudinal ligament and in the ventral epidural space.

Discussion: In adults, diskitis and spinal osteomyelitis may be the result of hematogenous, contiguous, or ascending spread. Direct inoculation may follow surgery. The incidence of spinal infections is greater in patients with AIDS, immunosuppression, advanced age, or after genitourinary surgery/manipulation. In adults the infection generally begins in the end-plate and then extends to the disk and involves the lumbar region. In children, the infection begins in the disk and then extends to the end-plates. In adults the most common organisms involved are staphylococcus aureus, enterobacter species, E. coli, tuberculosis, klebsiella, and salmonella. The latter two are relatively more common in patients with sickle cell disease. In children, the most common organisms found are staphylococcus aureus and streptococci. Symptoms are generally present 2–4 weeks before the patient seeks medical attention. Approximately 90% of bacterial spinal infections resolve after a 4-week course of antibiotics.

Radiographs of the spine are not sensitive for the early detection of spinal infections. MR imaging findings reflect the presence of edema in the vertebrae and disks, and enhancement is variable and remains for several weeks or even months. Appropriate response to antibiotics is evidenced by resolution of the soft tissue abnormalities, which accompanies the diskitis/osteomyelitis. Late healing is evidenced by diminishing contrast enhancement and restoration of the normal high T1 signal intensity in the marrow of the vertebral bodies. Up to one-half of the patients may demonstrate involvement of several disk levels.

CASE 2

Clinical History: 25-year-old male with a history of intravenous drug use, neck pain for 2 weeks, and fever.

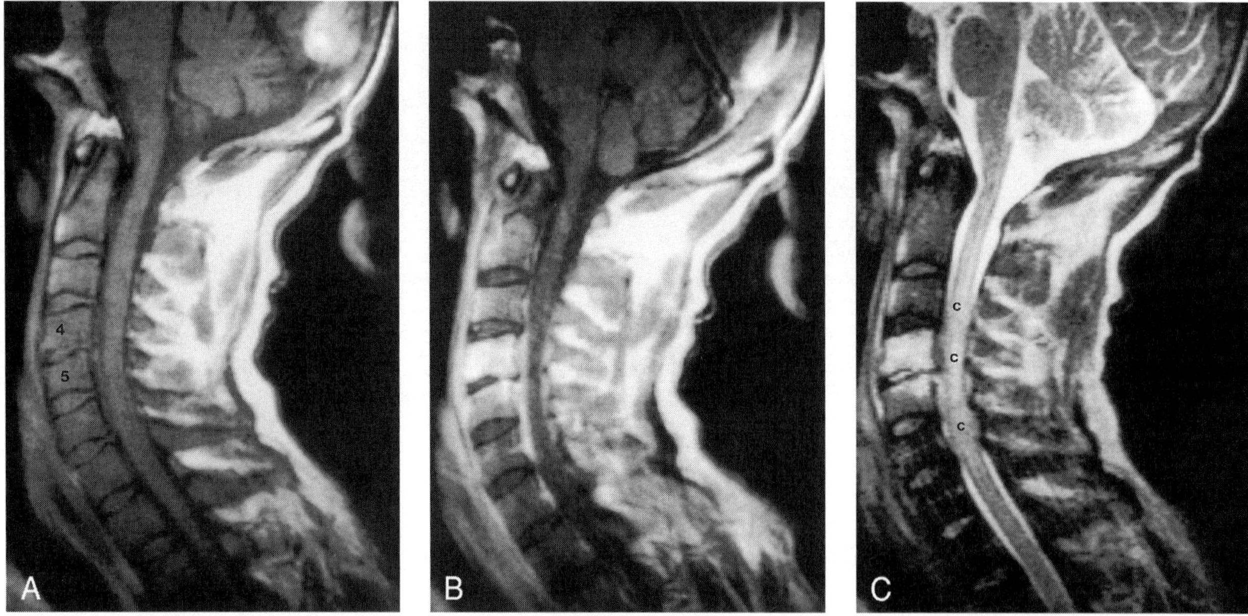

| Figure 2.2 A | Figure 2.2 B | Figure 2.2 C |

Findings: Midsagittal precontrast MR T1-weighted image (Fig. A) shows subtle irregularities in the inferior end plate of C4 (4) and decreased height of the C4-C5 (5) disk. Corresponding postcontrast image (Fig. B) shows significant enhancement of the C4 and C5 vertebral bodies. Note abnormal enhancement and thickening of the epidural space (anterior > posterior) from C3 to C6. The spinal cord is compressed. Corresponding T2-weighted image (Fig. C) shows hyperintense C4 and C5 and the disk. There is increased signal intensity in the precervical space. The spinal cord (c) is also hyperintense.

Diagnosis: Osteomyelitis and diskitis of C4 and C5. Epidural phlegmon. Spinal cord hyperintensity, which may be related to edema secondary to partial obstruction of the draining veins.

Discussion: Cervical spinal infections are rare, accounting for less than 10% of all spinal infections and one in 70,000–400,000 hospital admissions. Most involve the C4-C6 levels. Generally, 2–4 levels are involved. Cervical spinal infections are clinically aggressive processes leading to spinal cord compression in almost 75% of patients. The imaging features of this disease are similar to those of lumbar spine infections (see Case #1). A unique MR imaging feature is that of increased signal intensity in the spinal cord. High T2 signal intensity is seen in almost 65% of these patients and generally extends above and below the site of infection. There is thrombosis of extra- and intramedullary blood vessels resulting in edema and spongiform changes within the spinal cord. Other complications of cervical diskitis/osteomyelitis are infarction and direct infection of the spinal cord.

CASE 3

Clinical History: Three cases of the same disease involving the cervical (Fig. A), thoracic (Fig. B), and lumbar spine (Fig. C).

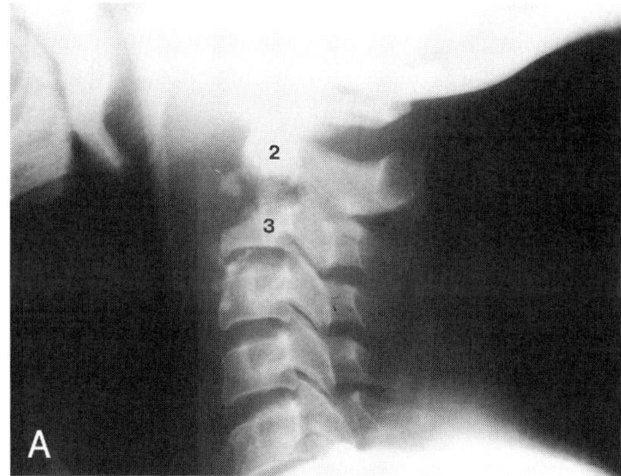

Figure 2.3 A

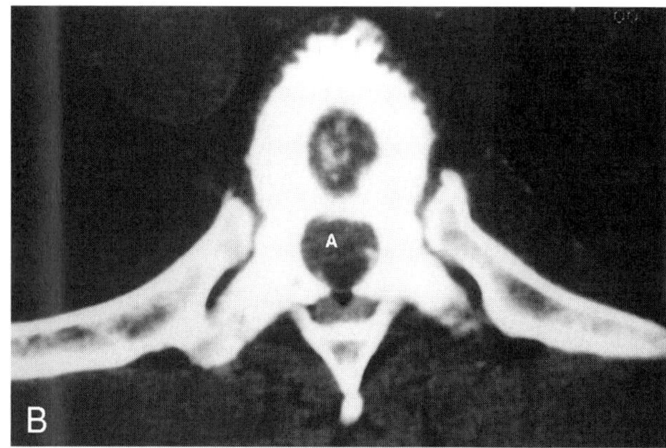

Figure 2.3 B

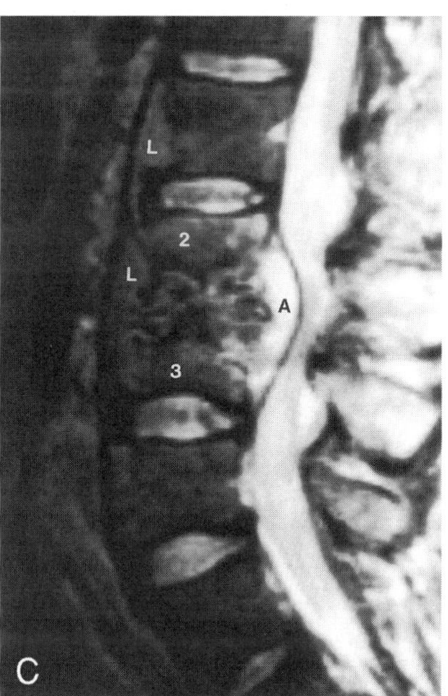

Figure 2.3 C

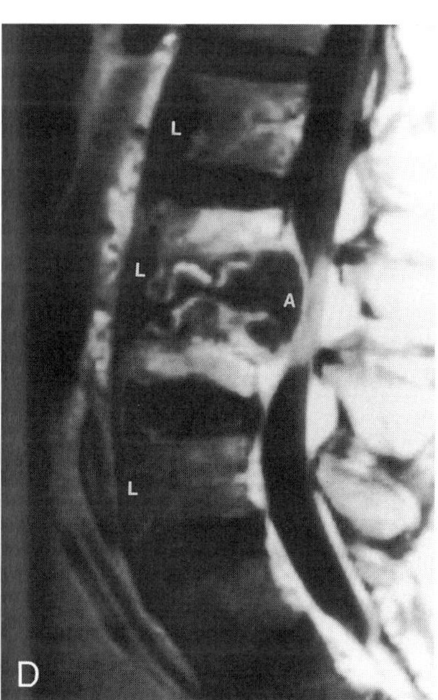

Figure 2.3 D

Findings: Lateral radiograph of the cervical spine shows destruction of the inferior and anterior aspect of C2 (2) and superior and anterior aspect of C3 (3). Note calcifications in the C3-C4 disk space and in the region of the anterior longitudinal ligament. The precervical soft tissues are increased in size. In a different patient, axial CT (Fig. B) of the midthoracic spine shows lucency with central bony sequestrum in a vertebral body. There is extension of the process into the anterior epidural space (A) and cord compression. In a third patient, midsagittal MR postcontrast T1-weighted image (Fig. C) shows destruction of L2 (2) and L3 (3), an anterior epidural abscess (A), and extension of the process (L) under the anterior longitudinal ligament. Corresponding postcontrast image (Fig. D) shows marked enhancement of L2 and L3, abscess in the anterior epidural space (A) and extension under (L) the anterior longitudinal ligament.

(continued)

Diagnosis: Spinal tuberculosis.

Discussion: Although rare, spinal tuberculosis is reemerging in developed countries secondary to migratory influx and an increase in the AIDS population. In the spine, tuberculosis involves the thoracic, lumbar, cervical, and, lastly, sacral regions. The infection begins in the anterior vertebral bodies and spreads into the disk and under the anterior and posterior longitudinal ligaments. Skip lesions are common, and collapse of vertebral bodies results in a gibbus deformity. At diagnosis, there is commonly severe involvement of the vertebrae, disks, and paraspinal tissues. CT demonstrates not only the bone destruction but also the common paraspinal abscess. In the lumbar region, psoas and flank abscess are common, whereas in thoracic spinal tuberculosis, mediastinal involvement may occur. MR imaging is helpful by demonstrating the extension under the ligaments and the degree of cord compression. The presence of a thick rim of enhancement around the paraspinal and intraosseous abscesses is typical of tuberculosis. Atypical presentations include isolated involvement of the posterior elements and destruction of one vertebra without soft tissue abnormalities. In both instances, the diagnosis may only be made histologically.

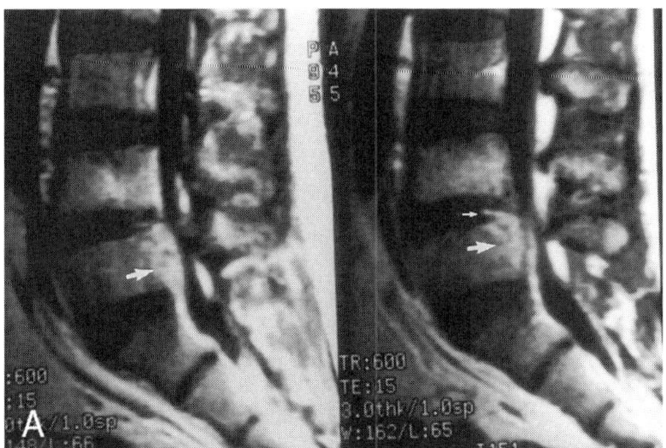

Figure 2.4 A

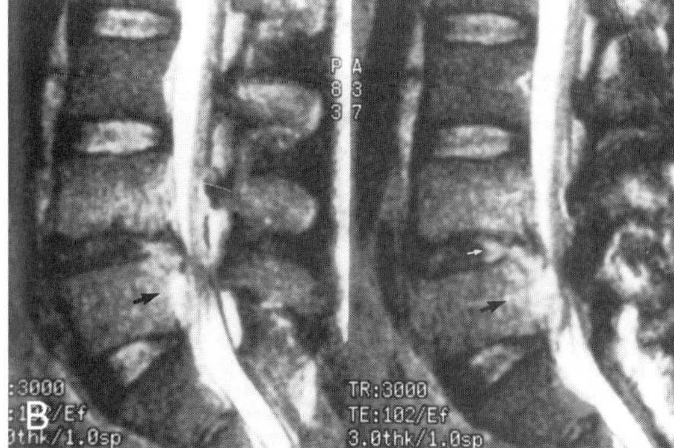

Figure 2.4 B

Clinical History: 27-year-old male with low back pain and fever. Two months before presentation he visited a farm in Mexico and drank goat's milk.

Findings: Mid- and para-sagittal postcontrast MR T1-weighted images (Fig. A) show abnormal enhancement (larger arrow) of the posterior aspect of L5 and some prominence of the ventral epidural space at this level. There is also enhancement (tiny arrow) of the L5-S1 disk posteriorly. Corresponding T2-weighted images show the abnormal areas in the posterior aspect (larger arrows) of L5 and disk (tiny arrow) to be hyperintense (Fig. B).

Differential Diagnosis: Bacterial and tuberculous diskitis and osteomyelitis, spinal brucellosis.

Diagnosis: Spinal brucellosis.

Discussion: Brucellosis is a granulomatous infection most commonly encountered in the Middle East but also in Latin America. It is found in young-to-middle aged patients and is extremely unusual in children. It is caused by the abortus, suis, canis and melitensis species of Brucella. Brucellosis most commonly targets the musculoskeletal system. Clinically and by imaging it is very difficult to differentiate it from tuberculosis. Brucellosis is diagnosed by means of positive serologic tests and positive blood cultures. A percutaneous biopsy is of limited use because isolating the organism from tissue samples is extremely difficult. Surgery is generally not needed because the response to antibrucellar chemotherapy is usually excellent.

Imaging shows two types of spinal brucellosis. In the focal type, one disk space and the adjacent superior (and generally anterior) end-plate of the vertebral body below are involved. In the diffuse type, in addition to disk space involvement, the adjacent vertebrae are diffusely involved. The most commonly affected segment is L4. MR images that may help to differentiate brucellosis from tuberculosis are involvement of only the lower lumbar region, near-normal appearing vertebral bodies, intact posterior elements, mild-to-moderate epidural space involvement, normal paraspinal soft tissues, and absent gibbus.

CASE 5

Clinical History: 48-year-old female undergoing immunosuppressive treatment for a recent kidney transplant presents with low thoracic pain and mild fever.

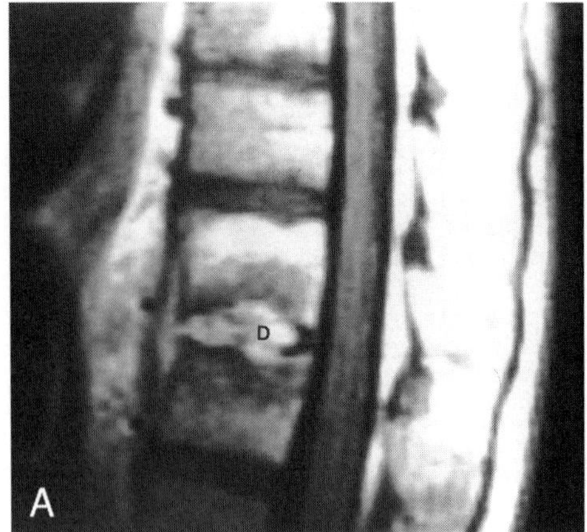

Figure 2.5 A

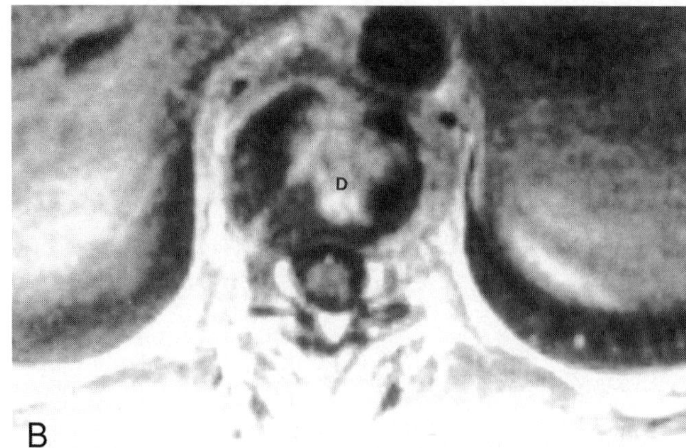

Figure 2.5 B

Findings: Postcontrast midsagittal MR T1-weighted image (Fig. A) shows enhancement of the T12-L1 disk (D). Abnormal disk enhancement (D) is also seen on an axial T1-weighted image (Fig. B). Note small amount of abnormal soft tissue surrounding the diseased disk space.

Differential Diagnosis: Bacterial diskitis, Candida diskitis.

Diagnosis: Candida diskitis.

Discussion: Spinal fungal infections are rare. Most causes are blastomycosis, coccidioidomycosis, candidiasis, and aspergillosis. Candida and aspergillus infections generally are found in immunocompromised patients or in those harboring indwelling catheters. Candidiasis is commonly caused by hematogenous spread, whereas aspergillosis is commonly secondary to direct extension. Blastomycosis is seen in the south central and midatlantic regions of the United States. More than 50% of patients infected with this microorganism develop some form of bone disease. Involvement of a disk space and adjacent rib suggests blastomycosis. Coccidioidomycosis typically involves several vertebrae but preserves the disk. Paraspinal abscesses are common. Contrary to blastomycosis and coccidioidomycosis, the imaging findings produced by spinal candidiasis and aspergillosis are nonspecific and identical to those resulting from the more common bacterial infections. Diagnosis requires demonstration of the microorganism.

CASE 6

Clinical Histories (Two Cases):

The first patient (Figs. A and B) is 40-year-old male status post-open heart surgery 3 weeks previously now presenting with low pain and fever.

The second patient (Figs. C and D) is a 50-year-old female in whom a lumbar puncture was done and now has back pain and lower extremity weakness but no fever.

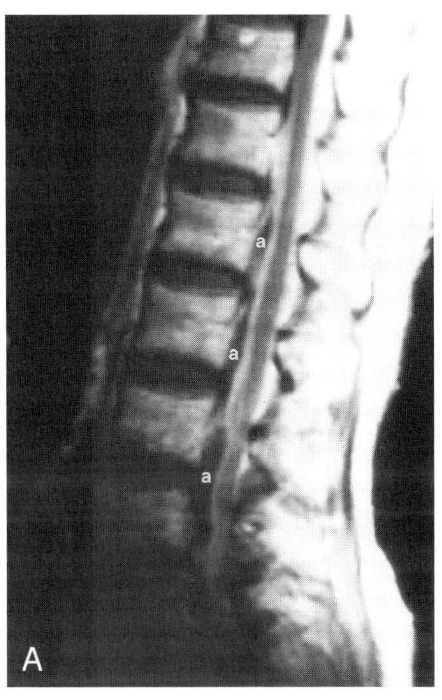

Figure 2.6 A

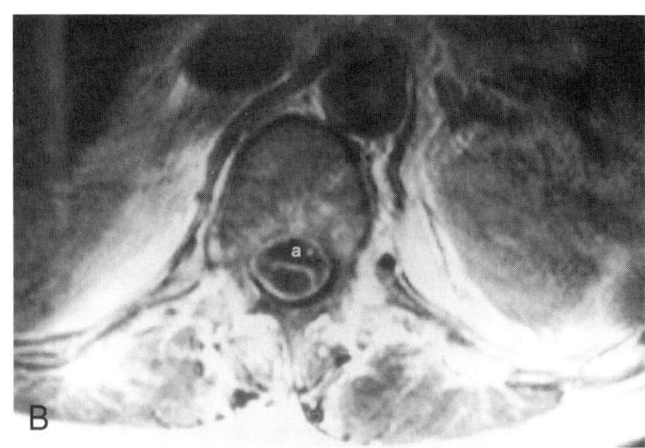

Figure 2.6 B

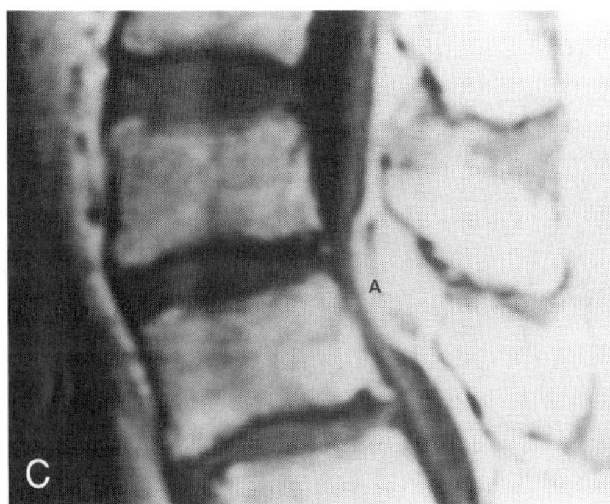

Figure 2.6 C

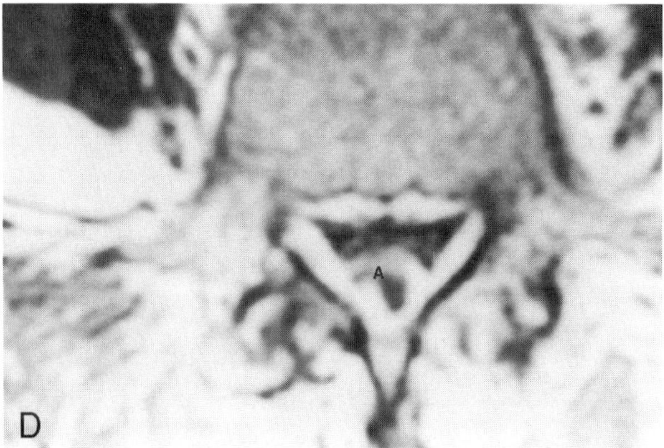

Figure 2.6 D

Findings: Midsagittal postcontrast MR T1-weighted image (Fig. A) shows a nonenhancing collection (a) of low signal intensity in the ventral epidural space. Note marked enhancement of the dura, compression of the thecal sac, and normal appearing disks and vertebrae. Axial postcontrast T1-weighted image (Fig. B) in the same patient clearly shows the abnormality (a) compressing the sac. In the second patient, midsagittal postcontrast MR T1-weighted image (Fig. C) shows an enhancing collection (A) with a low signal intensity center in the posterior epidural space at the L4-L5 level. Axial postcontrast image (Fig. D) shows the collection (A) and a diffusely thick and enhancing epidural space.

(continued)

Diagnosis: Epidural abscess, most likely from hematogenous origin (first case). Infected epidural hematoma from prior lumbar puncture (second case).

Discussion: Most epidural abscesses are secondary to diskitis and osteomyelitis but may also occur secondary to facet joint infections, posterior paraspinal abscess, urinary and respiratory tract infections, and retroperitoneal abscesses. However, up to 20% of them may be isolated. Isolated epidural abscesses are more common in the thoracic and lumbar regions. Most affected patients are middle aged, and predisposing factors include diabetes, intravenous drug use, trauma, renal insufficiency and hemodialysis, dental surgery, and epidural catheters. In a significant number of patients, the abscesses may be considered diffuse because they involve several segments. The most common microorganism is *Staphylococcus aureus*. When the abscesses occur in the cervical and thoracic regions, patients present with spinal cord compression symptoms. When they occur in the lumbar spine, a cauda equina syndrome is a common presentation. The inflammation within the epidural space may lead to thrombophlebitis if the veins are contained in it and this may result in venous infarction of the spinal cord. Imaging findings in epidural abscesses include intervertebral disk and vertebral enhancement, diffuse enhancement of a thickened epidural space, peripheral enhancement surrounding pus, and engorgement of the venous epidural plexus. After initiation of appropriate antibiotic therapy, some improvement should be noted within 5–10 days. Treatment for most epidural abscesses is, however, surgical.

CASE 7

Clinical History: 7-year-old female with chronic cough, fever, cervical pain, and weakness in the lower extremities.

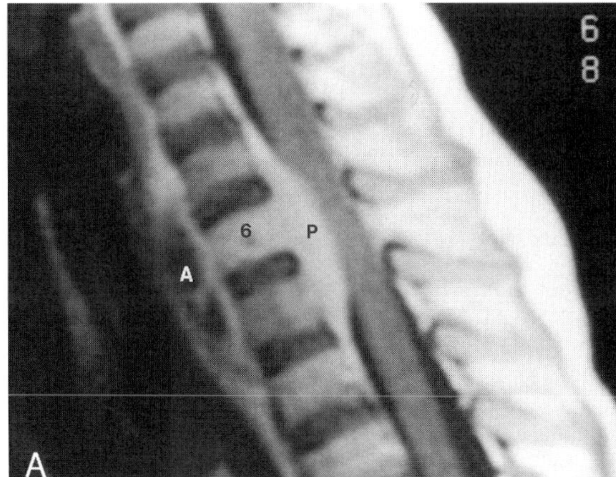
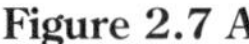

Figure 2.7 A

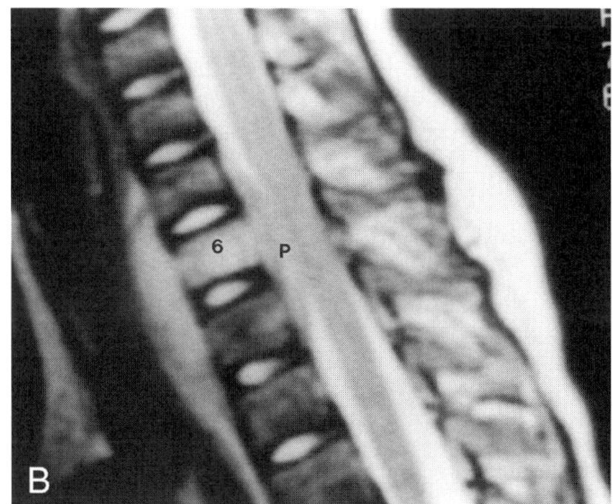

Figure 2.7 B

Findings: Midsagittal postcontrast MR T1-weighted image (Fig. A) shows marked enhancement of the C6 (6) vertebral body. There is a solidly enhancing mass (P) in the ventral epidural space at that level with compression of the spinal cord. Under the anterior longitudinal ligament there is an abscess (A). Corresponding MR T2-weighted image shows high signal intensity from C6 (6) and abnormalities in the ventral epidural space (P) and precervical space (Fig. B).

Differential Diagnosis: Bacterial and fungal diskitis/osteomyelitis, eosinophilic granuloma, metastatic disease; C6 osteomyelitis, epidural space phlegmon, and precervical abscess secondary to tuberculosis.

Diagnosis: C6 osteomyelitis, epidural space phlegmon, and precervical abscess secondary to tuberculosis.

Discussion: MR imaging is the most sensitive imaging test for the diagnosis of epidural abscesses (see Cases #2 and 6). In more than one-half of all patients, a source cannot be identified. Chronic epidural abscesses are the result of extension from diskitis/osteomyelitis. Acute epidural abscesses are generally of hematogenous origin. Tuberculosis generally results in osteomyelitis affecting the anterior vertebrae with subsequent disk space involvement and subligamentous spread. However, single vertebral body involvement without paraspinal abnormalities is a well-known atypical presentation of this disorder. MR imaging with contrast should be obtained if an epidural abscess is considered. Postcontrast fat suppression imaging helps to identify epidural abscesses by decreasing the high signal intensity of the surrounding epidural fat. In addition, contrast enables one to distinguish between a true abscess and a phlegmon or collection of chronic granulation tissue. This differentiation is important because surgery is almost always performed for true abscesses but not always done for solid nonpurulent collections.

Clinical History: 24-year-old male with AIDS and fever and pain in the left lower thoracic region.

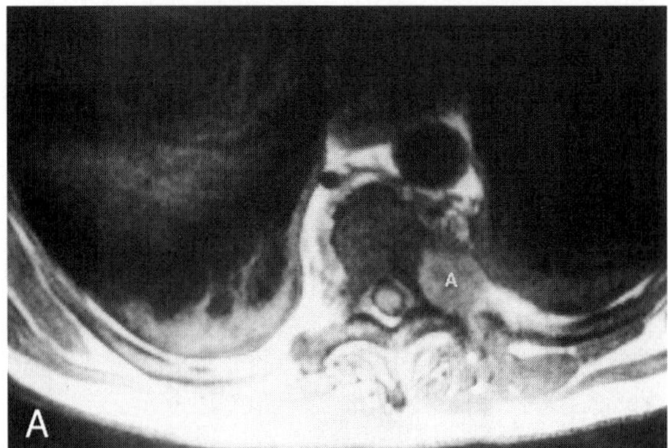

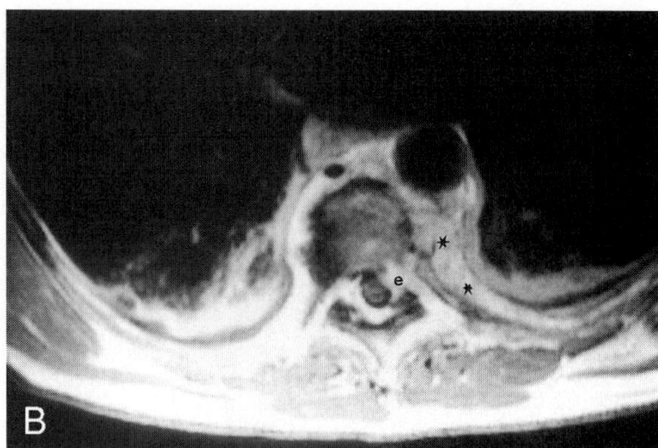

Figure 2.8 A   **Figure 2.8 B**

Findings: Axial precontrast MR T1-weighted image (Fig. A) shows an abnormal soft tissue mass (A) in the right paraspinal region where the 10th left rib joins the transverse process. After contrast administration (Fig. B), there is enhancement of enlarged soft tissues (*) anterior to the 10th left rib and epidural (e) extension of the process resulting in compression of the spinal cord. There are bilateral pleural reactions.

Diagnosis: Septic arthritis (caused by *Staphylococcus aureus*) of the left 10th costotransverse joint with epidural involvement and spinal cord compression.

Discussion: Infections of the costotransverse joints are unusual and are seen in patients with AIDS or intravenous drug abusers. Most of these infections are pyogenic but they may also be fungal in nature, particularly secondary to blastomycosis (see Case #5). Although the diagnosis may be aided by CT, MR imaging allows evaluation of adjacent spinal canal. Processes that may also affect the costotransverse synovial joints include arthritis (osteoarthritis, rheumatoid arthritis, and ankylosing spondylitis), diffuse idiopathic skeletal hyperostosis (DISH), synovial chondrometaplasia, fibrous dysplasia, and fractures. Tumors that may arise in this region are aneurysmal bone cysts, sarcomas, and, on rare occasions, metastases.

CASE 9

Clinical History: 27-year-old male with chronic nonspecific low back pain.

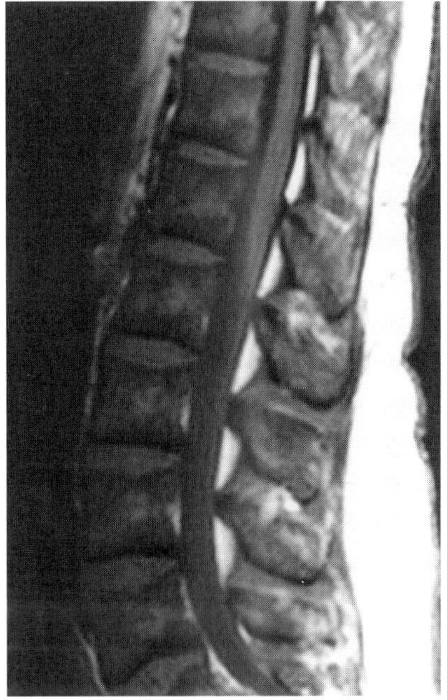

Figure 2.9

Findings: Midsagittal noncontrast MR T1-weighted image shows marked and diffused hypointensity in the bone marrow of the lumbar vertebral bodies.

Differential Diagnosis: Chronic anemia, diffuse marrow replacement with metastatic disease, multiple myeloma (but patient is too young for the latter), hypointense spine of AIDS.

Diagnosis: Hypointense spine of AIDS.

Discussion: Reversal of the normal T1 signal intensity in the bone marrow of the vertebral bodies is an abnormality seen in patients with AIDS. On bone marrow aspirates, these patients show only an increase in stainable iron. There generally is no evidence of tumor, hypercellularity, infection, or fibrosis. The most likely explanation for this MR imaging finding is increased iron retention in the bone marrow secondary to anemia of chronic disease. However, similar findings may be noted in patients who have undergone multiple blood transfusions, which lead to secondary siderosis. In these patients, iron is captured by the reticuloendothelial system and released very slowly or not at all. Hemosiderin, which contains iron, is paramagnetic and results in shortening of the T2 relaxation time. In large concentrations, both the T1 and T2 relaxations times are shortened, leading to low signal intensity in both types of sequences.

CASE 10

Clinical History: Patient with long-standing renal insufficiency treated with hemodialysis now presents with a 1-month history of cervical pain, decreased range of motion, and weakness in all extremities.

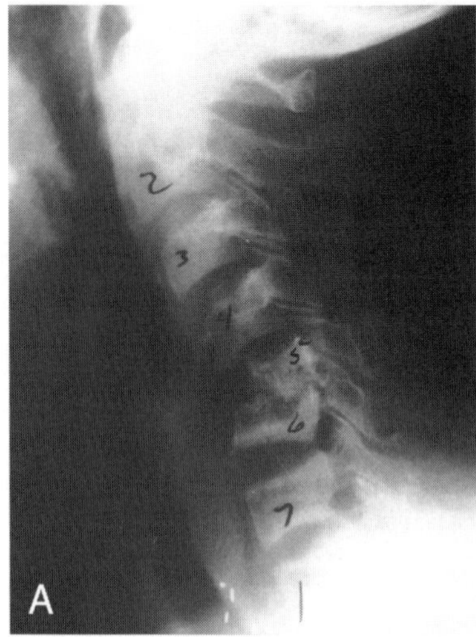

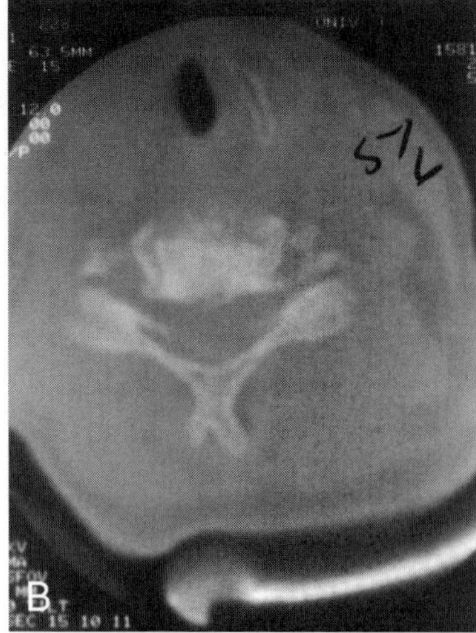

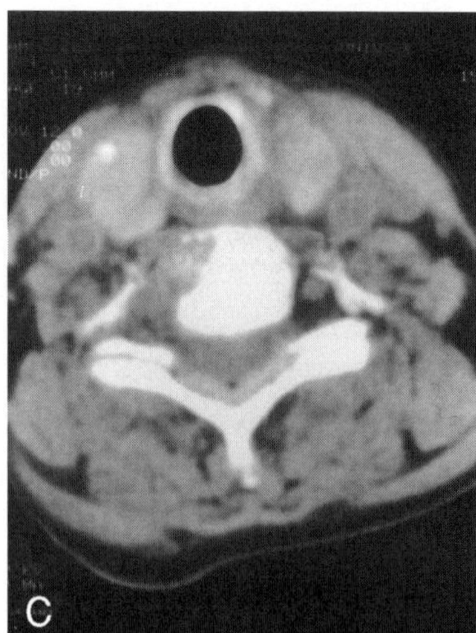

| Figure 2.10 A | Figure 2.10 B | Figure 2.10 C |

Findings: Lateral radiograph (Fig. A) shows destruction of C5 and C6 centered at the disk space. There is reverse angulation at this level and slight kyphosis. Axial CT, bone window setting (Fig. B) at the C5-C6 disk level shows destruction of the anterior aspect of C6. Axial CT, soft tissue window setting (Fig. C) shows destruction of the lateral aspect of C6.

Differential Diagnosis: Bacterial diskitis/osteomyelitis, tuberculosis, fungal infection, amyloidosis, neurogenic (Charcot's) spine, vertebral body osteochondrosis, hemodialysis-related destructive spondylitis.

Diagnosis: Hemodialysis-related destructive spondylitis.

Discussion: Destructive spondyloarthropathy may occur in patients who have undergone hemodialysis for many years. It is more common in middle-aged and older individuals. Usually there is no evidence of hyperparathyroidism. Histologically there are no microorganisms. There is significant ligamentous laxity in these patients. Increased amyloid deposition is commonly found in the spinal lesions. The cervical and lumbar regions are affected more than is the thoracic spine. Involvement of the craniocervical junction may be indistinguishable from severe rheumatoid arthritis. MR imaging may be used to differentiate hemodialysis-related destructive spondylitis from an infection. In the former, T2-weighted sequences show the vertebrae and disk to be of low signal intensity contrary to the high signal intensity expected with infection.

Clinical History: You are shown three different patients. The first patient (Fig. A) presented with a myelopathy. The second patient (Fig. B) presented with a cauda equina syndrome and hydrocephalus. The third patient (Figs. C and D) presented with seizures and bilateral lower extremity weakness. All patients were Latin American immigrants.

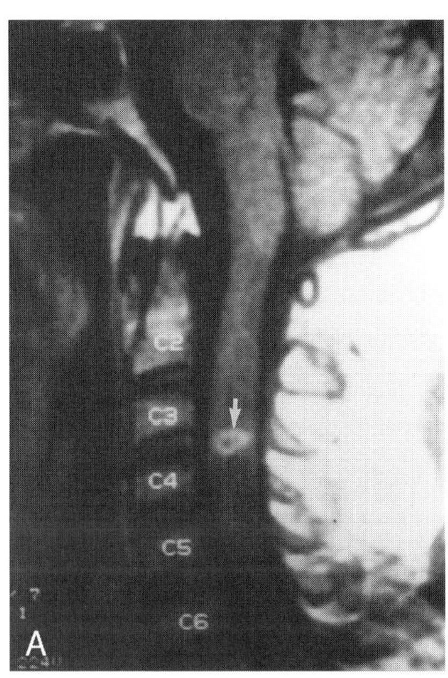

Figure 2.11 A

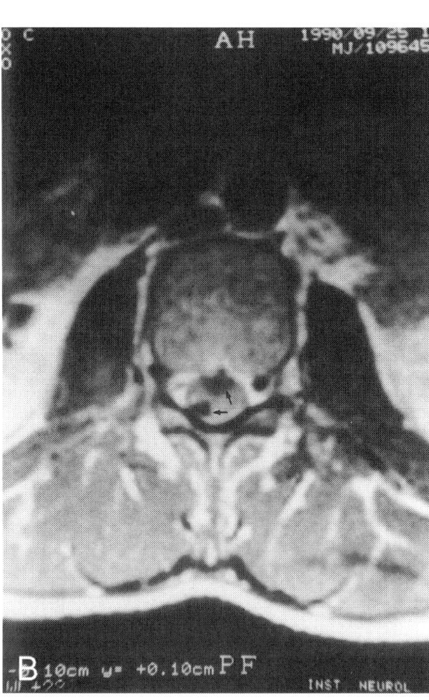

Figure 2.11 B

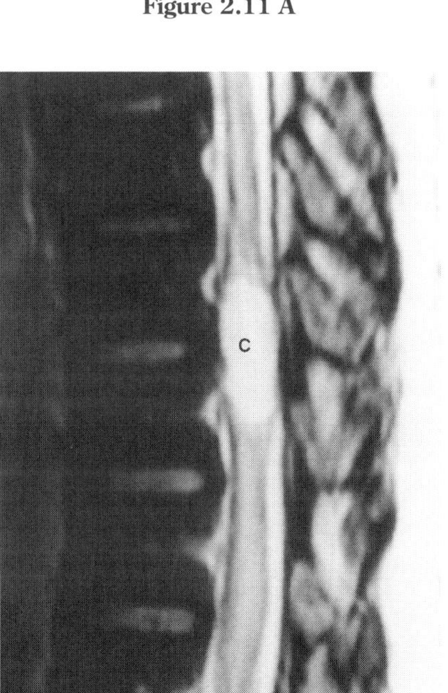

Figure 2.11 C

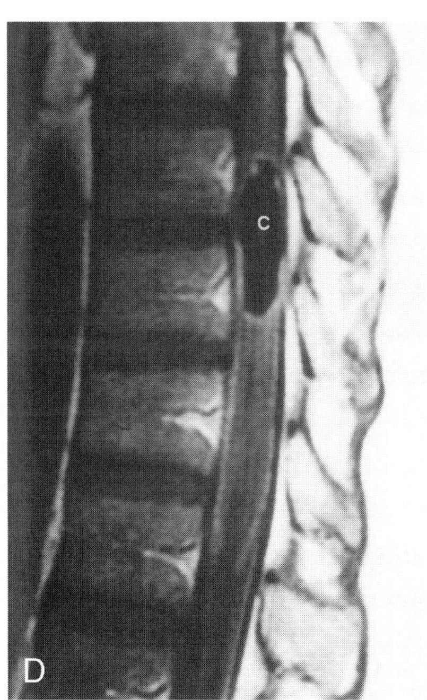

Figure 2.11 D

(continued)

Findings: Midsagittal postcontrast MR T1-weighted image (Fig. A) shows an intramedullary spinal cord ring enhancing lesion (arrow) at the C3-C4 level. Axial postcontrast MR T1-weighted image (Fig. B) in different patient shows two intradural lesions (arrows) compressing the cauda equina. In a third patient, midsagittal MR T2-weighted image (Fig. C) shows an intramedullary lesion (C) of high signal intensity in the distal thoracic spinal cord. Corresponding postcontrast MR T1-weighted image (Fig. D) shows the lesion (C) to be of signal intensity similar to CSF and to have peripheral enhancement. There is also enhancement of the surfaces of conus medullaris.

Diagnosis: Intramedullary (Figs. A, C, and D) and subarachnoid (Fig. B) cysticercosis.

Discussion: Neurocysticercosis is the result of infection with the invasive larva of the pork tapeworm (Taenia solium). After the worm eggs are ingested, their capsule is digested in stomach enzymes. They hatch in the bowel, burrowing in its wall and disseminating hematogenously. Approximately 1% of all patients with neurocysticercosis develop lesions in the spinal cord and/or spine. Subarachnoid cysticercosis is more common than intramedullary disease. The cysts may migrate into the subarachnoid space, but because they induce an arachnoiditis they may lodge and result in compression of neural structures. Subarachnoid disease most commonly involves the lumbar and thoracic regions, and the lesions tend to be multiple. Intramedullary lesions are usually solitary. Enhancement of intramedullary lesions is common and is caused by breakdown of the cord-blood-barrier. The spinal cord may show focal expansion and edema. Accompanying spinal cord nonparasitic cysts in association with cysticerci have been described.

CASE 12

Clinical History: A 33-year-old female presents with new onset of right arm weakness and paresthesias. One month later, this patient developed optic neuritis.

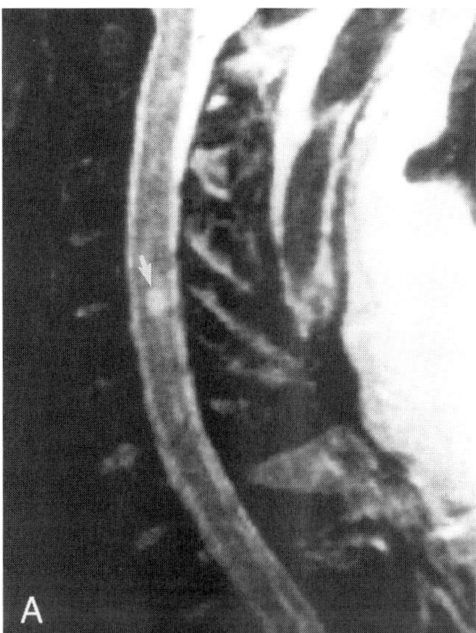

Figure 2.12 A

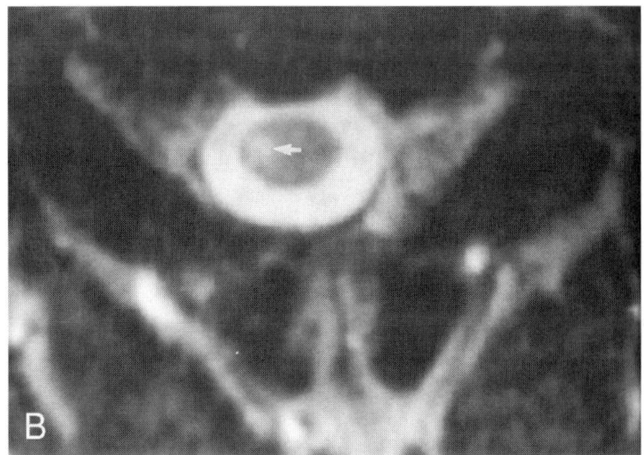

Figure 2.12 B

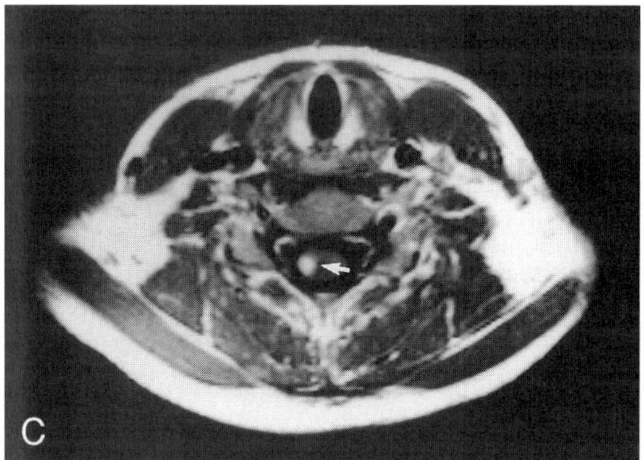

Figure 2.12 C

Findings: Slightly parasagittal MR T2*-weighted image (Fig. A) shows a focal abnormal area of hyperintensity (arrow) at the C4-C5 level. Axial MR T2*-weighted image (Fig. B) shows a lesion (arrow) in the right lateral aspect of the spinal cord. After contrast administration, axial MR T1-weighted image (Fig. C) shows the lesion (arrow) enhancing brightly.

Differential Diagnosis: Neoplasm, arterial or venous spinal cord infarctions, acute transverse myelitis (idiopathic), viral infections, acute disseminated encephalomyelitis, multiple sclerosis.

Diagnosis: Multiple sclerosis.

Discussion: Approximately 12% of patients who meet the clinical criteria for the diagnosis of multiple sclerosis show lesions confined to only the spinal cord. Most of these patients have only one or two lesions generally located in the cervical and upper thoracic regions. The number of lesions closely correlates with the degree of disability. The spinal cord is generally of normal diameter (no edema is present) when plaques are present. The length of a plaque is generally less than one vertebral segment. Transverse MR imaging shows that most plaques involve the lateral and posterior aspects of the spinal cord. Over 90% of patients with spinal cord lesions eventually show brain lesions.

Clinical History: 7-year-old boy with acute onset of seizures and weakness of all four extremities. Patient had a common upper respiratory tract infection 10 days previously.

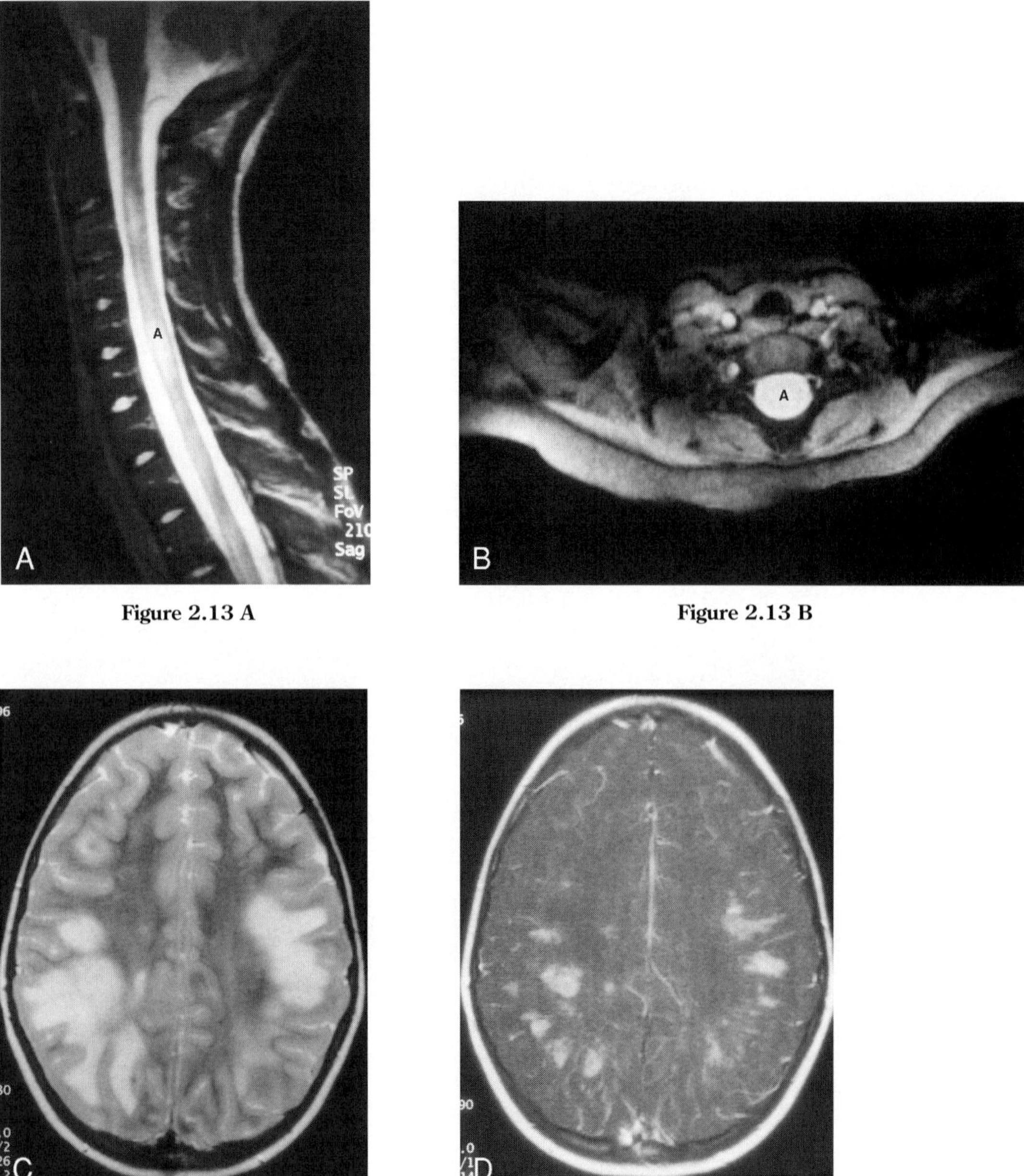

Figure 2.13 A

Figure 2.13 B

Figure 2.13 C

Figure 2.13 D

Findings: Midsagittal MR T2-weighted image (Fig. A) shows abnormal increased signal intensity (A) within the spinal cord at the C5-C6 levels and a smaller abnormal zone at C3. On an axial T2-weighted image (Fig. B), the entire cross-section of the spinal cord (A) is hyperintense and inseparable from surrounding CSF. Axial proton density image (Fig. C) of the brain shows abnormal hyperintense areas in the white matter with little mass effect. Corresponding postcontrast T1-weighted image (Fig. D) shows enhancement of most lesions.

(continued)

Diagnosis: Acute disseminated encephalomyelitis (ADEM).

Discussion: ADEM is probably an autoimmune reaction to viruses or viral particles similar to allergic encephalitis. This disorder generally manifests 2–3 weeks after measles, varicella, smallpox, mononucleosis, herpes zoster, mumps, influenza, and vaccinations. Prior subclinical infections are probably responsible for those cases in which no clear predisposing viral illness may be recalled. Most patients are between the ages of 6–10 years. The most common symptoms are seizures and altered mental status. Spinal cord lesions result in paraplegia, incontinence, and decreased or absent reflexes. ADEM is a monophasic disease resolving in 2–4 weeks. Approximately 80% of patients recover completely, 10% have residual sequelae, and 10% die. The lesions in the spinal cord are nonspecific but tend to involve long segments and produce expansion. Enhancement may occur but is not common.

Clinical History: 35-year-old African-American female presents with weakness and spasticity of all four extremities. This patient had an abnormal chest radiograph.

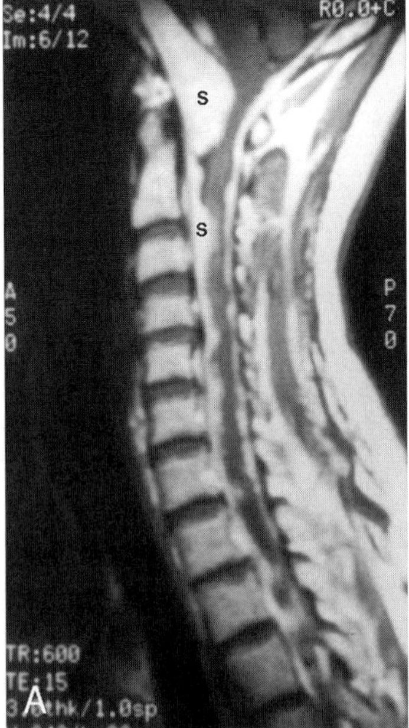

Figure 2.14 A

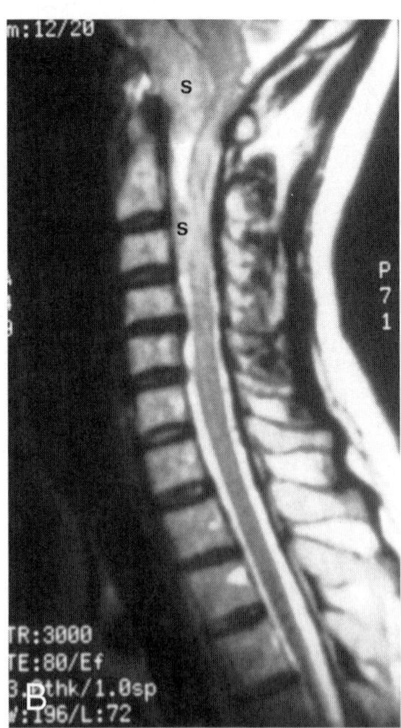

Figure 2.14 B

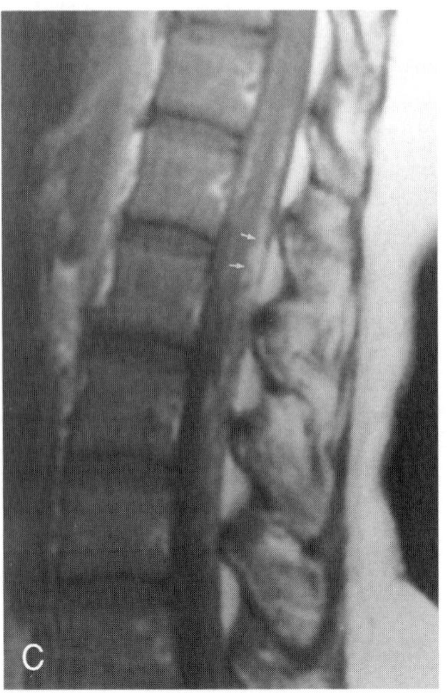

Figure 2.14 C

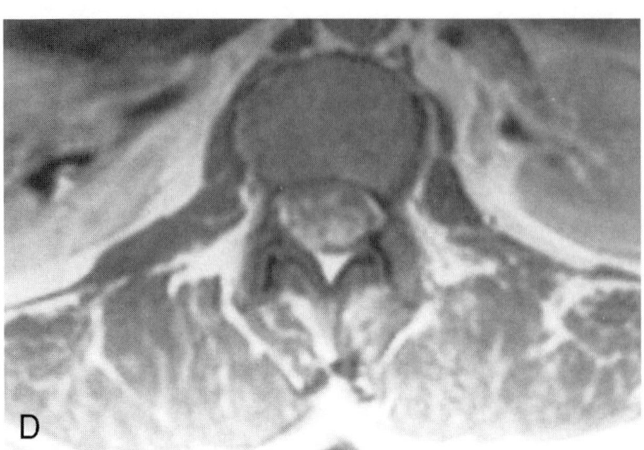

Figure 2.14 D

(continued)

Findings: Midsagittal postcontrast MR T1-weighted image (Fig. A) shows multiple extramedullary intradural masses (S) extending from the clivus to the thoracic region both anteriorly and posteriorly. There is significant compression of the spinal cord. Corresponding MR T2-weighted image (Fig. B) shows the masses (S) to be hypointense. Midsagittal postcontrast MR T1-weighted image (Fig. C) of the thoracolumbar region shows enhancement of surfaces of the conus medullaris (arrows) and of the cauda equina. Axial postcontrast image (Fig. D) shows the enhancement of the nerve roots in the cauda equina.

Differential Diagnosis: Metastases, lymphoma, tuberculosis, multiple meningiomas (for the lesions in the cervical region), sarcoidosis.

Diagnosis: Sarcoidosis.

Discussion: Involvement of the central nervous system by sarcoidosis occurs in approximately 5% of patients. The spinal cord is rarely affected. In almost two-thirds of patients with spinal cord disease, the diagnosis is unknown prior to the onset of symptoms. Spinal cord sarcoidosis may be intramedullary (35%), extramedullary (35%), or a combination of both (25%). The vertebrae may also be involved and may demonstrate lytic lesions. Sarcoidosis has also been reported to produce paraspinal soft tissue masses. The imaging findings may be indistinguishable from those produced by tuberculosis. Intramedullary lesions generally enhance and expand the spinal cord. Contrast enhancement is also necessary to visualize pial involvement. Occasionally sarcoidosis has imaging findings that may simulate a meningioma en plaque. Infarctions may also occur secondary to involvement of small vessels.

CASE 15

Clinical History: 50-year-old male with progressive mid-back pain and decreased deep tendon reflexes in both lower extremities.

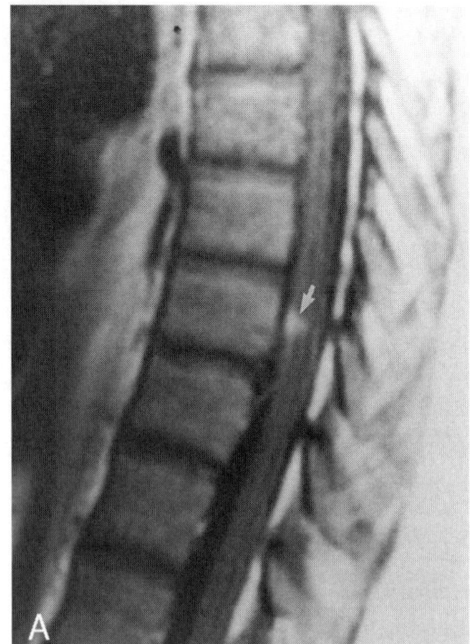

Figure 2.15 A

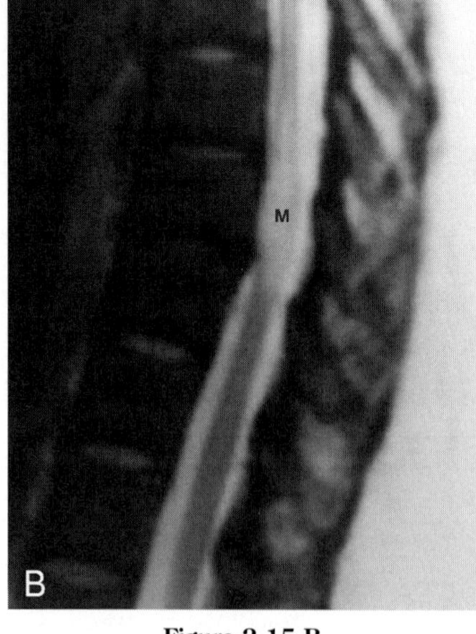

Figure 2.15 B

Findings: Midsagittal postcontrast MR T1-weighted image (Fig. A) shows a focal abnormal area (arrow) of intramedullary spinal cord enhancement at the T8 level. Corresponding MR T2-weighted image (Fig. B) shows the abnormal increased signal intensity (M) at the same level but more extensive than the area of enhancement. The spinal cord is slightly expanded.

Differential Diagnosis: Multiple sclerosis, acute disseminated encephalomyelitis, traumatic myelitis, infarction, idiopathic acute transverse myelitis.

Diagnosis: Idiopathic acute transverse myelitis.

Discussion: This inflammatory disorder of the spinal cord is probably autoimmune in nature. In many patients there is history of recent viral illness or vaccination. Most cases occur during the months of February to May. The symptoms include a rapid onset of bilateral motor, sensory, and autonomic dysfunction in the absence of spinal cord compression or a known neurologic disorder (such as multiple sclerosis). Idiopathic transverse myelitis is a diagnosis of exclusion. This disorder in found without any age or gender predilection. CSF analysis shows increased proteins and normal or increased white blood cells. The majority of patients improve with only supportive care. The thoracic spinal cord is involved more often than the cervical region. MR imaging shows cord swelling, low T1 signal intensity, and high T2 signal intensity. Involvement may vary from one level to the entire spinal cord. The pattern of contrast enhancement may be focal, diffuse and vague, peripheral, meningeal, or nodular.

CASE 16

Clinical History: 35-year-old female with a long-standing history of a multisystem autoimmune disorder presents with a 6-month history of progressive lower extremity spasticity.

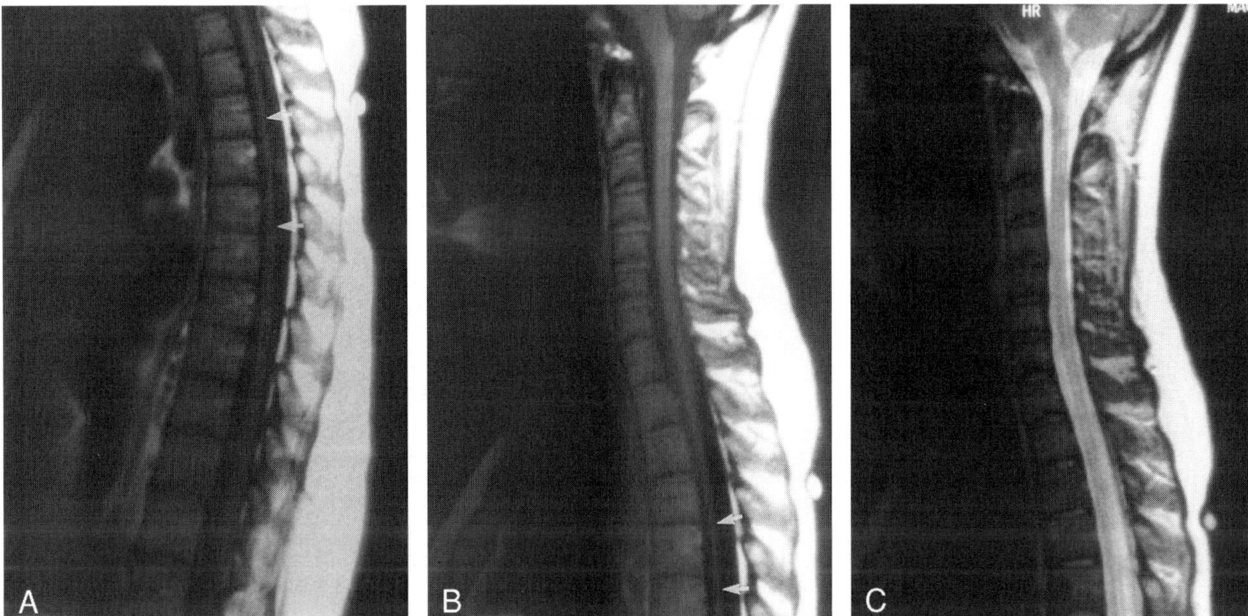

Figure 2.16 A   Figure 2.16 B   Figure 2.16 C

Findings: Midsagittal noncontrast MR T1-weighted image (Fig. A) shows marked atrophy of the thoracic spinal cord (arrows). Midsagittal T1-weighted image (Fig. B) of the cervicothoracic region shows that the atrophy involves the thoracic region (arrows) and spares the cervical cord. Corresponding T2-weighted image (Fig. C) shows no abnormal signal intensity from the spinal cord. No abnormal contrast enhancement was noted.

Diagnosis: Lupus myelopathy.

Discussion: Lupus erythematosus is a multisystem disorder leading to cerebral infarctions in about 50% of all patients. Infarctions are multifactorial and are caused by endocarditis, coagulopathy, and antiphospholipid syndrome. True lupus vasculitis is rare. Lupus myelopathy generally becomes apparent years after the onset of the disease, although rarely it is the presenting manifestation. It may either follow a rapid progressive course or be relapsing–remitting. In most cases, the disease predominantly affects the thoracic spinal cord. Acutely, the lesions are caused by coagulative and/or liquefactive necrosis that eventually leads to destruction of axons and myelin.

CASE 17

Clinical History: 5-year-old boy with ascending bilateral lower extremity weakness progressive over a 1-week period.

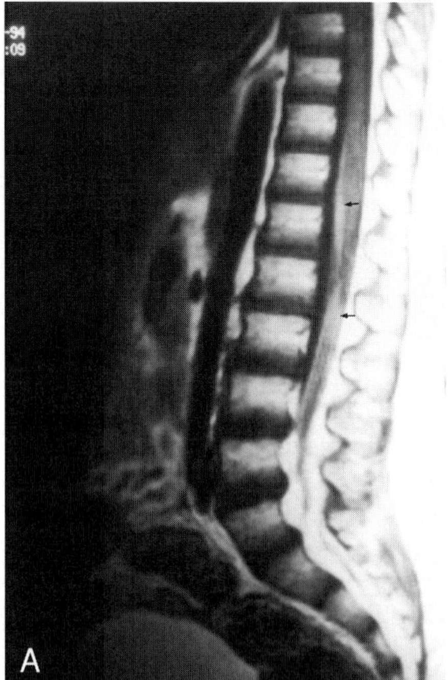

Figure 2.17 A

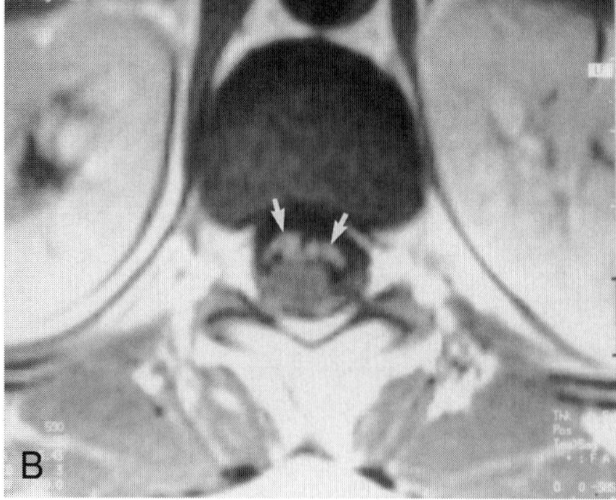

Figure 2.17 B

Findings: Midsagittal postcontrast MR T1-weighted image (Fig. A) shows abnormal enhancement (arrows) in the ventral aspect of the conus medullaris and in the cauda equina. Axial postcontrast image (Fig. B) shows swelling and marked enhancement (arrows) of the ventral rootlets of the cauda equina. There is mild enhancement of the dorsal rootlets.

Differential Diagnosis: Viral polyradiculitis (such as cytomegalovirus, other herpes viruses, and AIDS-related myelopathy), tuberculosis, metastases, lymphoma/leukemia, Guillain-Barré syndrome.

Diagnosis: Guillain-Barré syndrome.

Discussion: Guillain-Barré is an autoimmune inflammatory disorder predominantly affecting the peripheral nervous system. It may be preceded by a viral clinical illness in 65% of cases generally 3–6 weeks before the onset of neurologic symptoms. Guillain-Barré is usually monophasic. It occurs in approximately 1 in 100,000 individuals younger than 18 years of age. The symptoms are progressive and may lead to bulbar palsy. CSF analysis is nonspecific. Approximately 80% of patients have an excellent prognosis. Administration of corticosteroids is of uncertain benefit, but early plasmapheresis may shorten the course and severity of the disease. Pathologically there is demyelination and inflammation. Alteration of the nerve-blood-barrier is responsible for the enhancement seen on MR imaging. When enhancement of the spinal cord is present (as in the case shown here), the disease probably represents a combination of Guillain-Barré and idiopathic transverse myelitis (see Case #15).

CASE 18

Clinical History: 1-year-old boy with weakness in all extremities 2 weeks after receiving oral polio vaccine.

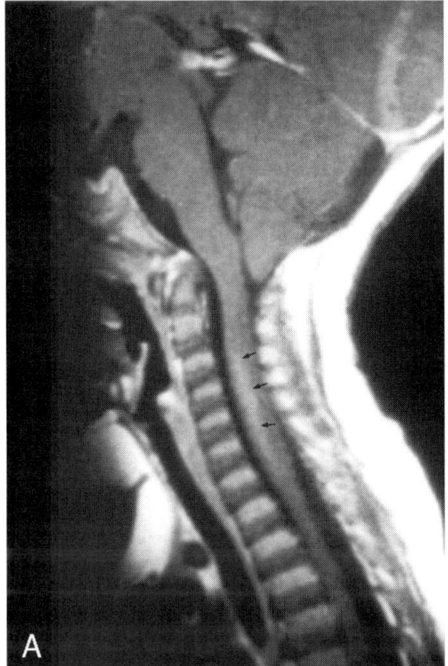

Figure 2.18 A

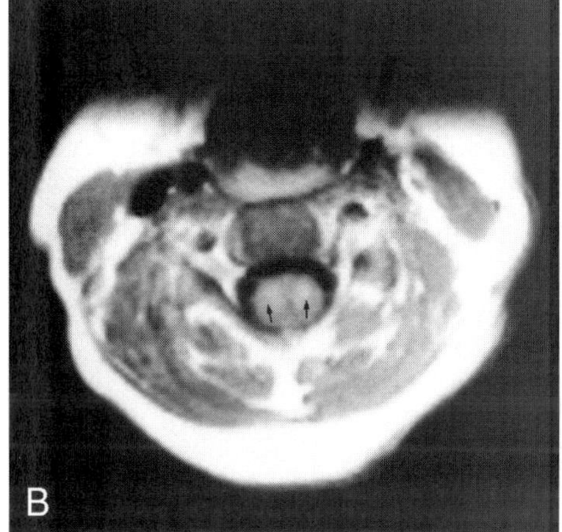

Figure 2.18 B

Findings: Midsagittal postcontrast MR T1-weighted image (Fig. A) shows subtle enhancement (arrows) in the anterior aspect of the cervical spinal cord. Note incidental Chiari type 1 malformation. On an axial postcontrast image (Fig. B), the enhancement (arrows) appears to be confined to the region of the anterior gray matter horns.

Differential Diagnosis: Acute disseminated encephalomyelitis, idiopathic transverse myelitis, probable postvaccination poliomyelitis.

Diagnosis: Probable postvaccination poliomyelitis.

Discussion: Poliomyelitis is a viral disorder affecting the lower motor neurons, specifically the anterior gray matter horns in the spinal cord. This disease is limited to humans and transmitted via fecal–oral route. It predominantly affects children and is generally a nonspecific febrile illness. In some cases, polioviruses induce an aseptic meningitis and only rarely do infections result in paralysis. Since the mid-1960s, this disease has been considered basically eradicated. Most cases of poliomyelitis are now the result of oral vaccination or caused by exposure of immunocompromised individuals to the virus (generally in the form of contact with recently vaccinated patients). Symptoms include flaccid paralysis, hypotonia, areflexia, decreased superficial reflexes, fever, nuchal pain and rigidity, and muscular fasciculations. CSF analysis is generally nonspecific, showing increased proteins and white blood cells. The virus may be cultivated from the CSF. The treatment is mostly supportive and, if the brainstem is involved, mechanical ventilation may be needed.

CASE 19

Clinical History: Patient with AIDS and a 3-day history of bilateral lower extremity weakness and urinary/fecal incontinence.

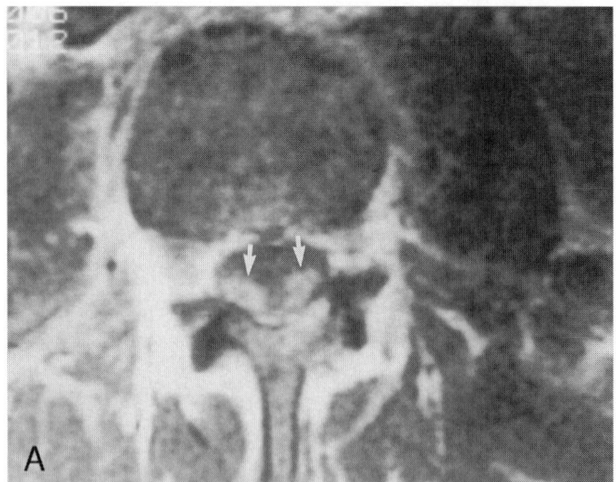

Figure 2.19 A

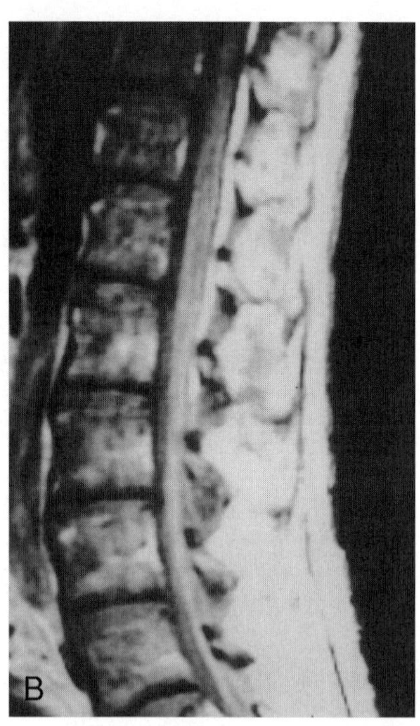

Figure 2.19 B

Findings: Axial postcontrast MR T1-weighted image (Fig. A) shows marked enhancement of all nerve roots (arrows) in the cauda equina. Midsagittal postcontrast MR T1-weighted image (Fig. B) shows enhancement of the cauda equina and questionable enhancement of the distal conus medullaris.

Differential Diagnosis: Guillain-Barré syndrome, lymphoma/leukemia, HIV radiculitis, tuberculosis, bacterial meningitis, metastases, cytomegalovirus (CMV) polyradiculitis.

Diagnosis: Cytomegalovirus (CMV) polyradiculitis.

Discussion: CMV polyradiculitis is relatively uncommon and occurs more often in patients with AIDS and other forms of immunosuppression. However, it may also occur in some immunocompetent patients. CMV is generally acquired from hematogenous dissemination. In the central nervous system it involves the brain, resulting in a hemorrhagic encephalitis. The cranial nerves and spinal cord and its nerve roots may also be affected. In patients with AIDS, CMV radiculitis may be isolated but may also be found in combination with HIV myelitis and syphilis. Symptoms include urinary retention, flaccid paresis, back and leg pain, and saddle-type anesthesia. CSF analysis tends to show abundant neutrophils and the virus may be cultivated from it. Treatment usually includes the administration of ganciclovir and foscarnet. On MR imaging, the rootlets of the cauda equina and conus medullaris are swollen. The nerves enhance markedly after contrast administration and may be clumped and adhere to the walls of the thecal sac.

Clinical History: 35-year-old female with atrophy and weakness of all extremities but more pronounced in the lower ones.

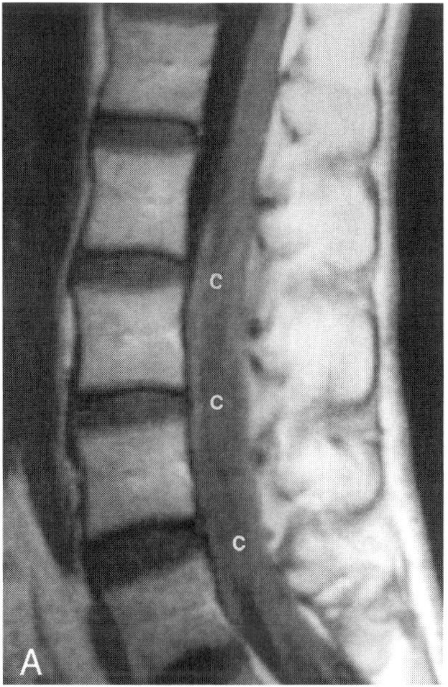

Figure 2.20 A

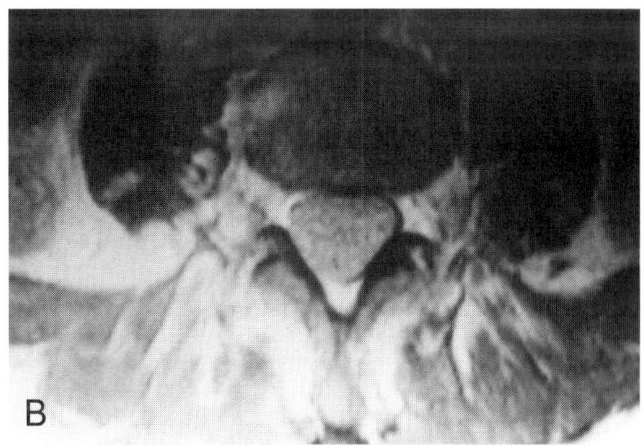

Figure 2.20 B

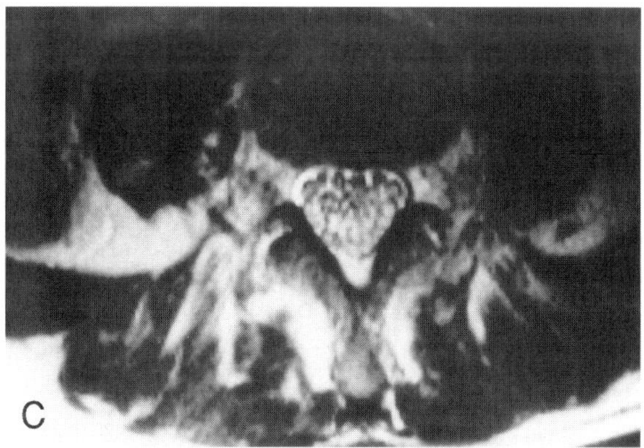

Figure 2.20 C

Findings: Midsagittal postcontrast MR T1-weighted image (Fig. A) shows enhancement and marked thickening of all lumbar nerve roots (C) and cauda equina. Axial postcontrast MR T1-weighted image (Fig. B) shows that the abnormal nerve roots completely fill the thecal sac. On a corresponding T2-weighted image (Fig. C), the nerve roots are of increased signal intensity.

Differential Diagnosis: Other hypertrophic polyneuropathies (i.e., Dejerine-Sottas disease, chronic inflammatory demyelinating polyradiculopathy, lead intoxication), viral polyradiculitis (see Case #19), Guillain-Barré syndrome (see Case #17), lymphoma/leukemia, metastases, tuberculosis, Charcot-Marie-Tooth (CMT) disease.

Diagnosis: Charcot-Marie-Tooth (CMT) disease.

Discussion: CMT disease is an inflammatory and hypertrophic polyradiculopathy. There is demyelination and remyelination leading to an onion bulb-like appearance of the nerves. It is usually diagnosed in young female patients and is a progressive disorder. Nerve degeneration leads to distal muscle atrophy beginning in the feet and extending to legs, arms, and trunk. Atrophy is more pronounced below the midthigh or elbow levels. Walking difficulties secondary to sensory ataxia and weakness are prominent. The peripheral nerves are commonly palpable at physical examination. There is no treatment.

Clinical History: You are shown imaging studies in four different young males, each with a chronic disorder. Fig. A is from a patient with back pain and arthralgias. Figs. B and C are from a patient with a similar history and also a cauda equina syndrome. Fig. D belongs to a different patient with a similar clinical history. Fig. E is from a patient after a recent fall.

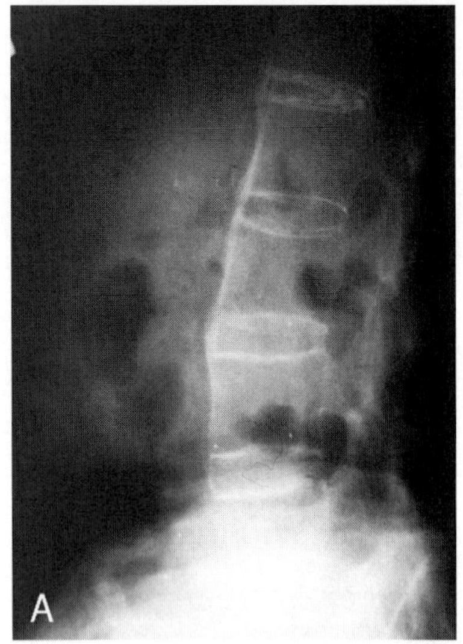

Figure 2.21 A

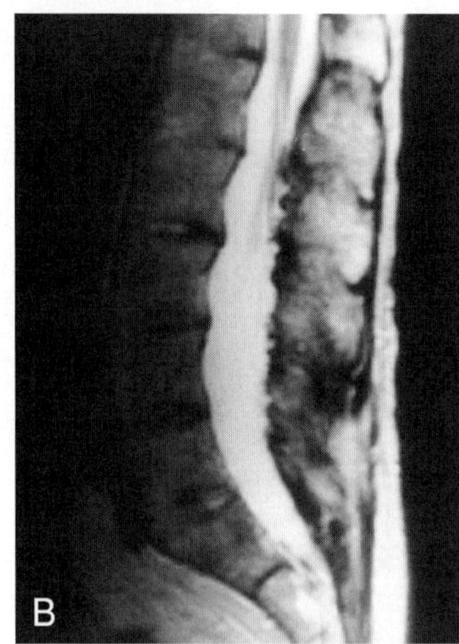

Figure 2.21 B

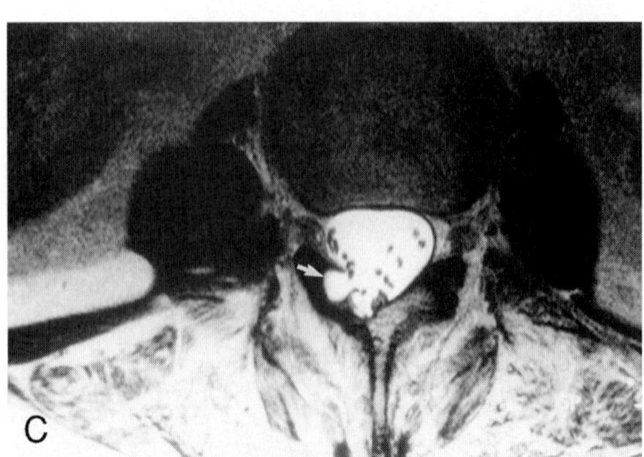

Figure 2.21 C

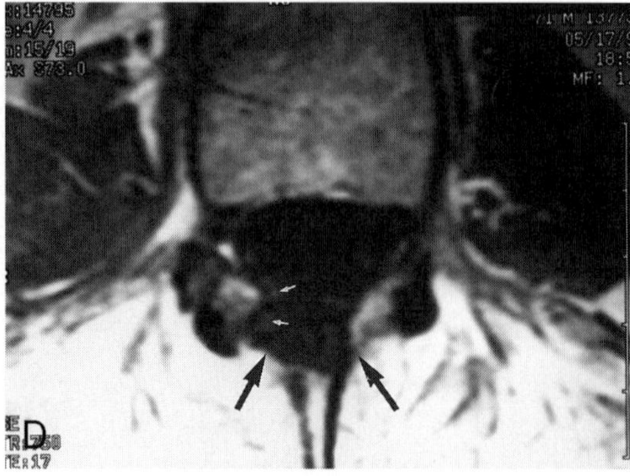

Figure 2.21 D

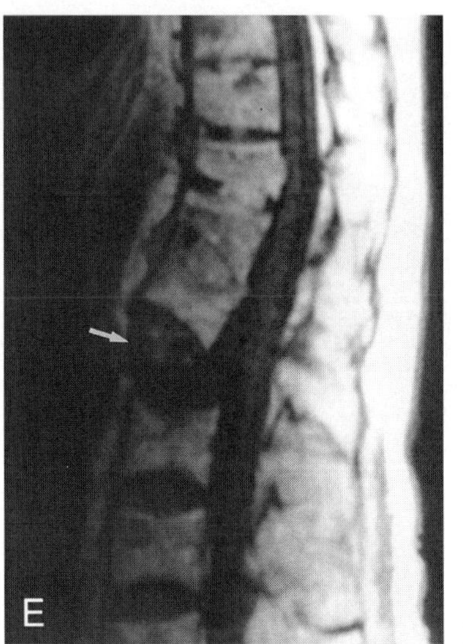

Figure 2.21 E

(continued)

Findings: In the first case, a lateral radiograph (Fig. A) of the lumbar spine shows anterior bridging syndesmophytes, squaring of the osteoporotic vertebral bodies, and calcification of the disks. In the second patient, a midsagittal MR T2-weighted image (Fig. B) shows indistinct disk spaces with fusion involving several vertebrae and a wide thecal sac containing multiple irregularities posteriorly. In the same patient, axial MR T2-weighted image (Fig. C) shows erosion of the bony spinal canal resulting in a dural diverticulum (arrow) and some matting of the nerve roots. In the third patient, an axial MR T1 weighted image (Fig. D) shows erosion of the posterior elements with a posterior dural diverticulum (arrows). Note that the nerve roots (tiny arrows) are matted and adherent to the lateral aspects of this diverticulum. Midsagittal MR T1-weighted image in a different patient (Fig. E) shows a fracture dislocation through a lower thoracic disk space (arrow). Note fusion of several vertebrae in the midthoracic region.

Diagnosis: Ankylosing spondylitis (AS). Fig. A shows the typical calcification of the anterior longitudinal ligament and squaring of the vertebral bodies. Figs. B, C, and D show AS with erosive dural ectasia and arachnoiditis. Fig. E is from a patient with AS and a fracture through a disk space.

Discussion: Ankylosing spondylitis, or Marie-Strumpell disease, is an inflammatory spondyloarthropathy associated with the histocompatibility antigen (HLA) B27. Most patients are males between the ages of 15–35 years. The most common symptoms at presentation are low back pain (80%) and pain over the sacroiliac joints. Initially, it affects the sacroiliac joints (bilateral symmetrical involvement) and then the spine and ligamentous insertions. Complications of ankylosing spondylitis are an adherent and erosive arachnoiditis, atlantoaxial subluxation, fractures, epidural hematoma, spinal cord compression, spinal stenosis, and a sterile diskitis (Anderson lesion). In cases of erosive arachnoiditis, there are dural ectasia and dural diverticula eroding the posterior vertebral elements. The nerve root sleeves may be dilated and rootlets of the cauda equina may be matted and adherent to the walls of the thecal sac. This arachnoiditis results in cauda equina syndrome. Fractures may occur through weakened vertebrae or the disk spaces. Fractures are more common in the cervical region but may occur anywhere. They may be single or multiple. Fractures alone or in combination with epidural hematomas may result in compression of the spinal cord. Epidural hematomas may also be spontaneous. Sterile destructive lesions may be localized to the central aspect of a vertebra or be extensive. These lesions occur more often in the thoracolumbar region. On T2-weighted images they are of low signal intensity, a feature that may be helpful in distinguishing them from a true infection.

CASE 22

Clinical History: 56-year-old female with a chronic disorder resulting in arthropathy and neck pain.

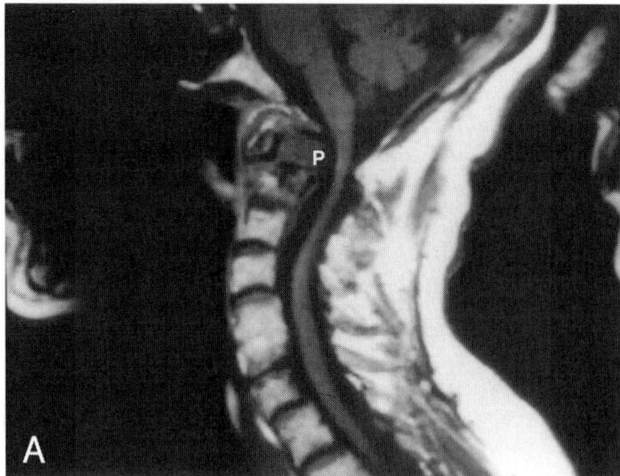

Figure 2.22 A

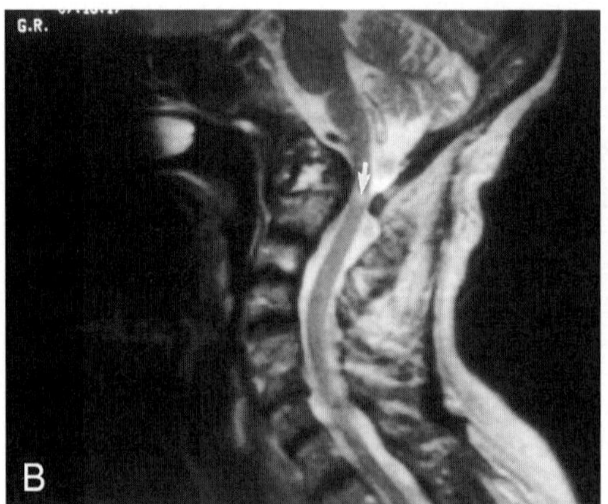
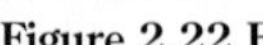

Figure 2.22 B

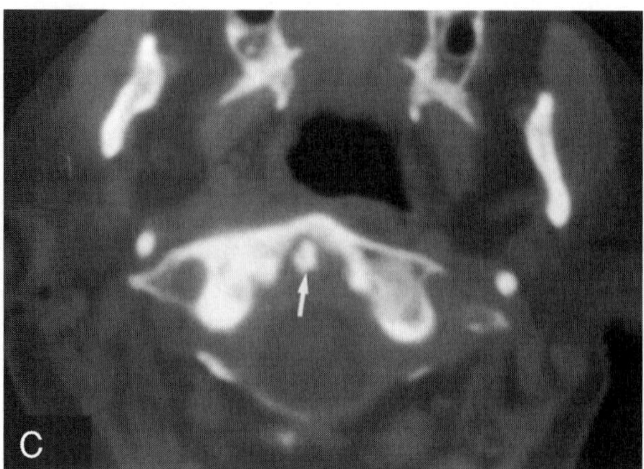

Figure 2.22 C

Findings: Midsagittal MR T1-weighted image (Fig. A) shows destruction of the dens and replacement by abnormal soft tissues (P). There is atlantoaxial subluxation with compression of the spinal cord at the cervico-medullary region. Note fusion of C5-C6. Corresponding MR T2-weighted image (Fig. B) shows similar findings. In addition, note the focal area of increased signal intensity (arrow) in the spinal cord probably related to myelomalacia. Axial CT section (Fig. C) shows extensive erosion of the dens (arrow) by surrounding pannus.

Diagnosis: Rheumatoid arthritis (RA) with atlantoaxial subluxation.

Discussion: This disorder is predominantly found in women between the ages of 25–55 years. RA affects the cervical region in 50–90% of all patients and results in atlantoaxial instability in approximately 25% of cases. About 5% of RA patients present with symptoms of compression of the high spinal cord secondary to this abnormality. Atlantoaxial subluxation results from laxity of the transverse ligament. Subluxation of more than 9 mm (width of the atlantoaxial interval) carries a poor prognosis. Surrounding pannus erodes the dens in 14–35% of patients. Pannus is of low density or soft tissue density on CT. On MR imaging, pannus is of intermediate T1 signal intensity and high T2 signal intensity, and it enhances after contrast administration. Atlantoaxial subluxation may result in a myelopathy or even sudden death. Other neurologic symptoms include paresthesias, paresis, and muscle wasting. Basilar invagination with superior protrusion of the dens into the foramen magnum occurs in 5–22% of cases. In the cervical region, RA predominantly affects the neurocentral joints of Luschka. This inflammation of the joints of Luschka may extend into the intervertebral disk space, producing erosive lesions of the end-plates, and eventually, fusion of the vertebral bodies.

Clinical History: You are shown three different patients who have developed changes and complications following a specific type of therapy.

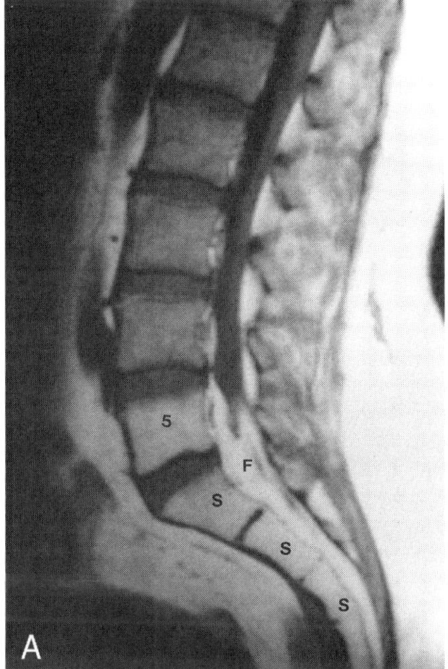

Figure 2.23 A

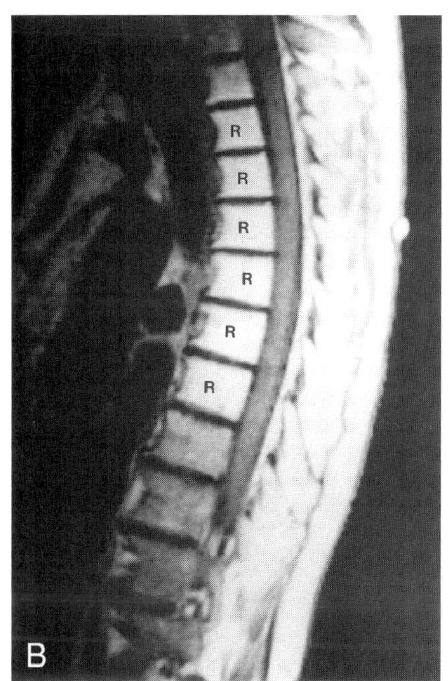

Figure 2.23 B

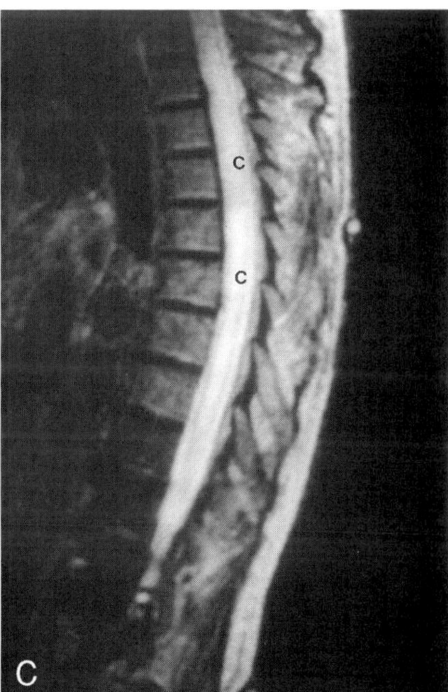

Figure 2.23 C

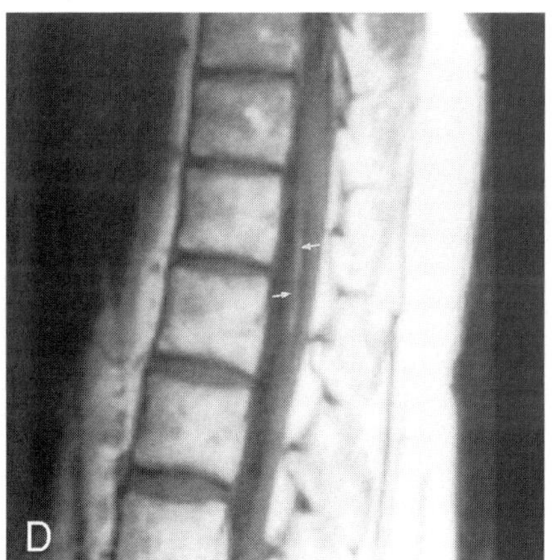

Figure 2.23 D

(continued)

Findings: Midsagittal noncontrast MR T1-weighted image (Fig. A) shows increased signal intensity at L5 (5) and the sacrum (S). Note increased amount of fat (F) in the distal epidural space. In a different patient, midsagittal noncontrast MR T1-weighted image (Fig. B) shows hyperintensity in the midthoracic vertebrae (R). The diameter of the spinal cord in slightly increased. Corresponding T2-weighted image (Fig. C) shows again hyperintensity in the vertebral body bone marrow and increased signal intensity in a swollen spinal cord (C). Midsagittal postcontrast MR T1-weighted image (Fig. D) in a different patient shows enhancement of a nerve root (arrows) that has been unchanged for more than 5 years after the patient's treatment.

Diagnosis: Postradiation changes. Fig. A shows fatty infiltration of the bone marrow and fatty proliferation in the epidural space. Figs. B and C show fatty bone marrow replacement and myelitis. Fig. D shows a radiculitis.

Discussion: The most common finding after radiation therapy is fatty replacement of hematopoietic bone marrow in the irradiated field. This is appreciated as increased T1 signal intensity corresponding to the radiation port. Postradiation myelitis is rare, occurring in less than 2% of all patients whose port included the spine. A minimum of 35 Gy are thought to be needed to produce spinal cord damage. A latency period of 6–24 months is common before the initiation of symptoms, which most commonly include dysesthesias and paresthesias. Spinal cord involvement is probably secondary to the development of a vasculitis. Vasculitis is also probably responsible for the associated radiculitis. On MR imaging, the affected spinal cord is swollen initially and may enhance after contrast administration. With time, the spinal cord atrophies.

CASE 24

Clinical History: 65-year-old man with mid- and lower-lumbar pain.

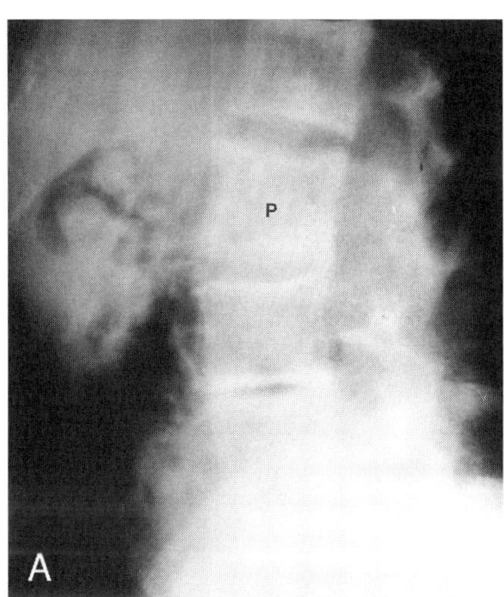

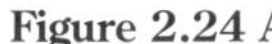

Figure 2.24 A

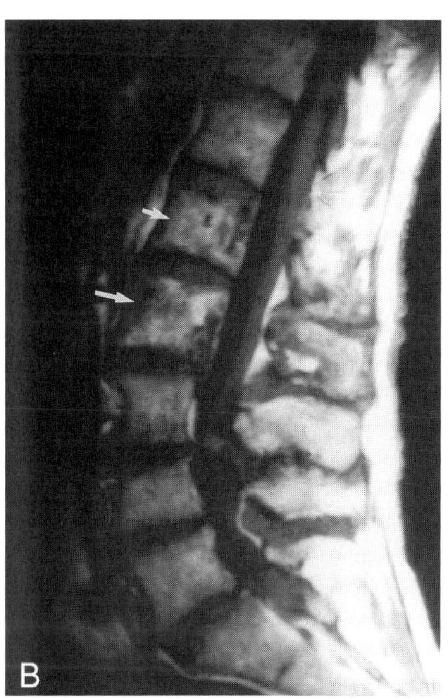

Figure 2.24 B

Findings: Lateral radiograph (Fig. A) of the lumbar spine shows increased density and enlargement of L2 (P). The bony trabeculae in this vertebra are coarse and enlarged. Midsagittal MR T1-weighted image (Fig. B) shows inhomogenous intensity from the L1 (smaller arrow) and L2 (larger arrow) vertebral bodies.

Differential Diagnosis: Osteoblastic metastases, hemangiomas, myelofibrosis (usually diffuse), Paget disease.

Diagnosis: Paget disease.

Discussion: Paget disease is generally found in individuals (approximately 3%) older than 40 years of age. The most common sites of involvement are the spine (75%), skull (65%), and pelvis (40%). The most common symptom is localized pain. Neurologic symptoms are the result of compression of the spinal cord and/or nerve roots by a remodeled or a fractured vertebra (e). Radiographs and CT demonstrate the bone changes of Paget disease. Initially there is bone lysis; then a mixture of lysis and zones of sclerosis ensues. The last phase of the disease is the sclerotic one. Sarcomatous degeneration occurs in a small number of patients. Onset of new pain in a bone known to be involved by Paget disease should raise the suspicion of sarcomatous degeneration. MR imaging also shows the bone marrow changes. In the initial phase of the disease, the vertebral bone marrow develops numerous vascular channels and is infiltrated by fibrous tissues. Cyst-like cavities and blood-filled sinusoids may be present. In the sclerotic phase of the disease, the bone marrow may return to normal. Hypertrophy of the vertebral bodies, particularly in the lumbar region, may result in central or lateral recess stenoses. In the craniocervical junction, softening of the base of the skull may lead to basilar invagination and compression of the spinal cord by a superiorly displaced dens.

Clinical History: This patient had a laminectomy for a herniated disk at L5-S1 3 years before this study. The patient has chronic low back pain. The previously operated level appeared normal.

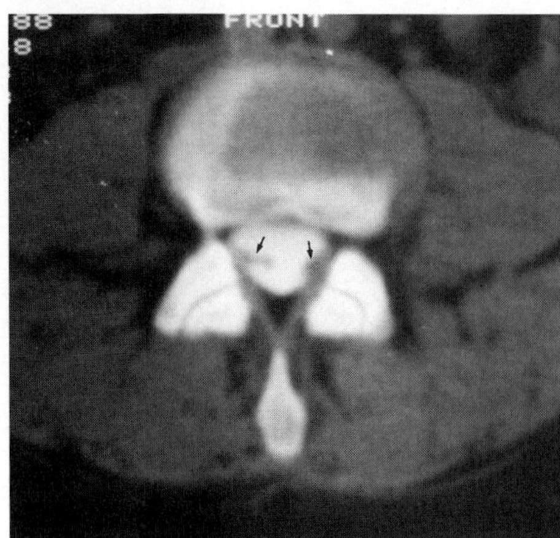

Figure 2.25

Findings: Postmyelogram axial CT section at L3-L4 level shows matted nerve roots (arrows) which are adherent to the walls of the thecal sac.

Diagnosis: Arachnoiditis (see Case #20, Chapter 1).

Discussion: Arachnoiditis refers to an inflammatory process affecting the dura, arachnoid, and pia. Initially there is a fibrous exudate covering the nerve roots. This exudate eventually develops into dense collagen adhesion, resulting in fixation of the nerve roots. The end result of this process is better termed "arachnoidal adhesions." Causes for arachnoiditis include prior surgery, pyogenic and granulomatous infections, trauma, subarachnoid hemorrhage, and instillation of spinal epidural anesthetics. Prior myelography is no longer a common cause because the contrast agents currently used result in little inflammatory reaction. Symptoms include chronic pain radiating to the lower extremities, hypesthesias, and paraparesis. MR imaging is slightly less sensitive than postmyelography CT in the identification of arachnoiditis. Abnormalities seen include clumping of the nerve roots, adherence of nerve roots to the walls of the thecal sac (empty sac sign), and soft tissue masses that may be large enough to obstruct the lumen of the thecal sac. The masses composed of fibrous tissues are generally hypointense on T2-weighted images. Arachnoiditis may result in enhancement of nerve roots. This abnormal enhancement should not be confused with enhancement of lumbar intradural veins. If more than one dose of MR contrast is administered, enhancement commonly occurs and should not be interpreted as representing arachnoiditis.

CASE 26

Clinical History: A 13-year-old male presents with mild-to-moderate back pain for 1 year and mild thoracic kyphosis.

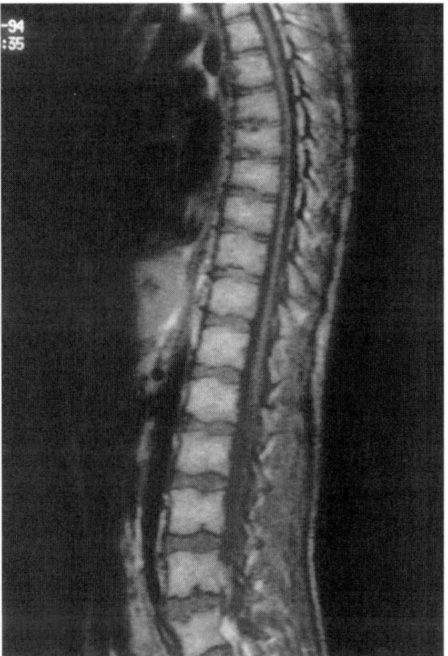

Figure 2.26

Findings: Midsagittal MR T1-weighted image shows irregular upper and lower end plates in all the vertebral bodies. There is mild wedge deformity of some upper- and mid-thoracic vertebral bodies and a mild kyphosis in this region.

Diagnosis: Scheuermann disease.

Discussion: Scheuermann disease, or progressive kyphosis, is a relatively common disorder affecting approximately 1% of individuals and is more common in males. The underlying etiology is probably related to mechanical stress upon the spine or to an osteochondrosis of the vertebral end plates. Histologically, there are zones of altered cartilage growth. The most common clinical manifestation is progressive kyphosis predominantly involving the thoracic region. The lumbar spine may also be affected. The main complaint of these patients is pain. Neurologic symptoms are distinctively absent of few. The initial examination of the spine should be done with radiographs. The radiographic criteria for the diagnosis of Scheuermann disease are: irregular upper and lower vertebral end-plates, apparent loss of disk space height, wedging of more than 5° in one or more vertebral bodies, and hyperkyphosis greater than 40° as measured by the Cobb method. This disease appears to be self-limiting in most patients, and when the kyphosis remains at less than 60°, most patients lead a normal life. Indications for surgery are a rapidly progressive kyphosis, severe pain, and respiratory compromise.

CASE 27

Clinical History: This 60-year-old male has a history of laryngeal carcinoma treated with radiation therapy 2 years previously. He now presents with spasticity and weakness predominantly in both lower extremities.

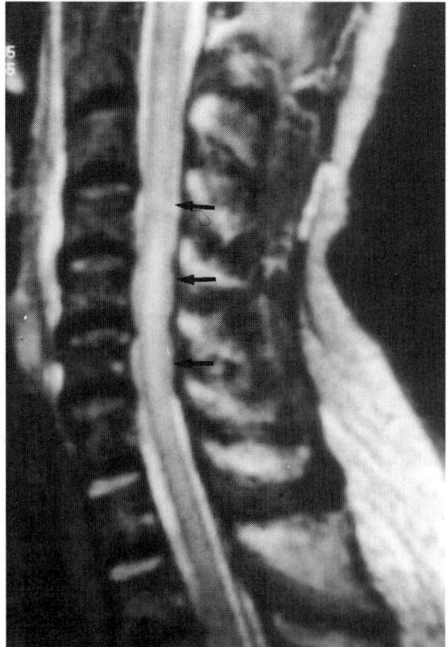

Figure 2.27

Findings: Midsagittal MR T2-weighted image shows an area of increased signal intensity (arrows) in the spinal cord extending from C4 to C6. There is no expansion of the cord, and the lesion did not enhance after contrast administration.

Diagnosis: Radiation-induced myelitis.

Discussion: Radiation therapy may result in several spinal complications (see Case #23). If it is delivered before spinal surgery, there is a 36% risk of acquiring an infection at the site of surgery. After radiation therapy, there is fatty infiltration of the bone marrow which is seen as increased signal intensity on MR T1-weighted images. This finding is usually limited to radiation port. Radiation myelitis is uncommon and is probably related to a vasculitis. It is more commonly encountered 6–24 months after termination of treatment and occurs in approximately 2–3% of all patients in whom the spinal cord was included within the port. MR is the imaging method of choice with which to evaluate these patients and shows only nonspecific increased T2 signal intensity corresponding to the port. There is no enhancement after contrast administration and no expansion of the spina cord. Radiation neuritis may occur and is seen as persistent enhancement of the nerve roots, particularly those of the cauda equina. When radiation to the spine is delivered in children, their growth is stunted. A rare and long-term complication of radiation to the spine is that of secondary sarcomas.

Clinical History: You are shown three cases. The first patient is a 4-year-old with low neck pain (Fig. A). The second patient is a 5-year-old male who presents with sudden onset of neck pain (Figs. B and C). Radiographs in the last patient were normal. The third case (Fig. D) is a young child with thoracolumbar pain which began abruptly.

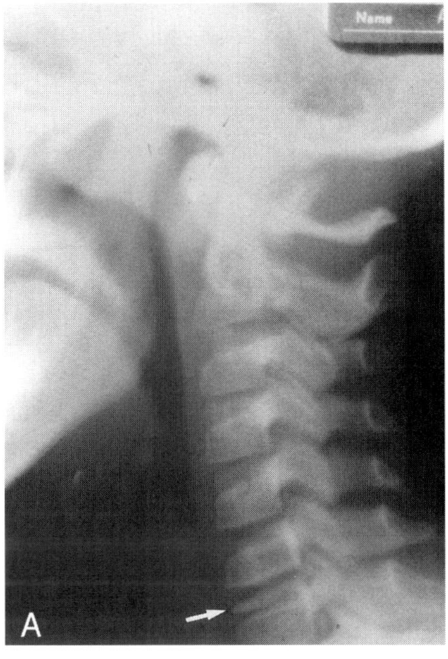

Figure 2.28 A

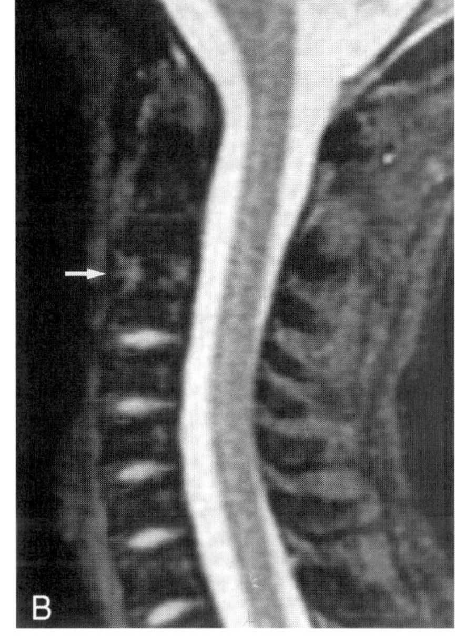

Figure 2.28 B

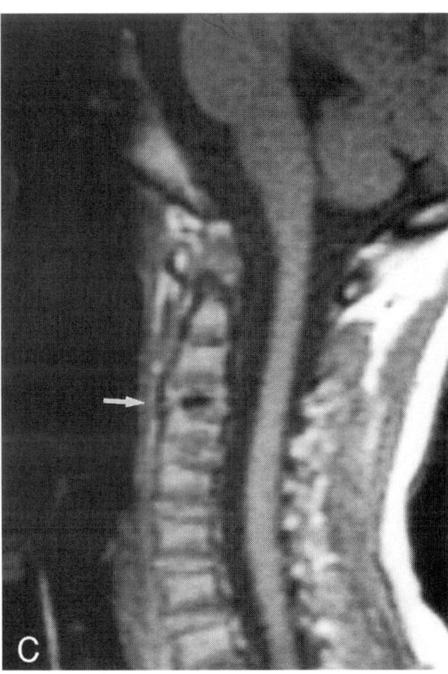

Figure 2.28 C

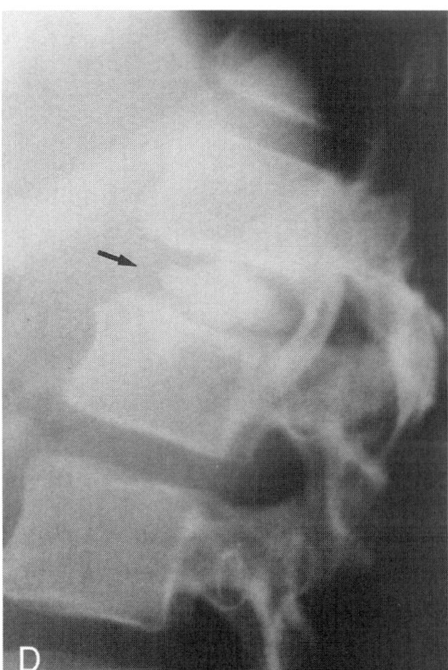

Figure 2.28 D

(continued)

Findings: Lateral radiograph of the neck (Fig. A) shows a disk calcification (arrow) at the C6-C7 level. In a different case, midsagittal MR T2-weighted image (Fig. B) shows widening of the C2-C3 disk space (arrow) and low signal intensity within it. Corresponding MR T1-weighted image (Fig. C) again shows a wide C2-C3 intervertebral disk space which contains some low signal intensity (arrow). In the last case, lateral radiograph (Fig. D) of the thoracolumbar junction shows disk calcification (arrow) at T12-L1 and slight widening of that disk space.

Differential Diagnosis (for all disk calcifications): Ochronosis, ankylosis spondylitis, gout, pseudogout, hemochromatosis, hyperparathyroidism, hypervitaminosis D, degenerative disease (all of these generally occur in adults), idiopathic disk calcifications.

Diagnosis: Idiopathic disk calcifications.

Discussion: In children, calcifications within an intervertebral disk are rare. They tend to be idiopathic and involve predominantly the cervical region but occasionally involve the thoracic and lumbar spine. Possible etiologies for these calcifications include microtrauma or a viral infection. Symptoms include neck pain and torticollis. The symptoms are generally self-limiting. Similarly, the radiographic findings may resolve. Disk calcifications may be accompanied by herniations which generally do not produce neurologic symptoms. MR imaging is more sensitive to these disk changes than are radiographs. Before calcification occurs, MR imaging may show widening and edema of the disk space(s), probably reflecting inflammation. MR imaging may also show low signal intensity within the disk space(s) in the absence of plain radiographic abnormalities.

TUMORS

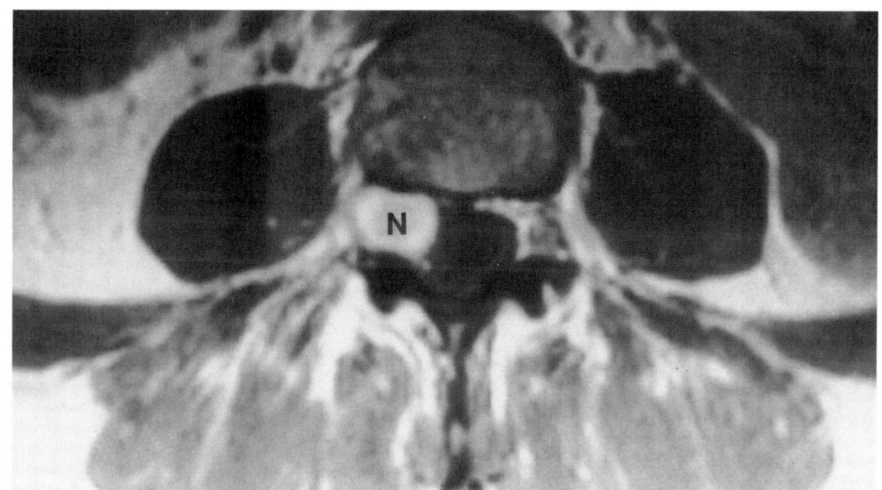

Clinical History: You are shown four cases. The first involves a patient (Figs. A and B) with a history of breast carcinoma who presents with sudden lower extremity paresis and a T11 sensory level. The second (Fig. C) also involves a patient with a primary breast carcinoma but who presents with only low back pain. The third patient (Fig. D) has a history of colon carcinoma and now has back pain. The last patient (Fig. E) has pain throughout her entire back and also a history of breast cancer.

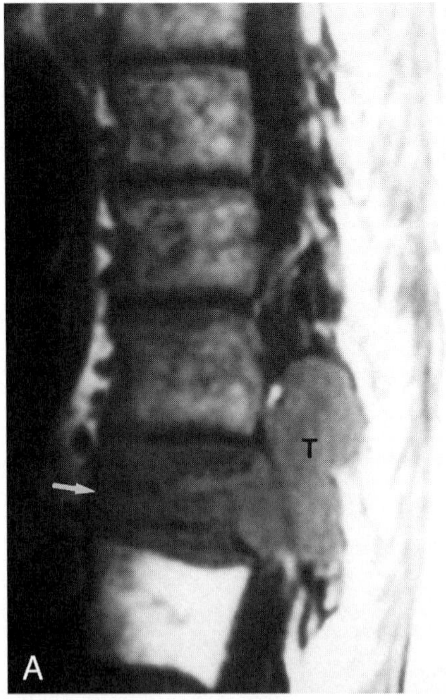

Figure 3.1 A

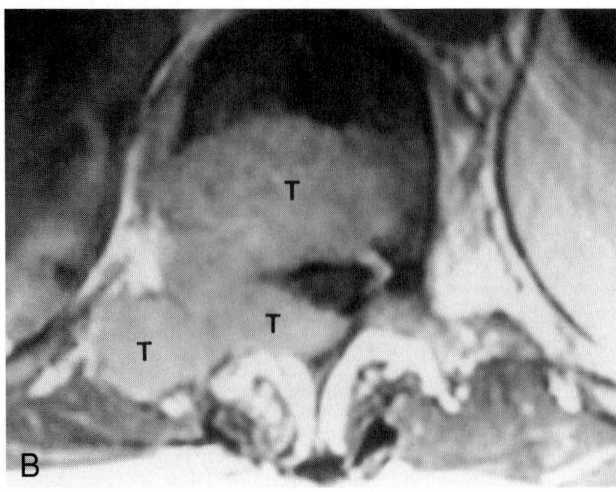

Figure 3.1 B

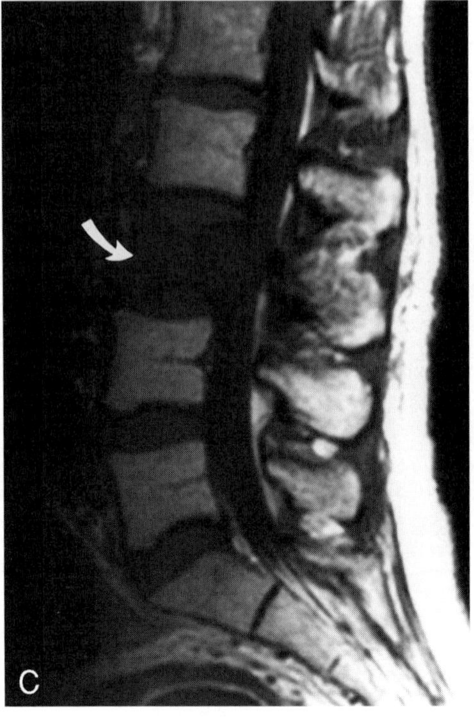

Figure 3.1 C

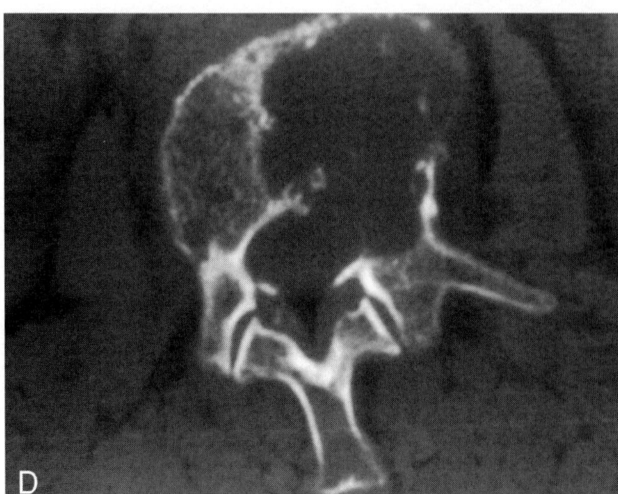

Figure 3.1 D

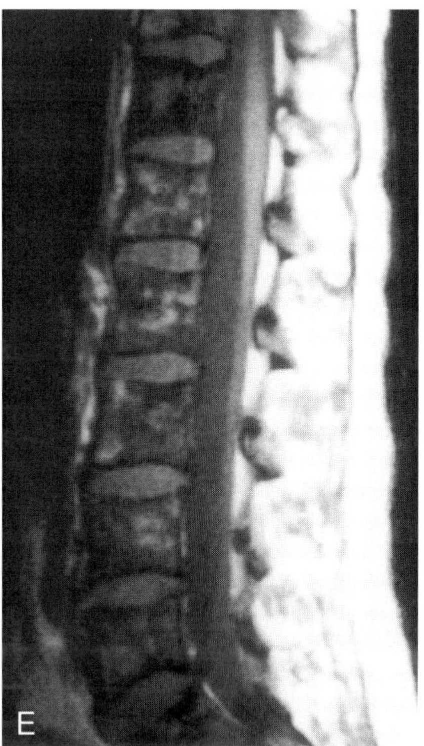

Figure 3.1 E

Findings: In the first patient, noncontrast midsagittal MR T1-weighted image (Fig. A) shows complete collapse of T11 (arrow), replaced by tumor. Tumor (T) also extrudes posteriorly and involves the vertebral neural arch, resulting in circumferential compression of the spinal cord. Note low signal intensity from metastatic disease infiltrating the other vertebral bodies. Postcontrast MR T1-weighted image (Fig. B) at T11 shows tumor (T) involving the vertebral body and right pedicle, lamina, and transverse process. The spinal cord is compressed. In the second patient (Fig. C), there is low signal intensity (arrow) replacing the bone marrow of the L3 vertebral body. There is only mild depression of the end-plates and no true compression fracture. The other vertebral bodies are bright secondary to prior radiation due to a second primary tumor in the uterus. In the third patient (Fig. D), axial CT section (bone window settings) shows a lytic lesion involving the body and left pedicle of L2. The image of the last patient (Fig. E) shows diffuse and patchy low signal intensity throughout the bone marrow of all the visualized vertebral bodies.

Differential Diagnosis: Metastases, multiple myeloma (and plasmacytoma), macroglobulinemia, histiocytosis, leukemia, lymphoma, disseminated infection.

Diagnosis: Metastases to the spine. In the first subject, there is compression of the spinal cord.

Discussion: Metastases to the vertebral bodies eventually occurs in approximately 5–10% of all cancer patients. At presentation, most lesions involve the osseous and epidural compartments producing compression of neural elements. The thoracic region is most commonly affected. Symptoms of metastatic spinal disease include pain, weakness, autonomic dysfunction, and sensory loss. Most metastases to the spine originate from primary tumors in the breast, prostate, lung, and uterus. They may also be caused by multiple myeloma and lymphoma. More than 90% of these patients demonstrate multiple sites of involvement at presentation. Intradural and intramedullary spinal cord metastatic disease is less common. MR is the imaging method of choice to evaluate these patients. On sagittal MR T1-weighted images, the involved vertebrae show low signal intensity representing tumor replacement of the normal fatty bone marrow. Epidural tumor is also well seen as masses of intermediate signal intensity that enhance after contrast administration. After contrast material is given, the lesions may become isointense with normal bone marrow making their identification difficult. However, postcontrast MR T1-weighted imaging with fat suppression clearly shows these metastases. Note that when diffuse, metastases to the vertebrae may initially be difficult to identify. Generally, on T1-weighted images, the disks are of lower signal intensity than the normal bone marrow. If the disks appear brighter than the bone marrow, then diffuse replacement of the marrow should be suspected.

CASE 2

Clinical History: 65-year-old male with a long-standing history of generalized back pain presents with lower extremity weakness, hyperreflexia, and a sensory level at T9.

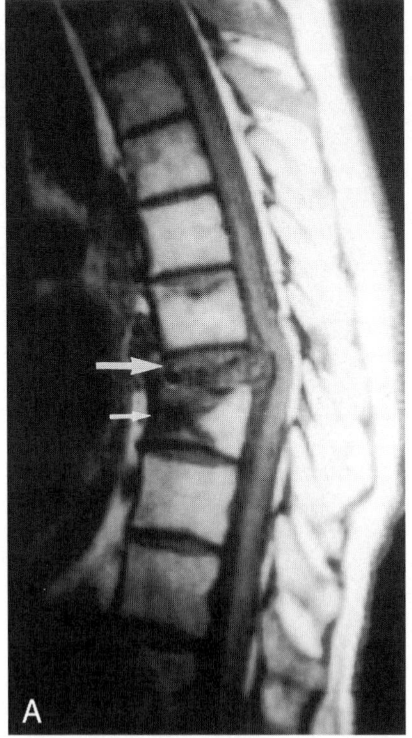

Figure 3.2 A

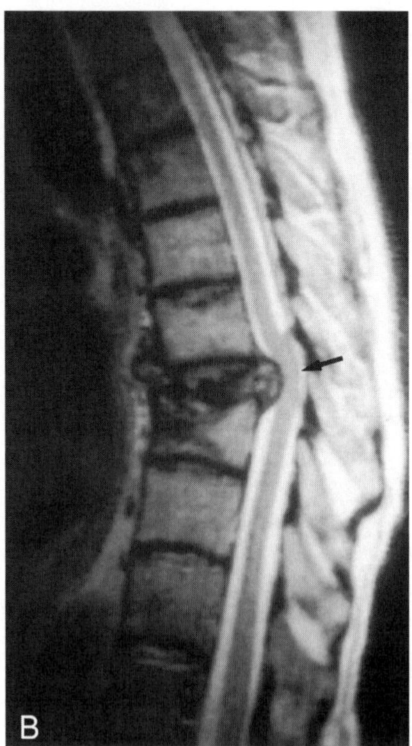

Figure 3.2 B

Findings: Midsagittal MR T1-weighted image (Fig. A) shows complete collapse of T7 (longer arrow) with posterior displacement of tumor resulting in compression of the spinal cord. The tumor has also involved the T8 vertebral body (shorter arrow). The signal intensity of several upper thoracic vertebrae is also abnormal, suggesting infiltration of the bone marrow. Corresponding T2-weighted image (Fig. B) clearly shows the compression of the spinal cord (arrow). There is abnormal low signal intensity in the upper thoracic vertebrae.

Differential Diagnosis: Metastasis, multiple myeloma, lymphoma, infection, pseudotumors of hemophilia and hyperparathyroidism, hemangioma, fibrous dysplasia, Paget disease, chordoma.

Diagnosis: Multiple myeloma, collapsed T8 resulting in spinal cord compression.

Discussion: Plasmacytoma is the solitary form of multiple myeloma. Serologic tests may be normal or abnormal in these patients. Plasmacytoma occurs in younger individuals more than does multiple myeloma. Most patients with plasmacytoma eventually develop diffuse disease. Plasmacytoma generally involves the vertebral body but may also affect the neural arch. This tumor tends to be lytic in appearance but occasionally it is sclerotic. Most patients complain of back pain and/or radiculopathies. Less common manifestations of plasmacytoma and multiple myeloma include polyarthritis, amyloidosis, gout, and infections. The imaging findings in plasmacytoma are nonspecific. T1-weighted images show replacement of the normal bright bone marrow by low signal intensity. Epidural extension with compression of the spinal cord or lumbar thecal sac is common. Most lesions are clearly seen on noncontrast MR images, and the administration of contrast generally does not show additional lesions. Contrast administration does, however, show decreasing enhancement in lesions responding adequately to therapy.

Clinical History: A previously healthy 7-year-old boy presents with severe thoracic back pain and no neurologic deficits.

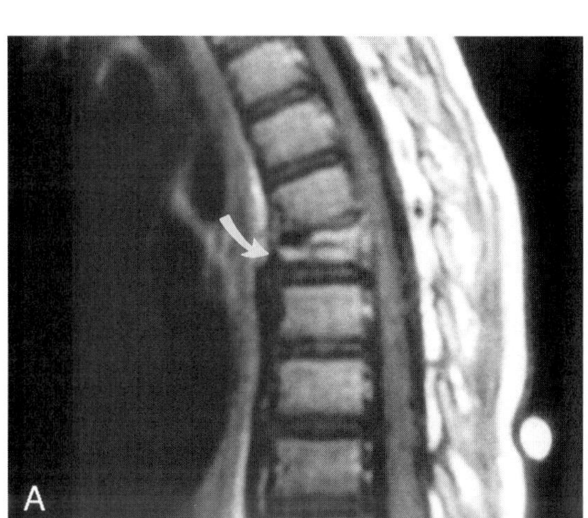

Figure 3.3 A

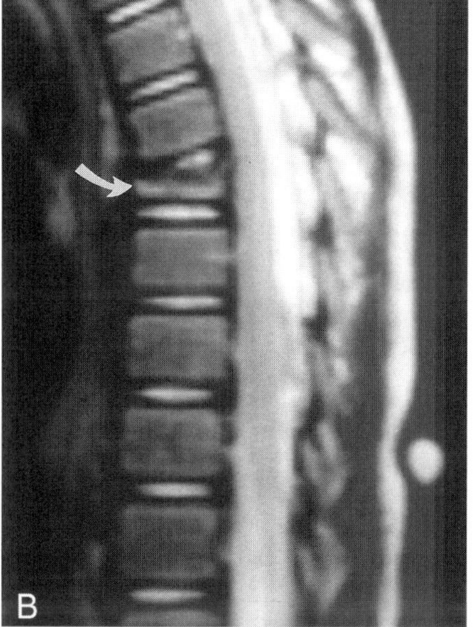

Figure 3.3 B

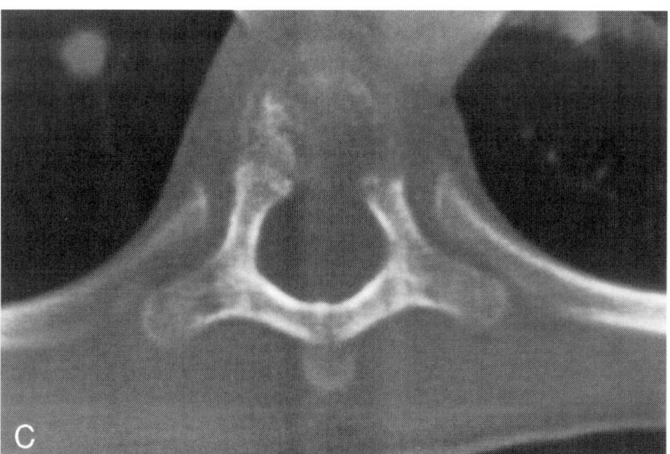

Figure 3.3 C

Findings: Midsagittal postcontrast MR T1-weighted image (Fig. A) shows complete collapse and abnormal enhancement of T6 (arrow). Note absence of associated soft tissue abnormality and no compression of the spinal cord. Corresponding T2-weighted image (Fig. B) shows slightly increased signal intensity from the collapsed vertebra (arrow). Axial CT (Fig. C) through T6 shows lytic lesion involving the vertebral body.

(continued)

Differential Diagnosis: metastasis, Ewing sarcoma, lymphoma, leukemia, granulomatous infection, eosinophilic granuloma producing collapse (vertebra plana) of T6.

Diagnosis: Eosinophilic granuloma producing collapse (vertebra plana) of T6.

Discussion: EG represents the localized form of the histiocytosis of Langerhans (histiocytosis X). Approximately 70% of patients with histiocytosis present with EG. It is more common in young white males. Approximately 10% of patients with EG eventually develop the diffuse form of the disease. The most common symptoms include localized pain, tenderness, swelling, a palpable mass, fever, and leukocytosis. The most common sites of involvement are the skull, mandible, spine, ribs, femur, and humerus. Radiographically, most lesions are lytic, slightly expansile, and have a well-defined border. Progressive involvement may lead to complete collapse of a vertebral body, resulting in the so-called "vertebra plana." The posterior elements may also be involved. The disk is preserved. The thoracic and lumbar regions are affected more commonly than is the cervical spine. Paraspinal soft tissue masses are small or absent. Spinal cord compression is not common. The lesion may be histologically confirmed by biopsy of curettage. The best treatment for eosinophilic granuloma is uncertain. Treatment involves immobilization and pain medication. Most of these lesions heal spontaneously; after the lesion has healed, kyphosis may result. Reconstitution of the vertebral height has been observed. Some advocate low-dose radiation when neurologic deficits are present.

CASE 4

Clinical History: You are shown a lesion that was found incidentally in a middle-aged female being evaluated for spinal cord symptoms from multiple sclerosis.

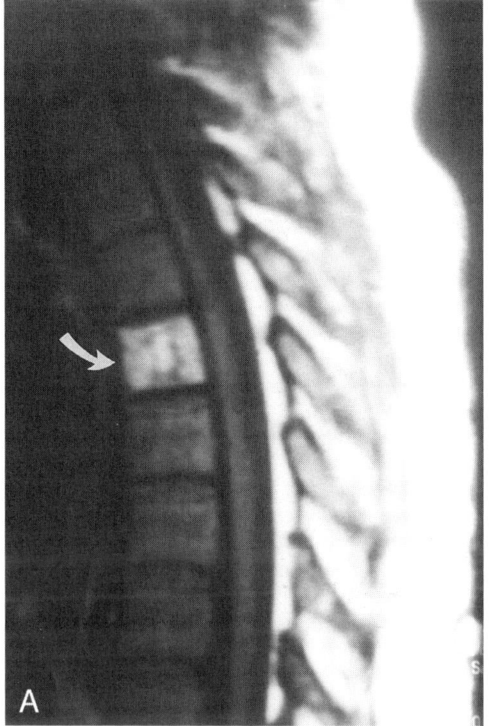

Figure 3.4 A

Figure 3.4 B

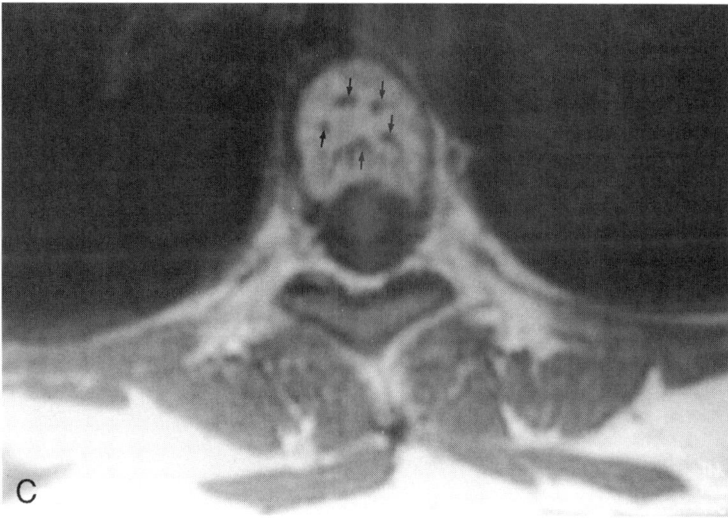

Figure 3.4 C

(continued)

Findings: Midsagittal noncontrast MR T1-weighted image (Fig. A) shows diffusely increased signal intensity in a thoracic vertebra (arrow) which is of normal height. The other vertebrae are normal. On a corresponding T2-weighted image (Fig. B), that vertebra (arrow) is also of increased signal intensity. Axial noncontrast T1-weighted image (Fig. C) shows that the abnormal vertebra is hyperintense but contains hypointense areas (arrows) which are thickened secondary trabeculae or large vascular channels.

Differential Diagnosis: Focal fatty replacement, metastasis, lymphoma, vertebral body hemangioma.

Diagnosis: Vertebral body hemangioma.

Discussion: Vertebral body hemangiomas are common lesions found mostly incidentally in approximately 11% of the general population. In more than 75% of cases the lesions are solitary, but multiple sites are not uncommon. Females are affected more often than are males (2:1). The most common sites of involvement are the thoracic and lumbar spine, followed by the cervical region. Approximately 75% of hemangiomas occur between T3 and T9. Histologically, these lesions are composed of thin-walled, blood-filled spaces lined by endothelium, which are traversed by thick, vertically-oriented, secondary, bony trabeculae. Thrombosis and regressive changes inside the lesion lead to fatty deposition. Occasionally, these hemangiomas become large enough to produce symptoms or may result in vertebral body fractures. Neuropathies and myelopathy are uncommon presentations. Some hemangiomas may undergo rapid expansion during pregnancy. Radiographs and CT show these lesions to be partly lytic and to contain thick trabeculae ("corduroy" appearance on plain radiographs and "polka dot" appearance on CT). On MR imaging, they are of high signal intensity on T1- and T2-weighted images. The enhancement is variable. Aggressive hemangiomas are of low signal intensity on T1-weighted images and hyperintense on T2-weighted sequences, thus indistinguishable from metastases.

CASE 5

Clinical History: You are shown two patients. The first one (Figs. A and B) is a 15-year-old male who presents with sacral pain of 6 months duration and radiculopathies involving S1-S5 on the left. The second patient (Figs. C and D) is a young male with pain in the mid-lumbar region.

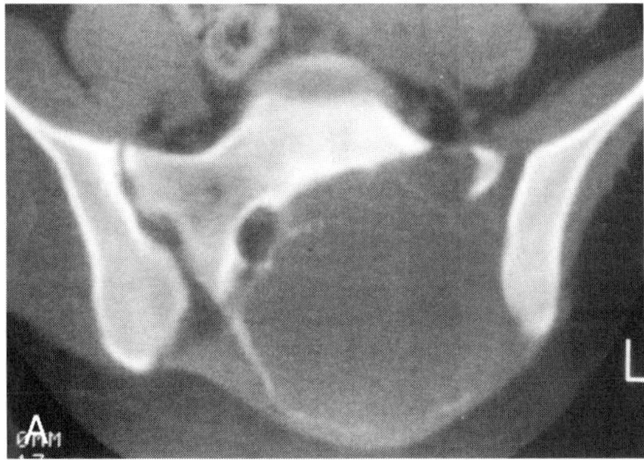

Figure 3.5 A

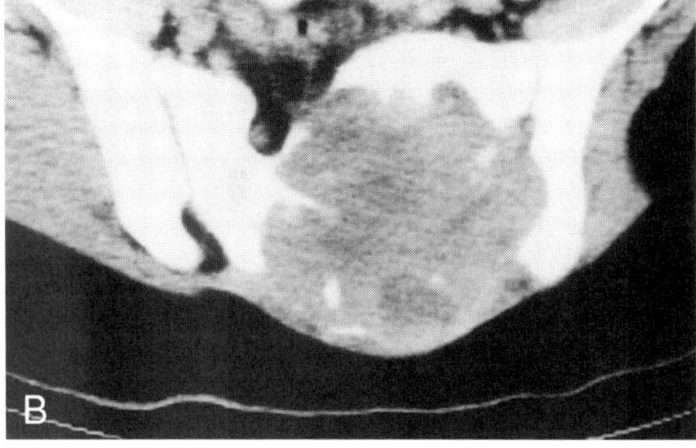

Figure 3.5 B

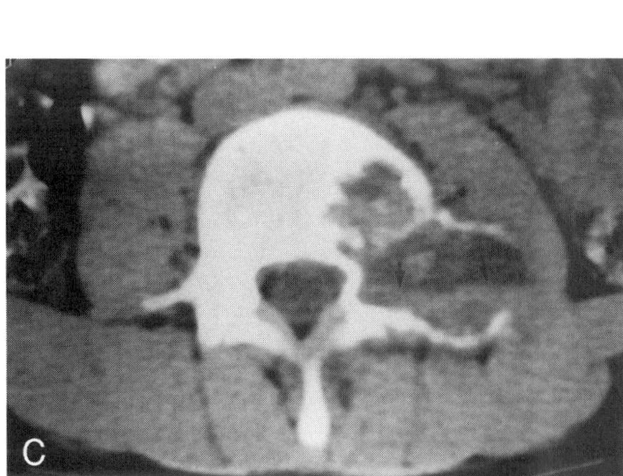

Figure 3.5 C

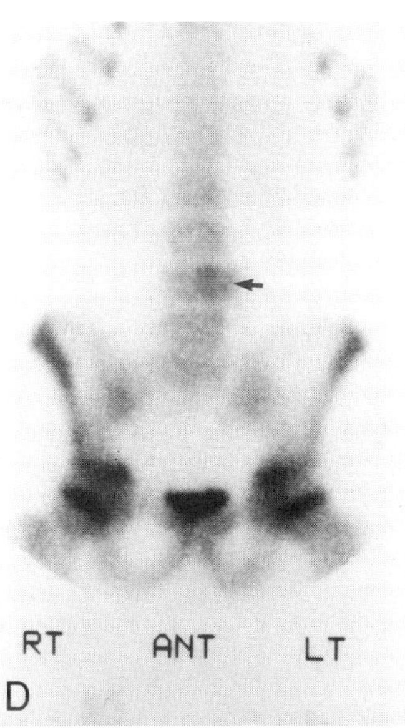

Figure 3.5 D

(continued)

Findings: Axial CT (Fig. A), bone window settings, shows an expansile, large, lytic lesion with a thin bone rim posteriorly involving the sacrum and widening the left sacroiliac joint. Axial CT (Fig. B), soft tissue window settings, obtained slightly above Fig. A shows the lesion to contain some areas of low density and some calcifications. In the second patient, axial CT (Fig. C) shows an expansile and lytic lesion involving the body, left pedicle, and transverse process of L2. Note fluid-blood levels (arrows) inside the lesion. In the same patient, radionuclide bone scan (Fig. D) shows increased uptake (arrow) at the level of the lesion.

Differential Diagnosis: Giant cell tumor, osteoblastoma, eosinophilic granuloma, posterior tuberculosis, pseudotumor of hyperparathyroidism, aneurysmal bone cyst.

Diagnosis: Aneurysmal bone cysts (ABCs).

Discussion: ABCs are generally expansile bone lesions filled with blood. More than 80% of these tumors are found in individuals younger than 20 years of age. Females are affected slightly more than males. The spine is involved in 10–30% of cases. The tumors may occur because of trauma, underlying tumors (such as giant cell tumor, osteoblastoma, chondrosarcoma, and osteosarcoma), and vascular malformations. However, most ABCs occur in the absence of an underlying lesion. Most occur in the thoracic spine, followed by the lumbar and cervical regions. Sacral involvement is rare. The most common symptoms are localized pain and neurologic deficits caused by compression of nerve roots and/or the spinal cord. In the spine, ABCs tend to be expansile lesions involving predominantly the posterior elements. In more than 75% of patients, the tumor extends into the vertebral body. Spinal ABCs also tend to extend to neighboring vertebrae, ribs, and paraspinal soft tissues. CT and MR imaging may show fluid-blood levels that are typical for this lesion. To visualize these levels, the patient should lie down at least 10 minutes before obtaining the images to allow the layers to settle. The MR imaging features of this lesion are complex due to the presence of blood of varying ages. After contrast administration, there is enhancement of the rim of the lesion. The treatment of the lesions consists of excision and curettage. The lesions tend to bleed during surgery, and preoperative embolization may be performed in large tumors. Radiation of these lesions generally yields poor results. Recurrence rates vary from 10–25%.

CASE 6

Clinical History: A 22-year-old male presents with lower lumbar pain that is worse at night.

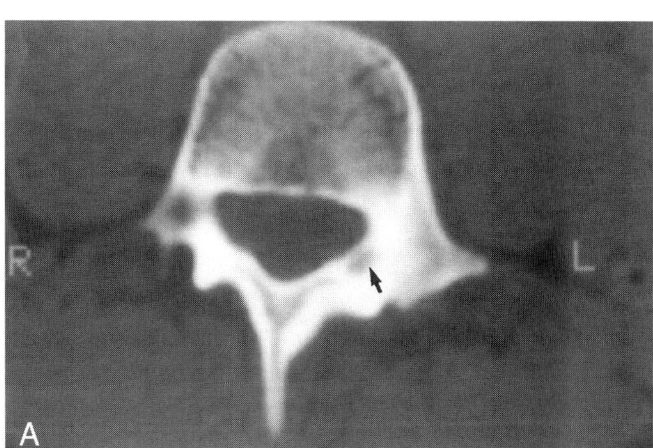

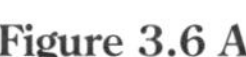

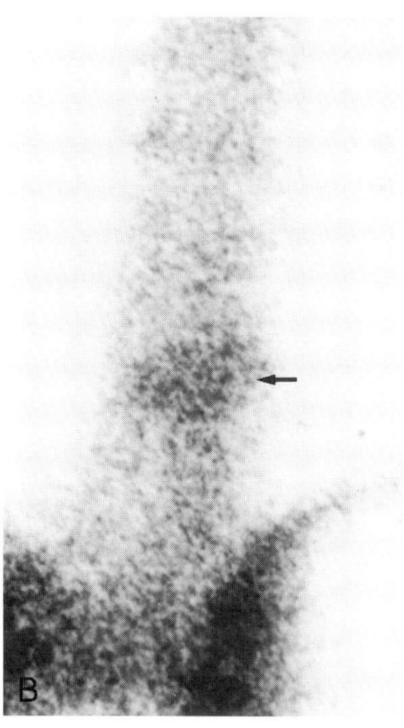

Figure 3.6 A   Figure 3.6 B

Findings: Axial CT (Fig. A) shows thick and sclerotic left pedicle and lamina of L4. Note the lucent nidus (arrow) amid the sclerotic zone. Oblique view of a radionuclide bone scan (Fig. B) shows increased uptake (arrow) in the lateral aspect of L4.

Differential Diagnosis: Osteoblastic metastasis, enostosis, unusual infection, lymphoma, pedicular sclerosis contralateral to spondylolysis or absent pedicle, osteoid osteoma.

Diagnosis: Osteoid osteoma.

Discussion: Osteoid osteomas comprise approximately 10% of all primary benign bone tumors, and 10% of them are found in the spine. Most patients become symptomatic between the ages of 6–17 years. Males are affected more commonly than are females. Osteoid osteomas are a relatively common etiology for painful, progressive scoliosis in adolescents. Other symptoms include localized pain (more severe at night and typically relieved by salicylates), radicular pain, gait disturbance, and muscle atrophy. Most osteoid osteomas arise in the pedicles, lamina, facet joints, and spinous processes. Less than 10% involve the vertebral body. The most commonly affected sites are the lumbar (60%), cervical (27%), thoracic (12%), and sacral (1%) regions. The tumors are small, generally measuring less than 1.5 cm in diameter. They are hypervascular. The nidus of the lesion is lytic and surrounded by reactive sclerosis. CT is most helpful in identifying the nidus. On MR imaging, the features of an osteoid osteoma are nonspecific with low-to-intermediate T1 signal intensity and high T2 signal intensity. Treatment of the lesion may be accomplished with long-term administration of anti-inflammatory drugs or surgical excision. The lesions generally resolve after 3 to 4 years of symptomatic treatment. En block resection results in resolution of the pain in more than 95% of patients. Scoliosis may occur due to the lesion or because of deformity after its resection. Radiation therapy is not indicated.

CASE 7

Clinical History: You are shown two patients. The first (Fig. A) is a 25-year-old male who presents with low thoracic pain, mild lower extremity weakness, and spasticity. The second (Fig. B) presents with a painful hard mass in the mid-lumbar back.

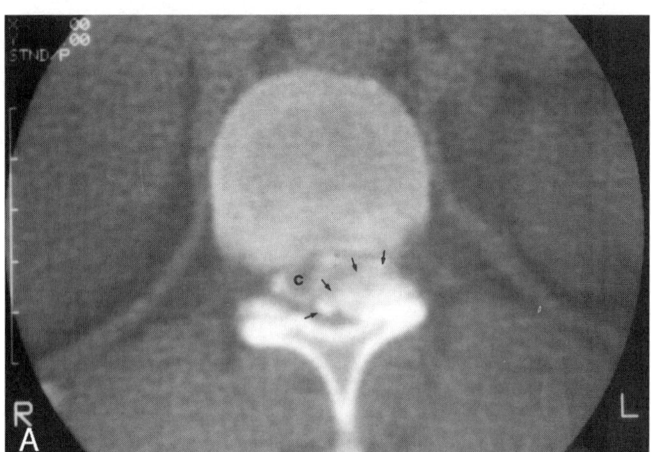

Figure 3.7 A

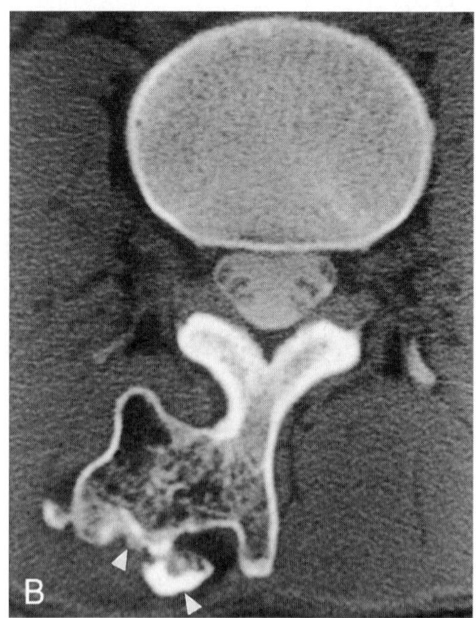

Figure 3.7 B

Findings: Axial CT (Fig. A) shows a bone excrescence (arrows) arising from the anterior aspect of the left facet joint at T11-T12. This study was obtained after a myelogram and shows that the lesion compresses the spinal cord (c). In the second subject, postmyelogram axial CT study (Fig. B), bone window settings, shows a bone excrescence arising from the left lateral aspect of the spinous process of L2. Note posterior cartilaginous cap (arrowheads).

Diagnosis: Osteochondromas.

Discussion: Osteochondromas (exostosis) are the most common of all benign bone tumors, accounting for approximately 40%. Only 1–4% of osteochondromas occur in the spine where they comprise 4% of all benign spinal tumors. In patients with multiple hereditary exostoses, only 9% are found in the spine. They are generally found in individuals aged 20–30 years. They are more frequent in males. Radiation is known to result in the formation of these masses. Osteochondromas are more common in the cervical spine and usually arise from the neural arch. Lesions that project into the paraspinal soft tissues are generally asymptomatic and are incidentally discovered. Lesions projecting into the spinal canal are symptomatic. Approximately 35% of patients present with a myelopathy. Trauma may precipitate the symptoms. These lesions are composed of normal bone and a cartilaginous cap. Degeneration into a sarcoma is extremely rare in spinal osteochondromas. In 21% of cases, the diagnosis may be reliably made on plain radiographs. CT is the imaging method of choice because it allows for exact measurement of the cartilaginous cap thickness. A cap thicker than 1–2 cm should be viewed with suspicion of malignant degeneration. The treatment of choice is surgical resection.

CASE 8

Clinical History: A 17-year-old male presents with upper thoracic pain and difficulty breathing.

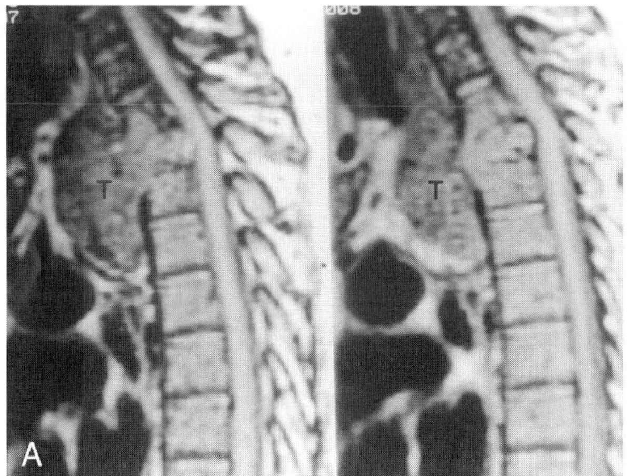

Figure 3.8 A

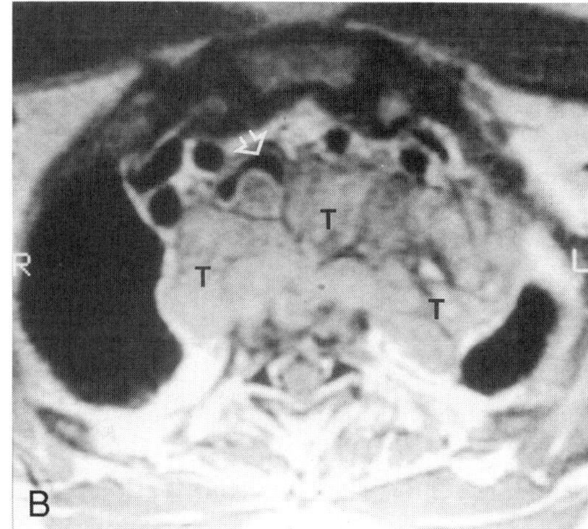

Figure 3.8 B

Findings: Two contiguous sagittal proton density MR images (Fig. A) show a large mass (T) arising from T4 and invading the lower aspect of T3 and superior aspect of T5. The mass projects mostly anteriorly, but there is an intraspinal component compressing the spinal cord. Axial postcontrast MR T1-weighted image (Fig. B) shows the large tumor (T) projecting mostly anteriorly and resulting in significant compression of the trachea (open arrow).

Differential Diagnosis: Osteoblastoma, aneurysmal bone cyst, metastasis, chordoma, giant cell tumor.

Diagnosis: Giant cell tumor.

Discussion: Giant cell tumors (GCTs) comprise approximately 4–5% of all primary bone tumors. Only 7% of them involve the spine. They are usually found after the second decade of life without a gender predilection. Most lesions are found in the sacrum, followed by the thoracic, cervical, and lumbar regions. The most common symptoms at presentation are radicular pain, weakness, and sensory deficits. Sudden enlargement of GCTs may be observed during pregnancy. The lesions are composed of giant osteoclastic cells amid a spindle cell stroma. Foci of hemorrhage (similar to those found in aneurysmal bone cysts) are common. Malignant degeneration is said to occur in 5–10% of all GCTs. They are expansile and lytic lesions with nonsclerotic borders. GCTs may contain internal calcifications, which are better seen on CT. The tumor may extend into the neighboring soft tissues. They arise more commonly in the vertebral body than in the neural arch. On MR imaging, its features are nonspecific with low T1 signal intensity and high T2 signal intensity. Their enhancement is variable and inhomogeneous. Areas of mixed signal intensities are probably related to the presence of hemorrhage. Trauma may result in collapse of the vertebrae and spinal cord compression. The prognosis of these patients is mixed because GCTs are locally aggressive and recurrences are common (40–60%).

CASE 9

Clinical History: A 25-year-old male presents with an enlarging lower extremity. The radiograph of this area shows multiple lytic lesions in the long bones. The patient also complains of back pain and is noted to have mild thoracic kyphosis.

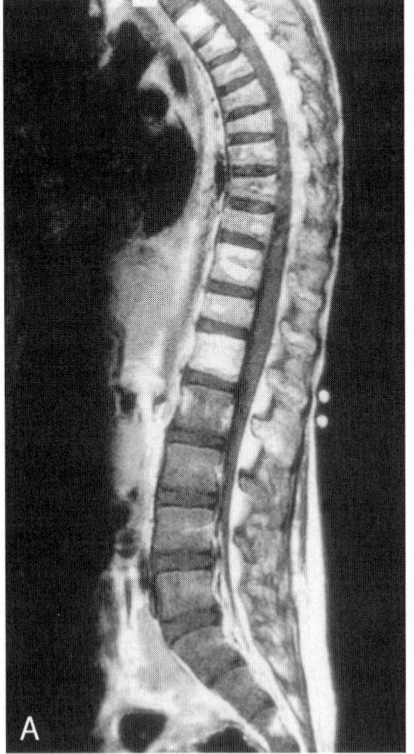
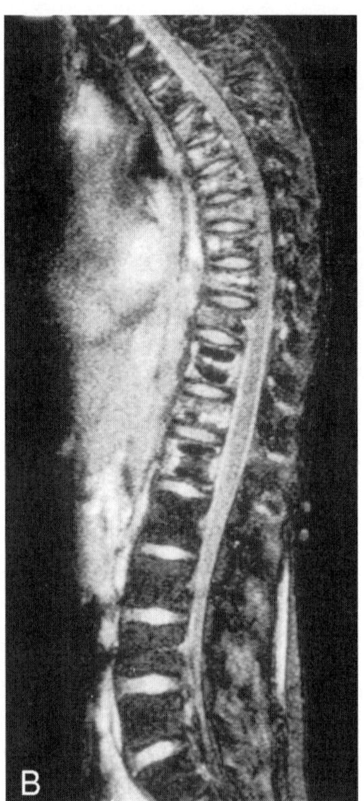

Figure 3.9 A   **Figure 3.9 B**

Findings: Midsagittal noncontrast MR T1-weighted image (Fig. A) shows that the bone marrow cavities in the vertebral bodies contain multiple areas of low, intermediate, and high signal intensity. There is mild compression of several mid-thoracic vertebrae and kyphosis. Corresponding MR T2-weighted image (Fig. B) shows multiple areas of increased signal intensity in the thoracic vertebrae.

Differential Diagnosis: Multiple hemangiomas, cystic angiomatosis, metastases, infection (particularly granulomatous), lymphangiomatosis.

Diagnosis: Lymphangiomatosis of bone.

Discussion: Lymphangiomas may be solitary or diffuse and aggressive (massive osteolysis of Gorham). Localized lesions are rare. Intraosseous lymphangiomas are more commonly found in children and adolescents. The vertebrae are the most common site after the long bones of the extremities. They may result in vertebral body collapse and compression of the spinal cord. Patients with multiple bone lymphangiomas may also have involvement of the viscera. Other clinical symptoms include local pain and swelling. They are composed of unilocular or multilocular spaces filled with a milky fluid. Their features are similar to those of cavernous hemangiomas. They are primarily osteolytic lesions that may contain thin septa. Otherwise, the imaging features of lymphangiomas are nonspecific. If lymphangiography is done, the diagnosis may be suggested with certainty because the contrast material tends to accumulate within the bone lesions.

CASE 10

Clinical History: You are shown two patients. The first is a 55-year-old female who presents with sacral pain and difficulty defecating (Figs. A–C). The second (Fig. D) is a 35-year-old male with difficulty swallowing, neck pain, and weakness in both upper extremities. The histologic diagnosis is the same for both patients.

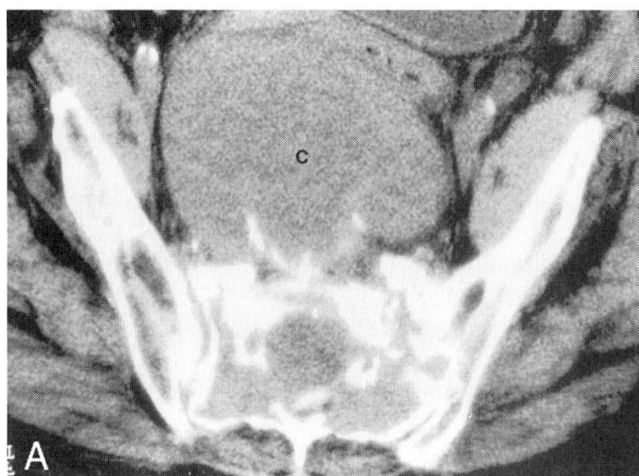

Figure 3.10 A

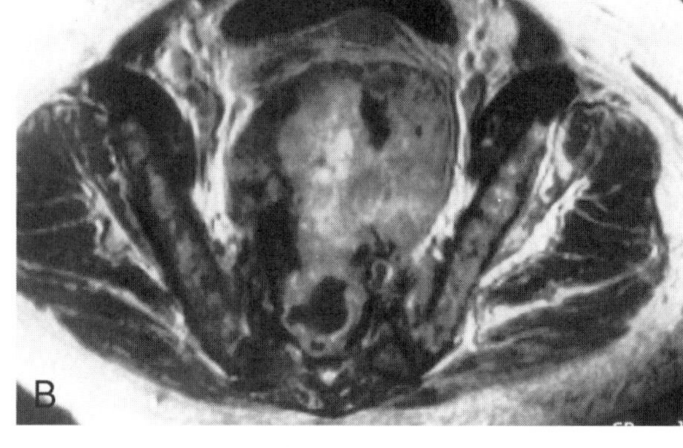

Figure 3.10 B

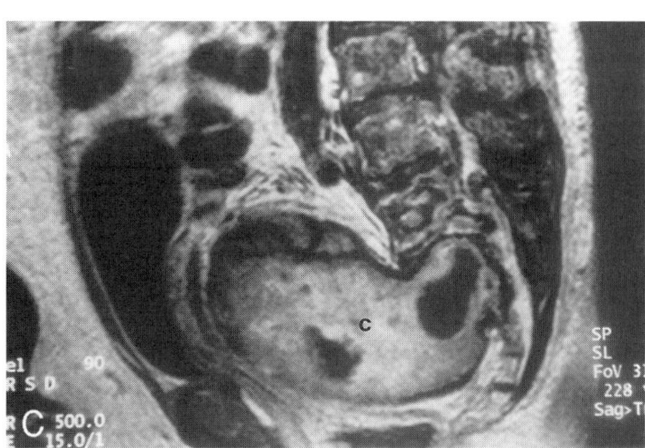

Figure 3.10 C

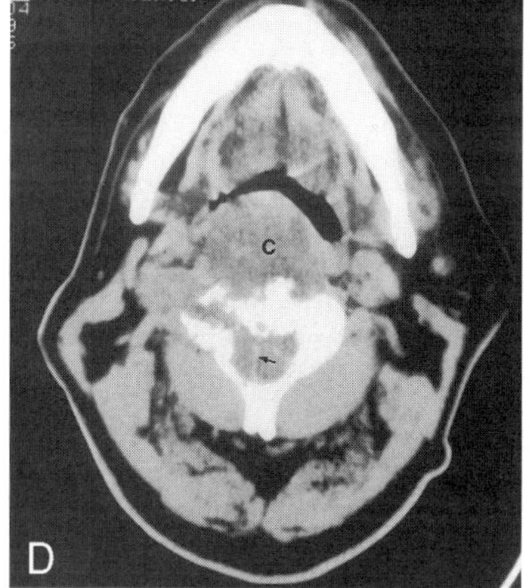

Figure 3.10 D

Findings: Axial CT of the pelvis (Fig. A) shows a destructive sacral lesion with a large soft tissue (C) component projecting into the pelvis. The tumor contains some calcifications. Axial noncontrast MR T1-weighted image (Fig. B) at a similar level as Fig. A shows the mass to be of heterogeneous signal intensity containing some cyst-like areas. Slightly parasagittal MR T1-weighted image (Fig. C) shows the mass (C) to compress the rectum, uterus, and bladder. Again, the tumor shows some cystic regions. In a different patient, noncontrast CT (Fig. D) shows a destructive lesion (C) involving C3. There is a large soft tissue component (C) in the precervical space, and the tumor extends into the spinal canal (arrow) via the right neural foramen.

(continued)

Differential Diagnosis: Metastasis, giant cell tumor, aneurysmal bone cyst, infection, chordoma.

Diagnosis: Chordoma involving the sacrum (first patient) and the cervical spine (second patient).

Discussion: Chordomas account for approximately 4% of all malignant bone tumors. They are believed to arise from remnants of the notochord resting in the intervertebral disk and vertebral bodies. More than 50% of chordomas arise in the sacrum, 35% in the clivus, and less than 15% in the spine. In the spine, the most commonly affected vertebra is C2. Involvement of the thoracic and lumbar spine is extremely rare. The most common age at presentation is 10–20 years and there is a second peak at 40–60 years. They are locally aggressive tumors and approximately 10–40% give rise to distant metastases. The most common symptoms at presentation are local pain, rectal dysfunction, and urinary incontinence. The tumor is filled with a gelatinous myxoid material and is surrounded by a fibrous pseudocapsule. It frequently (30–70%) contains calcifications that are better seen by CT. CT also identifies areas of low attenuation within the tumor. Sclerotic margins may be present. When a chordoma arises from the vertebral bodies or the disk spaces, it projects anteriorly as a large mass. On MR imaging, these tumors have low T1 signal intensity and high signal intensity on T2-weighted sequences. They may contain areas of hemorrhage, resulting in mixed signal intensities. They show variable and inhomogeneous enhancement after contrast administration. Contrast-enhanced MR imaging is needed to evaluate the degree of epidural extension. Recurrences are usually first identified in the pedicles and the posterior elements.

Clinical History: A patient with leukemia presents with bilateral lower extremity weakness and hyperreflexia.

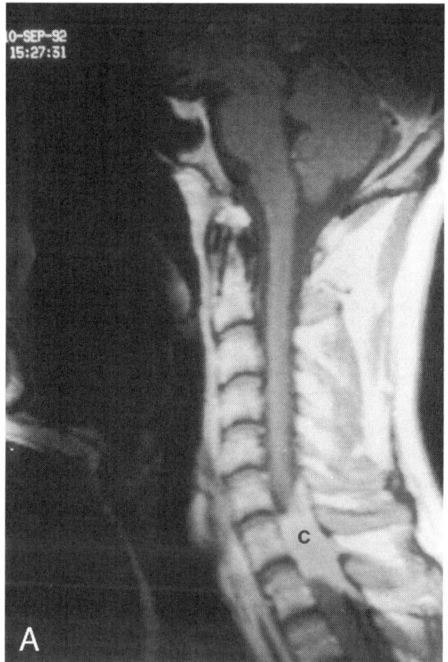

Figure 3.11 A

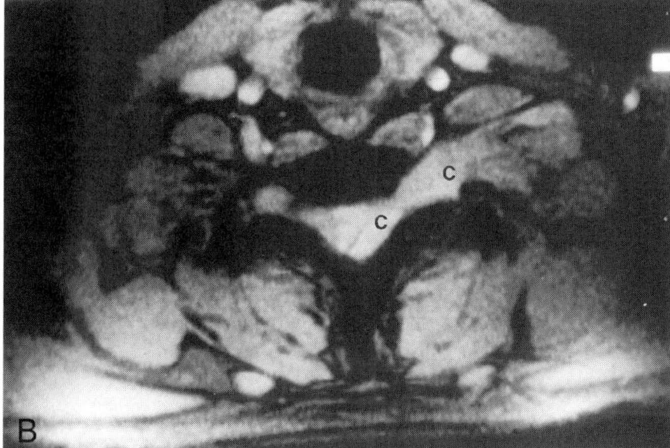

Figure 3.11 B

Findings: Midsagittal postcontrast MR T1-weighted image (Fig. A) shows an enhancing mass (C) projecting into the lower cervical spinal canal and resulting in significant compression of the cord. There is no bone destruction. Axial MR T2-weighted image (Fig. B) shows the lesion (C) extending along the left C7-T1 neural foramen into the spinal canal. This neural foramen is expanded.

Differential Diagnosis: Metastasis, lymphoma, meningioma, tumor of neural origin, sarcoma, chloroma (based on the clinical history).

Diagnosis: Chloroma.

Discussion: Chloroma (granulocytic sarcoma) is a focal mass comprised of immature granulocytes. It is most commonly seen in association with acute myeloid leukemia. Chloromas occur mostly in children and adolescents but may also be found in adults. Occasionally, they precede the onset of leukemia. Chloromas may be solitary or multiple. They are more often found in bone, periosteum, soft tissues, orbits, lymph nodes, and the skin. In bone, they produce lytic lesions predominantly affecting the axial skeleton. In the spine, they also present as paraspinal masses. Occasionally, they present as soft tissue lesions within the epidural space. Macroscopically, these tumors have a faint green color caused by myeloperoxidase in the tumor cells. By CT, they are predominantly of soft tissue density and do not have calcifications. On MR imaging, they are of low signal intensity on both T1- and T2-weighted images. This feature may reflect cellular compactness. They enhance homogenously after contrast administration. Thus, their imaging features are nonspecific and the diagnosis may be suggested only in the correct clinical setting.

Clinical History: A patient with a systemic lymphoma now presents with bilateral lower extremity weakness and bladder and bowel dysfunction.

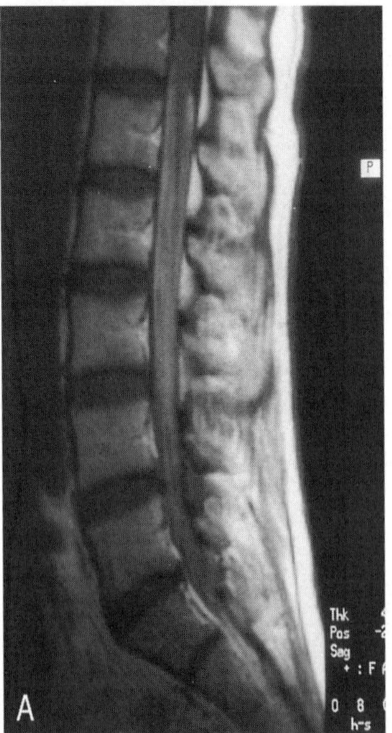

Figure 3.12 A

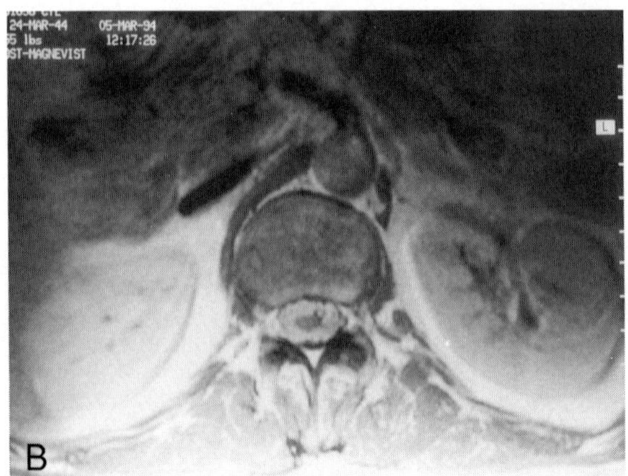

Figure 3.12 B

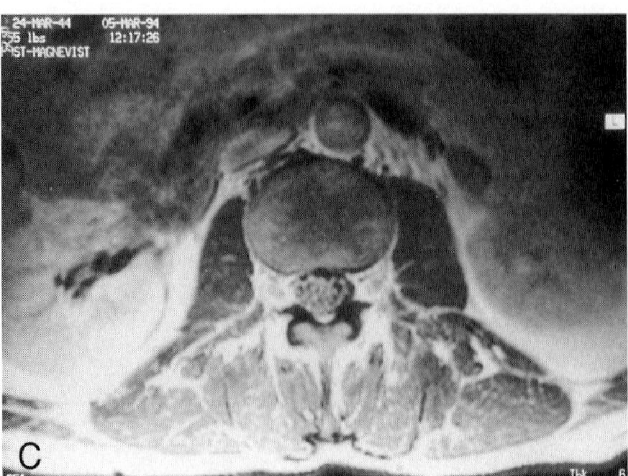

Figure 3.12 C

Findings: Midsagittal postcontrast MR T1-weighted image (Fig. A) shows diffuse enhancement of all nerve roots in the cauda equina. Axial postcontrast MR T1-weighted image (Fig. B) shows the abnormal enhancement of the proximal cauda equina. Note central nonenhancing tip of the conus medullaris. At a lower level, a postcontrast MR T1-weighted image (Fig. C) shows thick and enhancing nerve roots.

Differential Diagnosis: Metastases, lymphoma, leukemia, hypertrophic polyneuropathy, Guillain-Barré syndrome, lymphoma. (Rarely, some primary white matter disorders, such as metachromatic leukodystrophy and Krabbe, may present in children with similar findings.)

Diagnosis: Lymphoma.

Discussion: Both Hodgkin and non-Hodgkin lymphomas may involve the bones. Non-Hodgkin lymphoma is more common (and aggressive) than is Hodgkin disease. Lymphomas comprise approximately 5% of all primary malignant bone tumors and are found more often in older individuals. Between 10–50% of all lymphoma patients have bone involvement. In most cases of non-Hodgkin disease, the lesions are secondary to hematogenous dissemination of lymphoma. Lytic, moth-eaten lesions are common. Primary non-Hodgkin lymphoma is not common and spinal involvement is very rare. Hodgkin lymphoma usually represents secondary disease and has no specific imaging findings. Spine involvement is relatively common. Secondary Hodgkin lymphoma has a predilection for involvement of the epidural space, resulting in compression of the spinal cord. On MR imaging, there is replacement of the normal T1 signal intensity of the vertebral bone marrow by areas of low intensity. Lymphoma is relatively hypointense on T2-weighted images and enhances mostly homogenously after contrast administration. Contrast administration is essential in evaluating the epidural disease, and fat suppression aids in separating enhancing tumor from enhancing normal bone marrow.

CASE 13

Clinical History: A 6-year-old male presents with back pain, mild difficulty breathing, and low-grade fever.

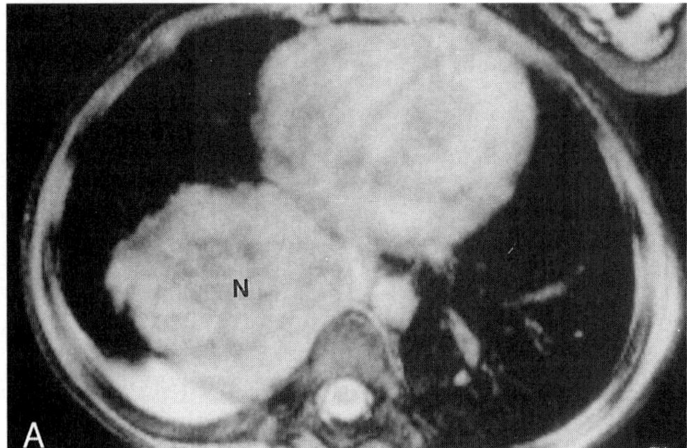

Figure 3.13 A

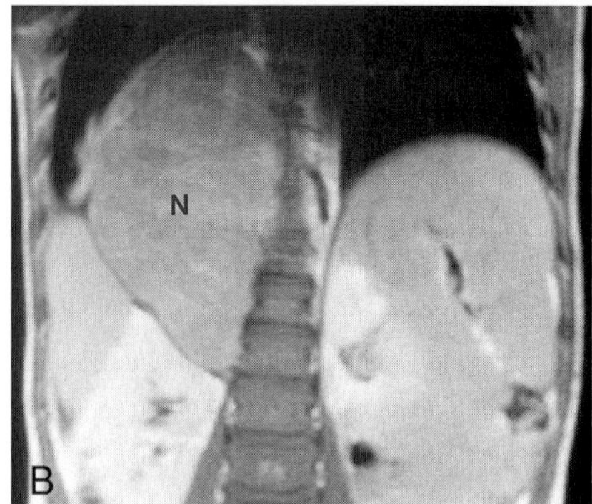

Figure 3.13 B

Findings: Axial MR T2-weighted image (Fig. A) shows a large right paraspinal mass (N) of intermediate signal intensity. There is a small right pleural effusion, and the spinal canal appears normal. Coronal postcontrast MR T1-weighted image (Fig. B) shows the mass (N) to enhance mildly and homogeneously.

Differential Diagnosis: Ganglioneuroma, ganglioneuroblastoma, neuroblastoma.

Diagnosis: Paraspinal neuroblastoma.

Discussion: Neuroblastomas are the most common solid tumors in children and the fourth most common childhood cancer. They are found most commonly in the abdomen, and they occur in the paraspinal regions in 25% of patients. These tumors are more common in males younger than 5 years of age. In a paraspinal location, they arise from the parasympathetic chain. Neuroblastomas are highly malignant and are composed of small, undifferentiated, round blue cells, necrosis, and hemorrhagic zones. These tumors may differentiate into ganglioneuroblastomas that are composed of immature neuroblasts and mature ganglion cells. Ganglioneuroblastomas may further differentiate into ganglioneuroma, which is mostly composed of mature ganglion cells. Both ganglioneuroblastoma and ganglioneuroma tend to occur in a paraspinal location, particularly in the thoracic region. Radiographs and CT show internal calcifications in 10–20% of these three tumors when they occur in the paraspinal regions. They may invade the vertebrae and ribs. They may also extend into the spinal canal and compress the cord. The MR imaging features of these lesions are nonspecific and their enhancement after contrast administration is variable.

CASE 14

Clinical History: You are shown two patients. The first (Figs. A, B) presents with sacral pain. The second (Fig. C) is known to have a primary bone tumor in the left distal femur and now presents with back pain and bilateral lower extremity weakness.

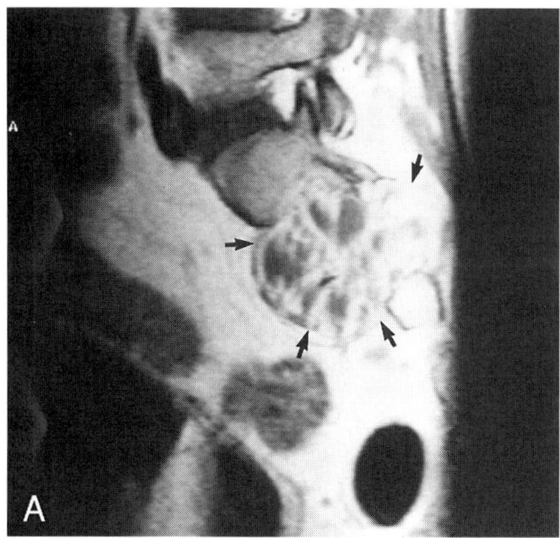

Figure 3.14 A

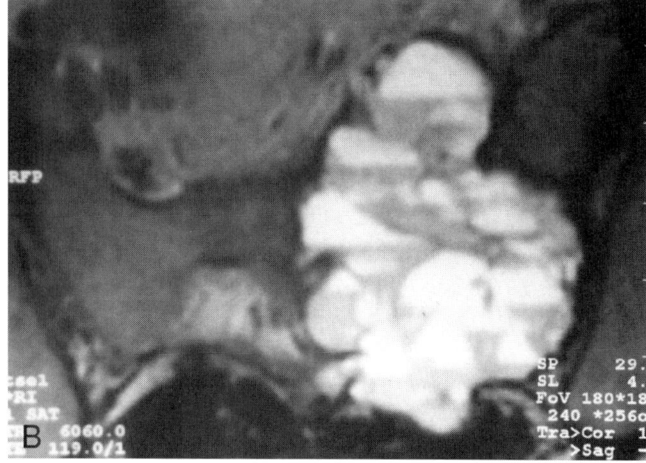

Figure 3.14 B

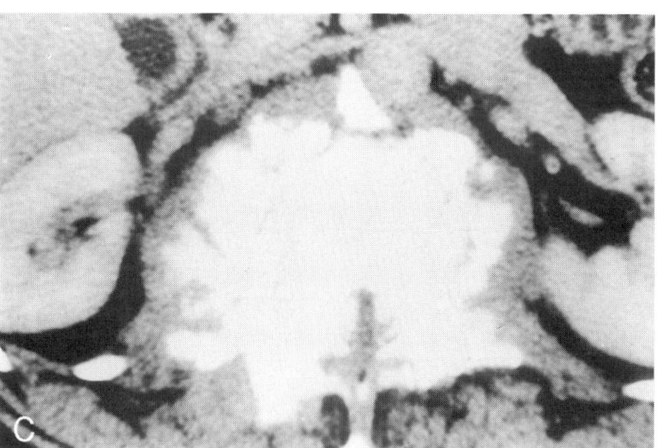

Figure 3.14 C

Findings: Parasagittal postcontrast MR T1-weighted image (Fig. A) shows a mass (arrows) arising from the superior aspect of the sacrum. Axial MR T2-weighted image (Fig. B) shows the tumor to contain multiple fluid levels reminiscent to those present in aneurysmal bone cysts. (Case courtesy M. Smith, M.D., Nashville, TN). In a different patient, axial CT (Fig. C) shows marked sclerosis and expansion of the L1. There is new bone formation in the anterior margins of the vertebral body and along the spinal canal. The latter formation results in compression of the conus medullaris. This patient had a similar lesion at T5.

(continued)

Differential Diagnosis: Because of the blood-fluid levels in the first case, aneurysmal bone cyst and giant cell tumor should be considered. In the second case, osteosarcoma, sclerotic metastasis, and an infection such as tuberculosis should be considered.

Diagnosis: Primary sacral osteosarcoma and a metastatic osteosarcoma to L1.

Discussion: Only 3% of all primary bone sarcomas arise in the spine. Metastases from these sarcomas to the spine are also rare. Most primary spinal sarcomas are found during the first decade of life. In older individuals, these sarcomas may be secondary to underlying Paget disease and prior radiation therapy (there is a latent period of 5 to 25 years). They are more common in males. Patients generally present with localized pain. Chondrosarcomas are much less common than osteosarcomas and generally occur in older patients. Osteosarcomas may arise in the vertebral body or its posterior elements. They are predominantly blastic lesions but commonly contain lucent areas. Chondrosarcomas usually arise in the region of the costotransverse joint. They are large masses that, on radiographs and CT, contain the so-called "popcorn" calcifications. They tend to invade the adjacent soft tissues. Both tumors are of intermediate T1 signal intensity and are bright on T2-weighted images. At times, the T2 signal is mixed. Extension into the spinal canal, resulting in compression of the spinal cord, is common with both tumors. Highly malignant chondrosarcomas demonstrate intense, diffuse, and homogeneous contrast enhancement contrary to less malignant ones, which show only septa of enhancement.

CASE 15

Clinical History: A young female (Figs. A,B) presents with a 2-month history of upper lumbar pain, low grade fevers, loss of weight, and lower extremity weakness.

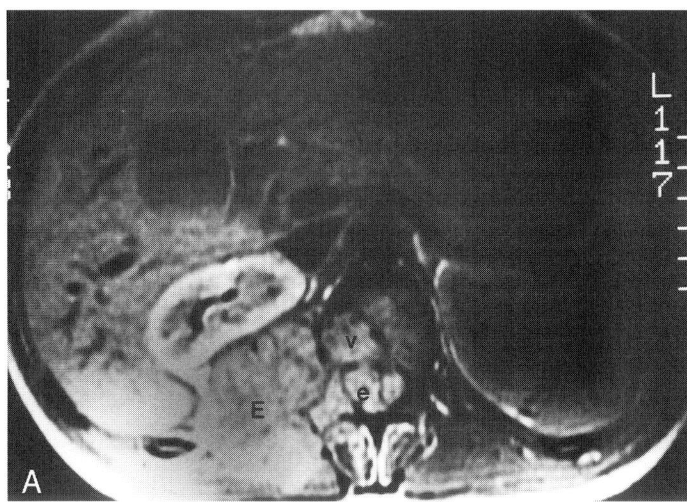

Figure 3.15 A

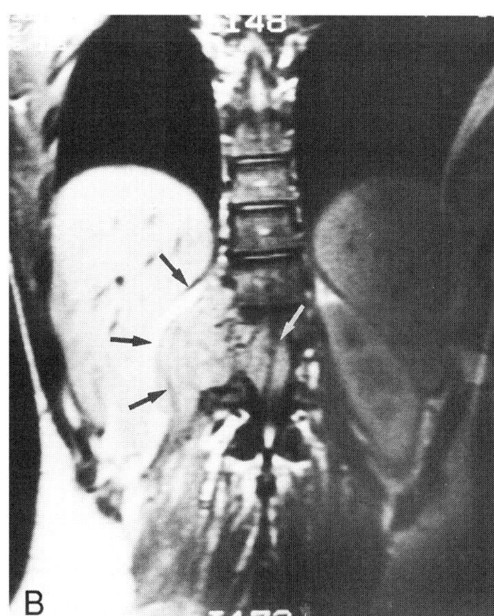

Figure 3.15 B

Findings: Axial postcontrast MR T1-weighted image (Fig. A) shows a right lumbar paraspinal mass (E) invading the adjacent vertebral body (v) and extending into the spinal canal (e). Coronal postcontrast MR T1-weighted image (Fig. B) shows the paraspinal component (black arrows) of the mass and its intraspinal component (white arrow). (Case courtesy of E. Palacios, M.D., Berwyn, IL.)

Differential Diagnosis: Chondrosarcoma, osteosarcoma, malignant fibrous histiocytoma, metastasis, lymphoma, plasmacytoma, Ewing sarcoma.

Diagnosis: Ewing sarcoma arising from the costovertebral region.

Discussion: The spine is the site of origin for approximately 3.5% of all Ewing sarcomas. In the spine, the sacrum is the most commonly involved region. Almost all cases of Ewing sarcomas are diagnosed before the age of 30 years. Males are affected more frequently than are females. Patients typically present with pain, rapidly progressing neurologic deficits, and systemic symptoms. Because fever tends to be prominent, the clinical differential diagnosis should include infection. Histologically, these tumors are composed of abundant, small, blue, round, and undifferentiated cells similar to those found in the primitive neuroectodermal tumors. Indeed, it is difficult to distinguish between Ewing sarcomas and primitive neuroectodermal tumors. Ewing sarcomas also contain hemorrhage and necrosis. These sarcomas produce partial or complete destruction of the bone they arise in. In the vertebrae, the lesion may be surrounded by a sclerotic rim. A paraspinal mass that extends into the spinal canal is a relatively common finding. The adjacent disk height may be reduced. Calcifications within these lesions are uncommon. CT clearly shows the bone features of the lesion, but MR imaging is needed to evaluate the intraspinal extension of the tumor.

CASE 16

Clinical History: A 45-year-old female presents with weakness in all extremities and hyperreflexia.

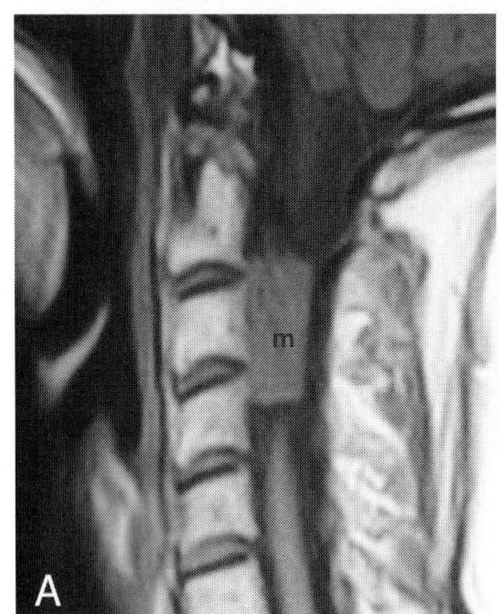

Figure 3.16 A

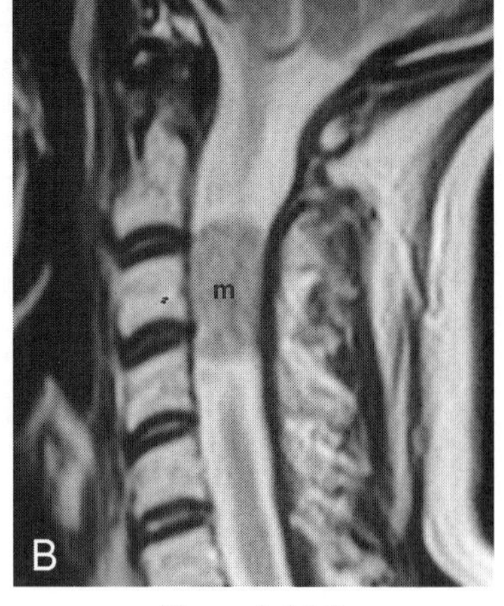

Figure 3.16 B

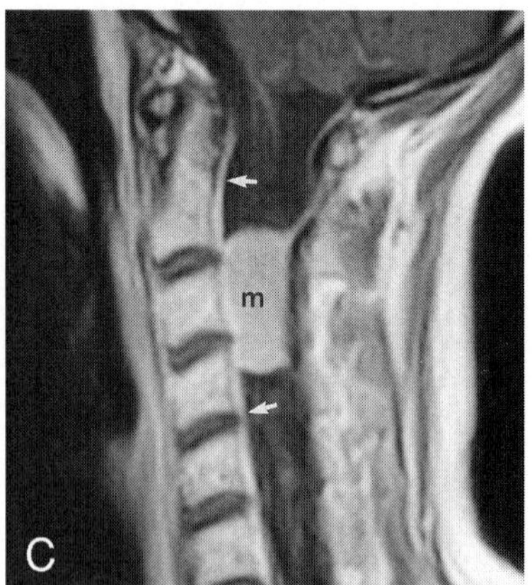

Figure 3.16 C

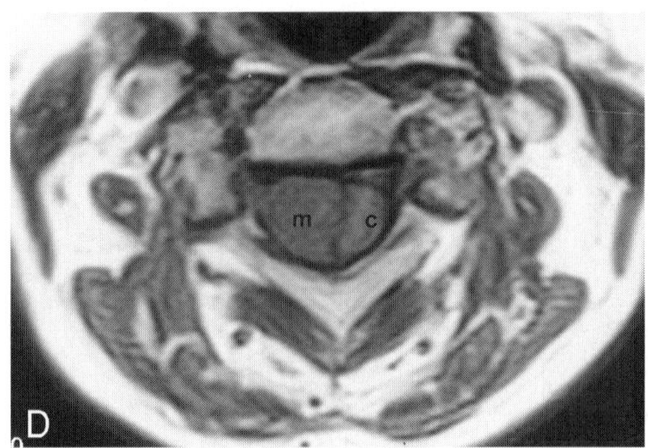

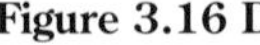

Figure 3.16 D

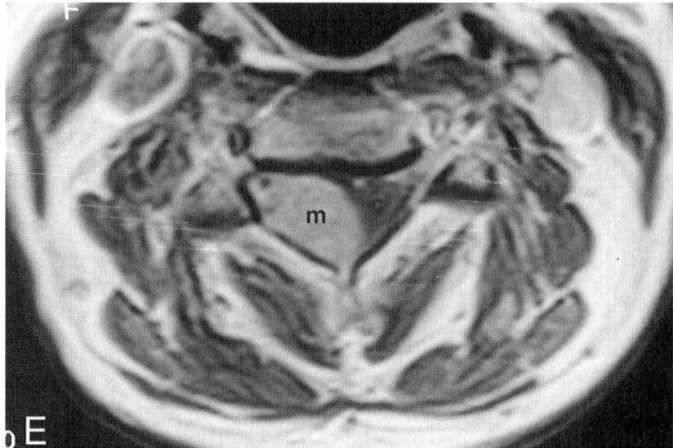

Figure 3.16 E

Findings: Parasagittal noncontrast MR T1-weighted image (Fig. A) shows an intraspinal mass (m) at the level of C3. Corresponding MR T2-weighted image (Fig. B) shows the mass (m) which is isointense to the spinal cord on both T1- and T2-weighted sequences. Corresponding postcontrast MR T1-weighted image (Fig. C) shows that the mass (m) enhances markedly and homogeneously. Note enhancement of thick adjacent dura (arrows). From these sagittal images, it is not possible to determine the exact compartment in which the lesion arises. Axial noncontrast MR T1-weighted image (Fig. D) shows the mass (m) to be intradural but separate from the spinal cord (c), thus extramedullary in location. Corresponding axial postcontrast MR T1-weighted image (Fig. E) shows the mass (m) to be clearly separable from the spinal cord (c).

Differential Diagnosis: Nerve sheath tumors, metastasis, lymphoma, meningioma, chloroma.

Diagnosis: Intraspinal meningioma.

Discussion: Meningiomas are the most common primary spinal tumors after schwannomas. Meningiomas represent 40% of intradural extramedullary masses. They are more common in middle-aged to older females. Most of them (80%) are found in the thoracic region, followed by the cervical spine (15–20%). In the cervical region, they usually arise at the cranial junction, particularly near the foramen magnum. Less than 5% of all spinal meningiomas occur in the lumbar region. Most spinal meningiomas are intradural (85%), but some (15%) are mixed (intradural–extradural) in location. Patients generally present with vague pain and/or progressive neurologic symptoms secondary to the compression of the spinal cord or the nerve roots. By CT, these masses enhance relatively homogeneously. Meningiomas are commonly located in the posterolateral aspects of the spinal canal and may contain calcifications (10%). On MR imaging, they tend to be isointense to the spinal cord in both T1- and T2-weighted images. Calcified meningiomas may be hypointense on both sequences. They enhance homogenously and markedly after contrast administration. Occasionally, spinal meningiomas are multiple and can be associated with neurofibromatosis type 2. Chronic compression of the spinal cord by a meningioma may result in the formation of the syringohydromyelia.

Clinical History: The first patient (Figs. A,B) is a 37-year-old man who presents with a right L2 radiculopathy. The second patient (Fig. C) has a systemic disorder.

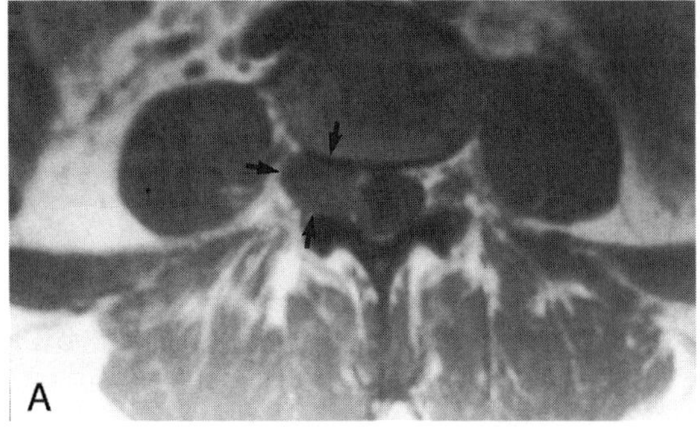

Figure 3.17 A

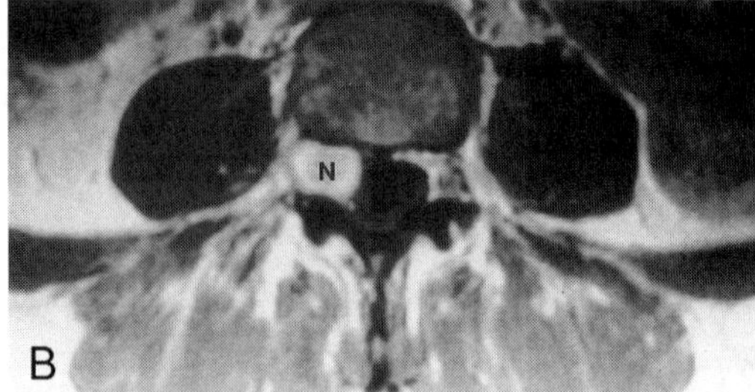

Figure 3.17 B

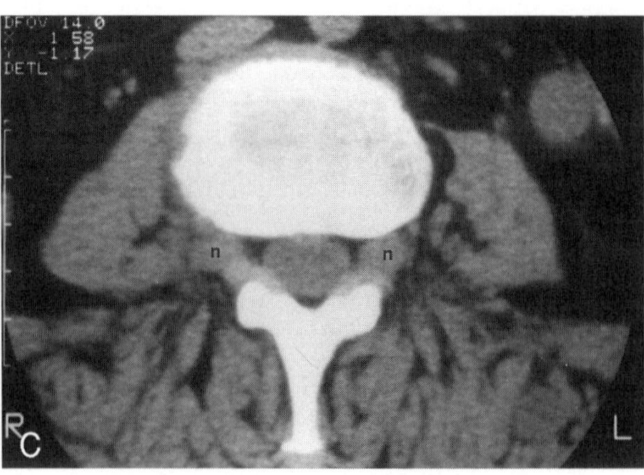

Figure 3.17 C

Findings: In the first patient, axial noncontrast MR T1-weighted image (Fig. A) shows a rounded mass (arrows) in the right L2-L3 neural foramen. There is expansion of this foramen. The mass is clearly extradural in location. Corresponding postcontrast MR T1-weighted image (Fig. B) shows the lesion (N) to enhance homogeneously. In the second patient, axial CT (Fig. C) shows masses (n) in both neural foramina.

Differential Diagnosis: Schwannoma, meningioma, metastasis, lymphoma, sequestered disk fragment, chloroma, neurofibroma.

Diagnosis: Isolated schwannoma in the first case, bilateral neurofibromata in a patient with neurofibromatosis type 1.

Discussion: Tumors originating from the nerve roots may be schwannomas (also called neurilemmomas and neurinomas) or neurofibromas. They are the most common primary spinal tumors, followed by meningioma (see Case #16). They tend to be more common in females aged 40–60 years. In males, they are usually found at a younger age. Contrary to meningiomas, neurofibromas are more commonly found in the lumbar spine and tend to be both extradural and intradural in location ("dumbbell" appearance). They arise mostly from the dorsal nerve roots. They may project into the spinal canal and become embedded within with spinal cord. They grow slowly and result in remodeling of the adjacent bone structures by pressure erosion. Erosion of the vertebral bodies may result in kyphoscoliosis. Spinal neurofibromas are more common in patients with neurofibromatosis type 1, whereas schwannomas (and meningiomas) are more common in patients with neurofibromatosis type 2. Paraspinal neurofibromas are common in patients with neurofibromatosis. Overall, spinal masses are more common in neurofibromatosis type 2. Intratumoral calcifications are rare. These tumors enhance by both CT and MR imaging. The enhancement is less homogeneous than that seen in meningiomas. These tumors may enhance in the so-called "target" fashion. Schwannomas may be cystic or hemorrhagic. Malignant degeneration into neurofibrosarcomas is uncommon in the absence of neurofibromatosis, but in its presence occurs in 4–11% of neurofibromas. Neurofibrosarcomas are found more often in females. Malignant degeneration of schwannomas is extremely rare.

Clinical History: A 4-year-old boy presents with a tumor in the cerebellum. He has no symptoms referable to the spine. This spine study was obtained as part of his staging.

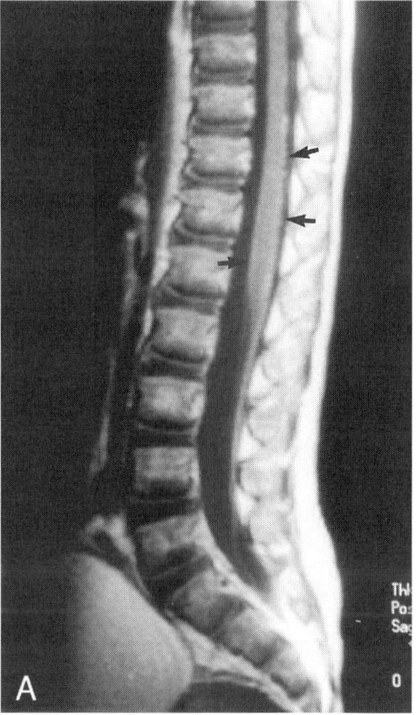

Figure 3.18 A

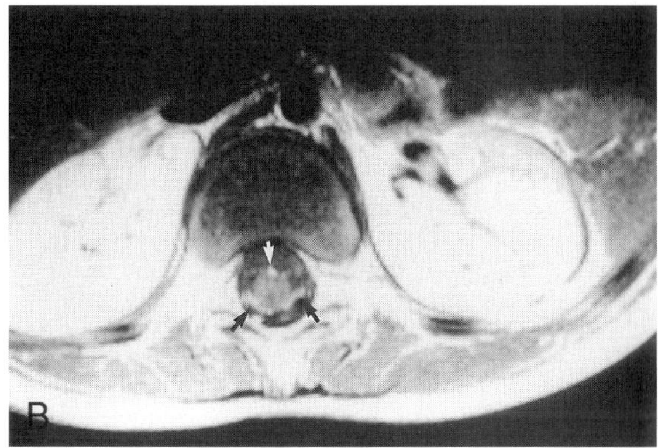

Figure 3.18 B

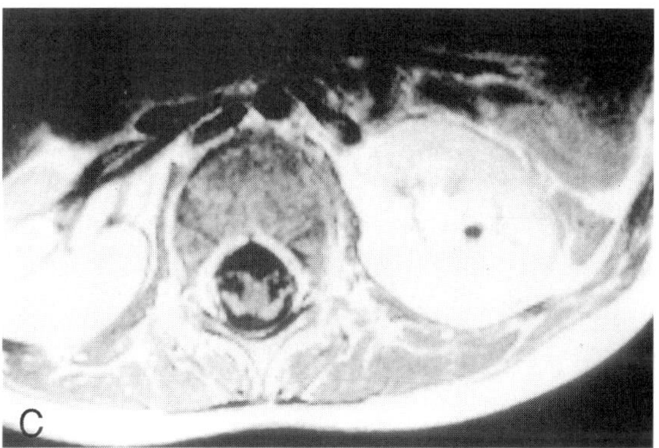

Figure 3.18 C

(continued)

Findings: Midsagittal postcontrast MR T1-weighted image (Fig. A) shows questionable enhancement (arrows) along the surfaces of the spinal cord and conus medullaris. The nerve roots also appear to enhance. Axial postcontrast MR T1-weighted image (Fig. B) shows enhancement (black arrows) of dorsal nerve roots and ventral surface (white arrow) of the conus medullaris. Axial postcontrast MR T1-weighted image (Fig. C) obtained slightly below Fig. B shows abnormal enhancing nerve roots. Note that the dorsal nerve roots are also thickened.

Differential Diagnosis: Guillain-Barré syndrome, lymphoma, leukemia, metastases, transverse myelitis, Refsum or Dejerine disease (hypertrophic polyneuropathies in childhood), spinal leptomeningeal (drop) metastases from medulloblastoma.

Diagnosis: Spinal leptomeningeal (drop) metastases from medulloblastoma.

Discussion: The term "drop" metastases refers to tumor deposits in the spinal subarachnoid space. These metastases generally lodge in the dependent portions of the lumbar thecal sac, thus the use of the term "drop." Drop metastases are more common with tumors arising within the central nervous system. Primary neoplasias that produce drop metastases include mainly primitive neuroectodermal tumors, germinoma, choroid plexus tumors, and astrocytomas. Meningeal carcinomatosis may also be produced by lymphoma, leukemia, melanoma, and primary tumors in the breast, lung, and gastrointestinal tract. Symptoms include back pain, sensory deficits in the lower extremities, polyneuropathies, cauda equina syndrome, and loss of bowel and bladder control. Analysis of the cerebrospinal fluid shows elevated proteins, normal-to-low glucose level, and malignant cells in approximately 75% of patients with drop metastases. Prognosis is poor, with most patients dying 4 to 6 months after the diagnosis. The most common sites for drop metastases are the lumbar spine, followed by the thoracic and cervical regions. MR with contrast is the imaging method of choice and shows clumping, crowding, and enhancement of the nerve roots. Nodular enhancement may be seen on the surfaces of the spinal cord. Patients with cerebral tumors who are prone to develop drop metastases should be imaged before surgery. If the patient is imaged immediately after surgery, false positive studies are not uncommon. If the spine was not studied before surgery, MR imaging should be delayed for 4–6 weeks to allow for inflammation and postoperative changes to subside.

CASE 19

Clinical History: You are shown three patients. The first (Figs. A and B) has neurofibromatosis type 2 and presents with bilateral lower extremity weakness and hyperreflexia. The second patient (Figs. C and D) is a 55-year-old male who presents with bilateral lower extremity weakness and bladder and bowel dysfunction. The third (Figs. E and F) presents with progressive quadriparesis and difficulty swallowing.

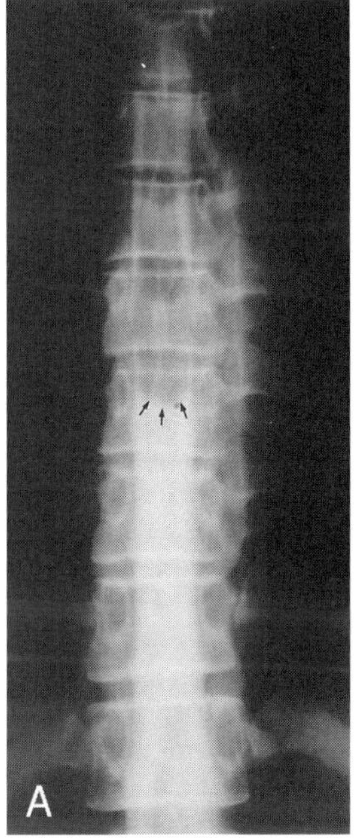

Figure 3.19 A

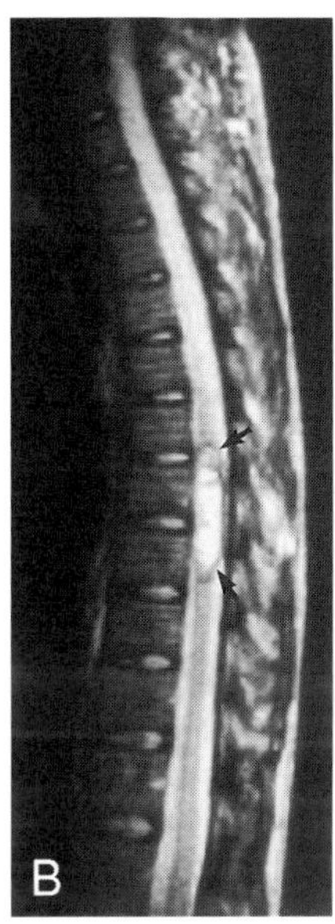

Figure 3.19 B

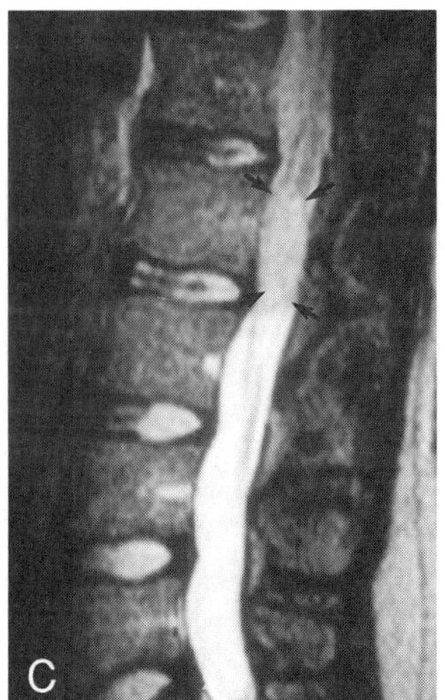

Figure 3.19 C

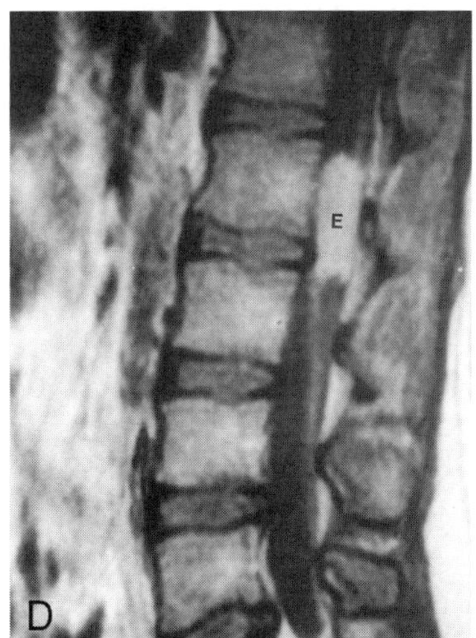

Figure 3.19 D

(continued)

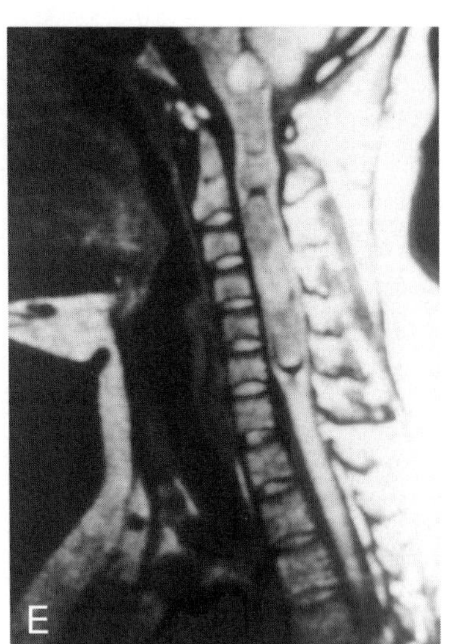

Figure 3.19 E

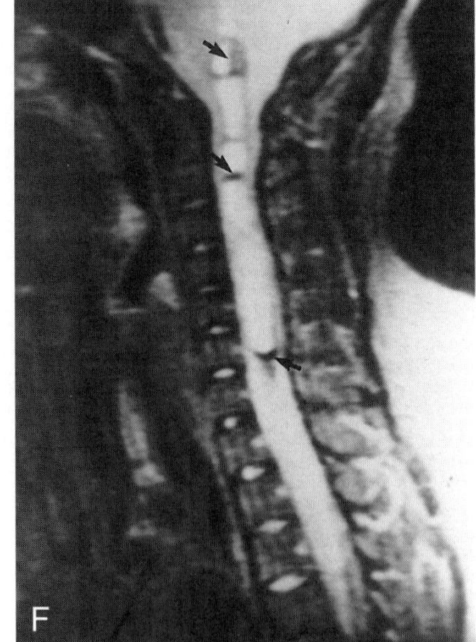

Figure 3.19 F

Findings: Frontal radiograph (Fig. A) from a myelogram shows a high-grade block to the flow of contrast material at T9. Note the lower border (arrows) of the lesion with a "meniscus" sign indicating the intradural and possibly intramedullary location of the mass. Midsagittal MR T2-weighted image (Fig. B) shows an intramedullary tumor of high signal intensity. Note that the borders (arrows) of this tumor are of low signal intensity, suggesting the presence of hemosiderin and/or ferritin (chronic blood products). In a different patient, a midsagittal MR T2-weighted image (Fig. C) shows an intradural lesion (arrows) at the L1 level. Corresponding postcontrast MR T1-weighted image (Fig. D) shows this tumor (E) to enhance. In the third case, a midline sagittal noncontrast MR T1-weighted image (Fig. E) shows a complex intramedullary tumor extending from the lower pons to the C6 level. Note that the tumor contains mixed signal intensity with some significantly hypointense regions suggesting the presence of chronic blood products. In a corresponding T2-weighted image (Fig. F), the tumor contains blood levels (arrows). (Case courtesy M. Smith, M.D., Nashville, TN.)

Differential Diagnosis: Astrocytoma, ependymoma, intramedullary metastasis, hemangioblastoma, ganglioglioma, paraganglioma (for ependymomas arising in the filum terminale).

Diagnosis: Spinal cord ependymoma (first and third cases), and ependymoma (myxopapillary type) arising in the filum terminale (second case).

Discussion: In adults, ependymoma is probably the most common spinal cord tumor, closely followed by astrocytoma. It occurs predominantly in the thoracic cord, conus medullaris, and in the filum terminale. It is found more commonly in females aged 40–60 years. Its incidence is also increased in patients with neurofibromatosis type 2. Patients commonly present with only nonspecific back pain but may also have weakness of the lower extremities and bowel and/or bladder dysfunctions. Most ependymomas arising in the filum terminale are of the myxopapillary type. These tumors tend to be well-encapsulated and often amenable to complete surgical excision. Invasion of the conus medullaris does, however, occur. Incomplete resection requires treatment with radiation. Ependymomas are slow-growing tumors that remodel the adjacent bone in 30% of cases. These tumors may attain a very large size before they are discovered. MR is the imaging method of choice. They are hypointense with respect to the spinal cord on T1-weighted images and hyperintense on T2-weighted sequences. Approximately 65% demonstrate inhomogeneous signal intensity secondary to prior hemorrhage. A rim of hemosiderin (marked hypointensity) may be present. Hemorrhage in a spinal tumor should always suggest ependymoma. Almost 50% of ependymomas harbor cysts. All tumors show some degree of contrast enhancement. Syringohydromyelia may be associated with these tumors. Myxopapillary ependymomas are elongated and enhance homogeneously after contrast administration.

Clinical History: You are shown two patients. The first (Figs. A and B) is a 7-year-old child who presents with back pain and weakness in all extremities. Hyperreflexia was present on physical examination. The second (Figs. C–E) is an adult with a similar clinical history. The third (Figs. F and G) is a college female student with mid-thoracic pain and lower extremity weakness of 1 month's duration.

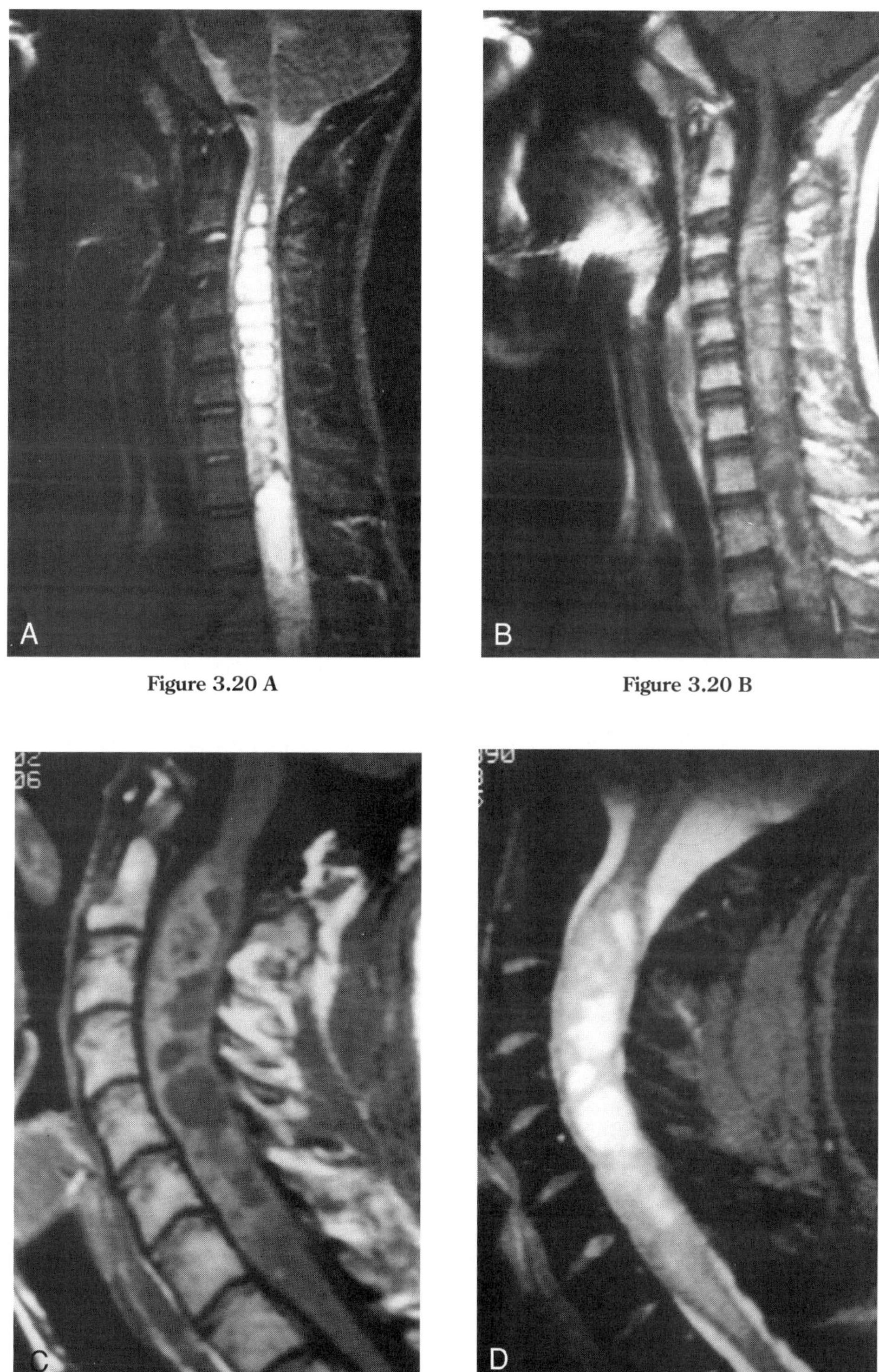

Figure 3.20 A

Figure 3.20 B

Figure 3.20 C

Figure 3.20 D

(continued)

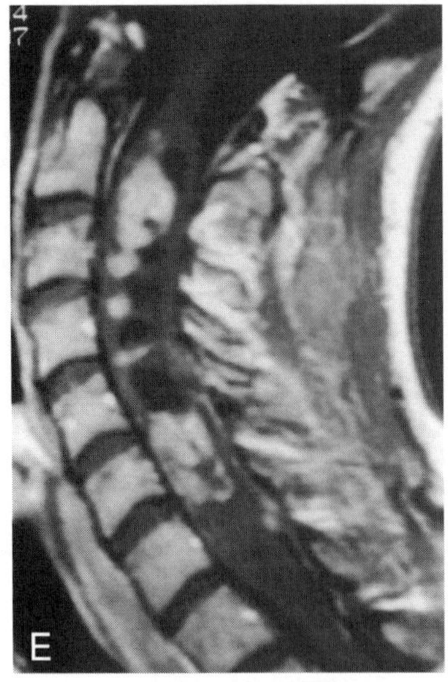

Figure 3.20 E

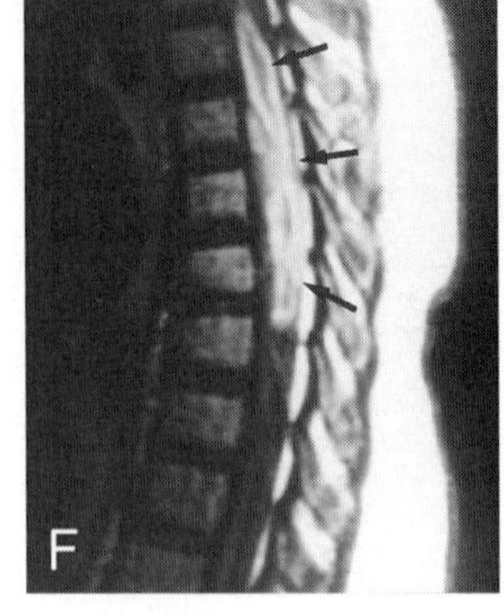

Figure 3.20 F

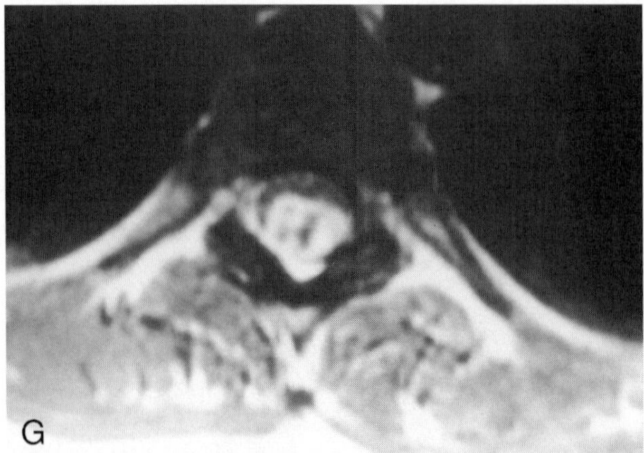

Figure 3.20 G

Findings: In the first case, a midsagittal MR T2-weighted image (Fig. A) shows a multiseptated mass of high signal intensity involving the cervical spinal cord and extending into the thoracic region. There is expansion of the cord. Corresponding postcontrast MR T1-weighted image (Fig. B) shows inhomogeneous enhancement of most of the lesion. Note that despite the "cystic" appearance of this mass on the T2-weighted image, the tumor is solid. In the second case, a midsagittal noncontrast MR T2-weighted image (Fig. C) shows significant expansion of the cervical spinal cord by a mass which contains focal areas of high signal intensity and some nodules of intermediate signal intensity. On a corresponding noncontrast MR T2-weighted image (Fig. D), the mass shows that it contains some nodules anteriorly which are somewhat hyperintense and some bright cyst-like areas dorsally. After contrast administration, a corresponding image (Fig. E) shows that the anterior nodules enhance markedly. The cysts are clearly seen. (Case courtesy M. Smith, M.D., Nashville, TN.) In the third patient, a midsagittal postcontrast MR T1-weighted image (Fig. F) shows an irregularly enhancing mass (arrows) in the midthoracic spinal cord. In the same patient, axial T1-weighted postcontrast image (Fig. G) shows the enhancing intramedullary lesion.

Differential Diagnosis: Ependymoma, astrocytoma, ganglioglioma, hemangioblastoma, transverse myelitis, metastasis, and occasionally spinal cord changes induced by an arteriovenous fistula.

Diagnosis: Spinal cord astrocytomas.

Discussion: Spinal cord astrocytomas are predominantly found in children and in adults aged 20 to 30 years. They are also more common in patients with neurofibromatosis type 1. They are more common in males. They are more commonly found in the cervical and thoracic regions and occasionally they may involve the entire length of the spinal cord (holocord astrocytomas). Histologically, the majority of spinal cord astrocytomas are Grades 1 and 2 but more malignant tumors may also be found. Benign astrocytomas are more common in adults (nearly 90%). Most astrocytomas expand the cord but rarely may be exophytic. Early symptoms are nonspecific and include back pain and progressive scoliosis. Astrocytomas are slow-growing tumors, producing bone remodeling in 50% of patients. MR is the imaging method of choice to evaluate these tumors. They are hypointense to the spinal cord on T1-weighted images and hyperintense on T2-weighted images. All enhance to some degree after the administration of contrast material. Cysts are found in 25–35% of these tumors. Associated syringohydromyelia is found in almost 40% of patients. Usually, the borders of these tumors are ill-defined. Gangliogliomas in the spinal cord are rare and are indistinguishable from the more common astrocytoma by imaging studies.

CASE 21

Clinical History: This patient presents with weakness in all extremities. He has a history of a cerebellar mass and a renal cell carcinoma.

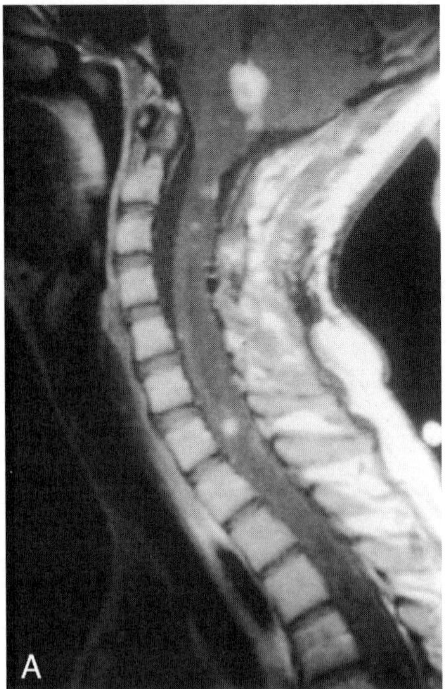

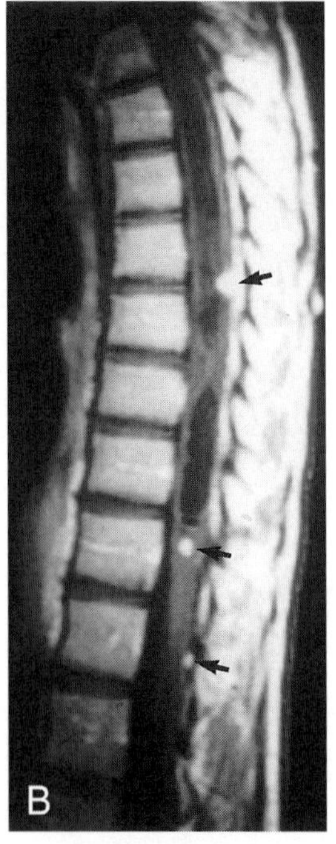

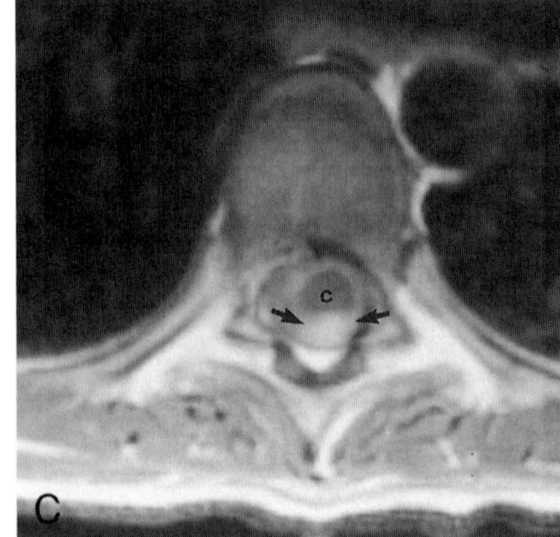

Figure 3.21 A   **Figure 3.21 B**   **Figure 3.21 C**

Findings: Midsagittal postcontrast MR T1-weighted image (Fig. A) of the cervicothoracic region shows multiple, solid, enhancing lesions within the spinal cord. The spinal canal is mildly expanded. Note enhancing tumor in cerebellum inferior to the fourth ventricle. Midsagittal postcontrast MR T1-weighted image (Fig. B) of the thoracic spine shows multiple enhancing tumor nodules (arrows) and cysts. Note the "peripheral " location of the enhancing lesions. Axial postcontrast MR T1-weighted image (Fig. C) at a mid-thoracic level shows the subpial location of an enhancing tumor nodule (arrows). Note cyst (c) anterior to the tumor.

Differential Diagnosis: Intramedullary metastases, astrocytoma, ependymoma, hemangioblastoma (rarely, sarcoidosis and fungal infections may result in a similar appearance).

Diagnosis: Spinal cord hemangioblastomas in a patient with Von Hippel Lindau disease (VHL).

Discussion: Spinal cord hemangioblastomas are tumors that are found more often in patients with VHL. Approximately 30% of hemangioblastomas are associated with VHL. They are usually found in individuals aged 20–40 years and in younger patients with VHL. Most of these lesions (60–80%) are solitary; multiple tumors are more common in the presence of VHL. There is no gender predilection. They are more commonly found in the cervical and thoracic regions. Typically, these lesions resemble those found in the cerebellum. MR is the imaging method of choice. They tend to be cystic and harbor an enhancing mural nodule. The nodule is generally subpial in location. Approximately 20–25% of spinal hemangioblastomas are solid and indistinguishable from other intramedullary tumors. Solid and multiple tumors are more common in patients with VHL. Hemangioblastomas tend to produce significant edema of the spinal cord. Associated syringohydromyelia is present in 40–60% of patients. Dilated, serpiginous vessels in the subarachnoid space adjacent to the tumor nodule are common. The tumor nodules enhance markedly and homogeneously.

Clinical History: A female with known primary carcinoma of the breast presents with sudden onset of bilateral lower extremity weakness.

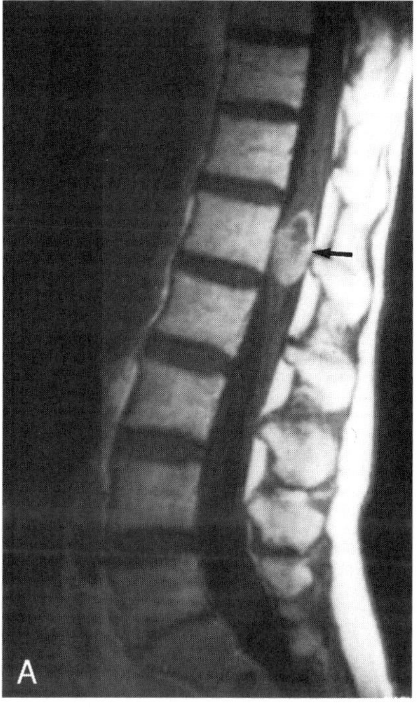

Figure 3.22 A

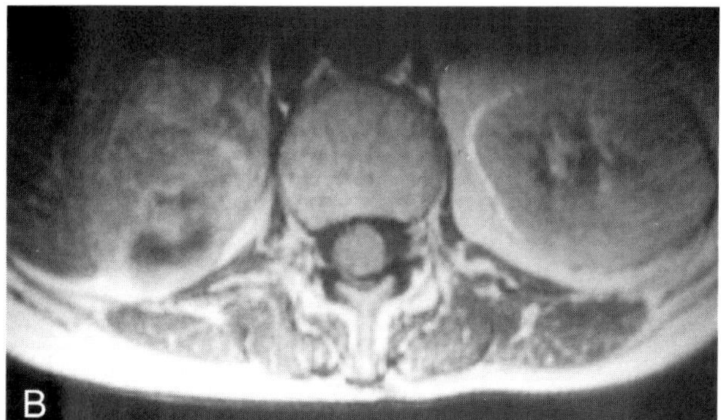

Figure 3.22 B

Findings: Midsagittal postcontrast MR T1-weighted image (Fig. A) shows an enhancing lesion (arrow) within the conus medullaris. Note partial central necrosis within the tumor. Axial postcontrast MR T1-weighted image (Fig. B) shows the enhancing lesion to involve the entire diameter of the conus medullaris.

Differential Diagnosis: Solid hemangioblastoma, ependymoma, astrocytoma, intramedullary metastasis.

Diagnosis: Intramedullary metastasis from primary breast carcinoma.

Discussion: Intramedullary spinal cord metastases are rare, occurring in less then 10% of patients with metastatic disease to the central nervous system. Of all cancer patients, fewer than 1% develop metastases to the spinal cord. Primary lung carcinoma accounts for more than 50% of spinal cord metastases, followed by tumors from the breast. Other primary neoplasias responsible for spinal cord metastases are lymphoma, melanoma, colorectal carcinoma, leukemia, and head and neck primaries. The thoracic spinal cord is affected more commonly. MR is the imaging method of choice in these patients. The spinal cord appears expanded in a fusiform fashion and, after contrast administration, the tumor nodule enhances markedly and has discreet borders. Central necrosis is not uncommon. T2-weighted images show surrounding edema. Most lesions are solitary. Associated cysts are not a feature of intramedullary spinal cord metastases. Hemorrhage is uncommon. Metastases from melanoma may be of increased T1 signal intensity before the administration of contrast material.

Clinical History: This 68-year-old female with a history of myelofibrosis presents with a 1-month history of increasing back pain and lower extremity sensory neuropathy.

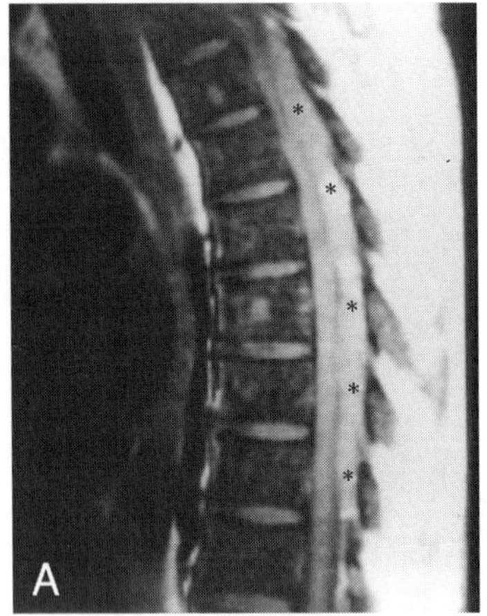

Figure 3.23 A

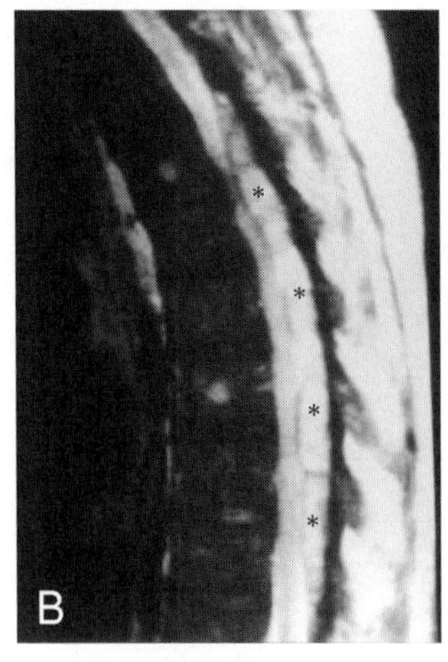

Figure 3.23 B

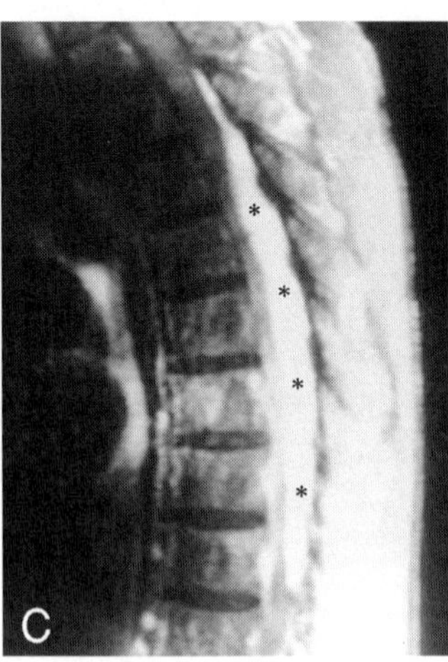

Figure 3.23 C

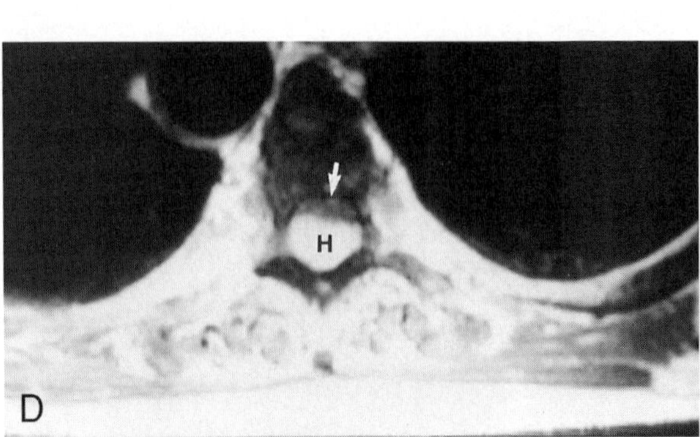

Figure 3.23 D

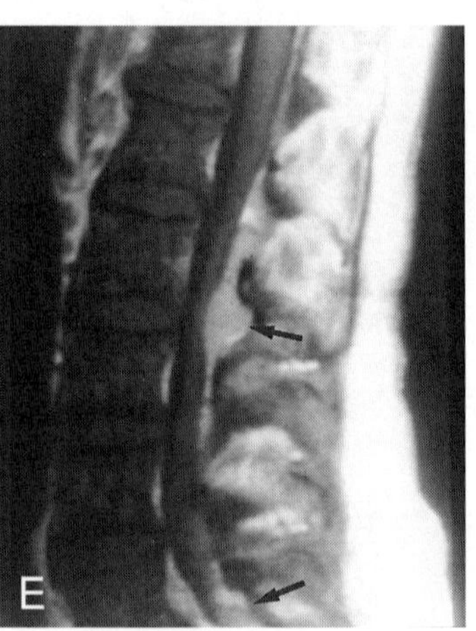

Figure 3.23 E

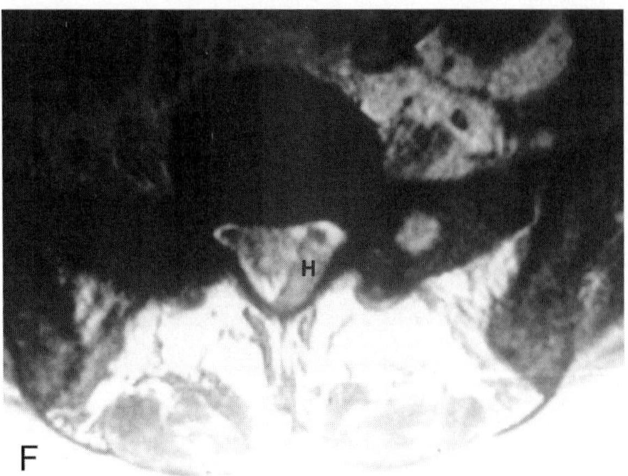

Figure 3.23 F

Findings: Midsagittal noncontrast MR T1-weighted image (Fig. A) shows a mildly hyperintense abnormality (*) in the posterior thoracic epidural space compressing the spinal cord. The bone marrow in the vertebral bodies is abnormally hypointense. Corresponding T2-weighted image (Fig. B) shows the abnormality (*) to be hyperintense. Corresponding postcontrast fat suppressed T1-weighted image (Fig. C) shows that the lesion (*) enhances markedly. Axial postcontrast MR T1-weighted image (Fig. D) shows that enhancing abnormality (H) results in marked anterior displacement and compression of the spinal cord (arrow). Noncontrast midsagittal MR T1-weighted image (Fig. E) in the lumbar region shows extradural lesions (arrows) of high signal intensity. Note again, the hypointense bone marrow. Axial noncontrast T1-weighted image (Fig. F) shows a lesion (H) in the epidural space with compression of the distal thecal sac.

Differential Diagnosis: Metastases, lymphoma, epidural hematoma (particularly in patients with a coagulopathy), epidural abscesses, extramedullary hematopoiesis, and chloromas.

Diagnosis: Extramedullary hematopoiesis.

Discussion: Extramedullary hematopiesis is rare and is associated with chronic anemias. Disorders known to result in extramedullary hematopoiesis include beta-thalassemia, myelofibrosis, polycythemia vera, and myelodysplastic syndromes. The most frequently involved organs are the spleen, liver, kidney, adrenal gland, heart, lymph nodes, and thymus. Involvement of the spinal epidural space is extremely rare. The epidural space becomes involved presumably because of extrusion of bone marrow from the surrounding vertebra. Extramedullary hematopoiesis may result in compression of the spinal cord, at which point treatment is indicated. Laminectomies have been used. The most popular form of treatment is relatively low-level radiation. The major risk of radiation therapy is in inducing even more myelosuppression in already anemic patients.

CONGENITAL DISORDERS

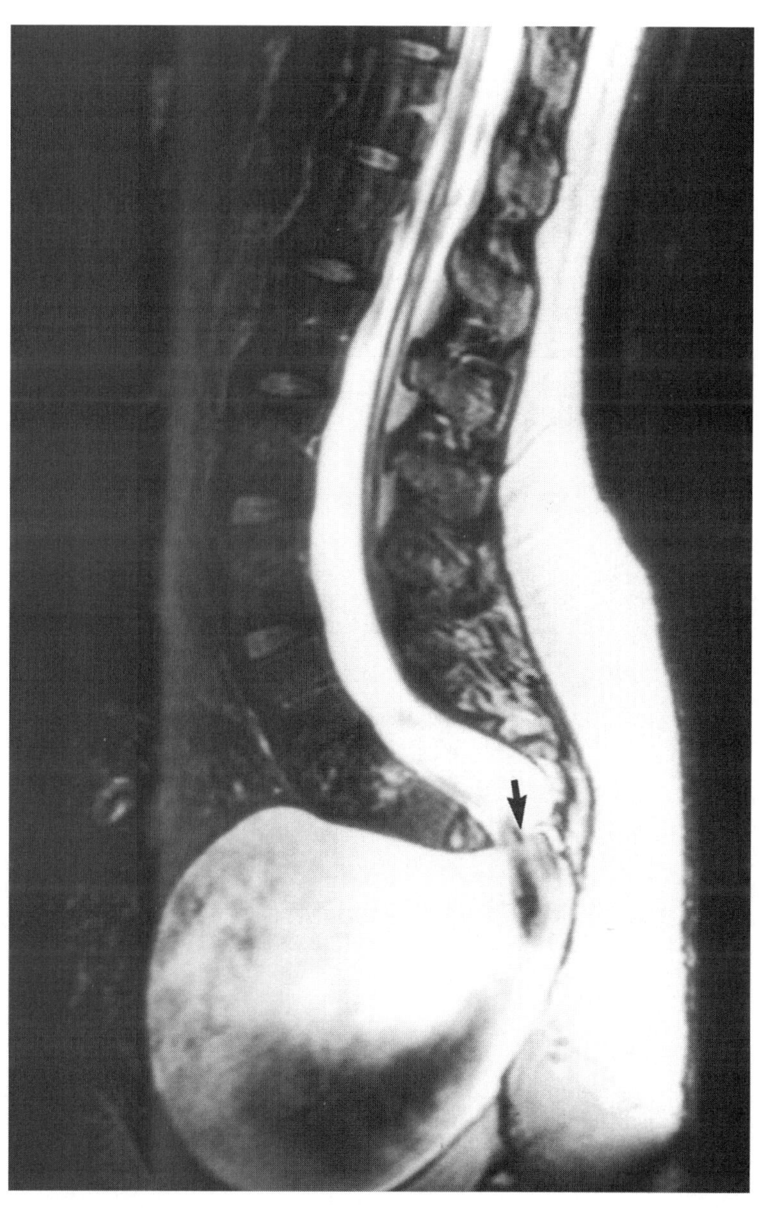

Clinical History: You are shown two patients. The first (Figs. A–C) is a 6-year-old undergoing a routine follow-up study of the spine because of a previously resected cerebellar medulloblastoma. The second patient (Fig. D) was noted to have this abnormality while being studied for a liver lesion.

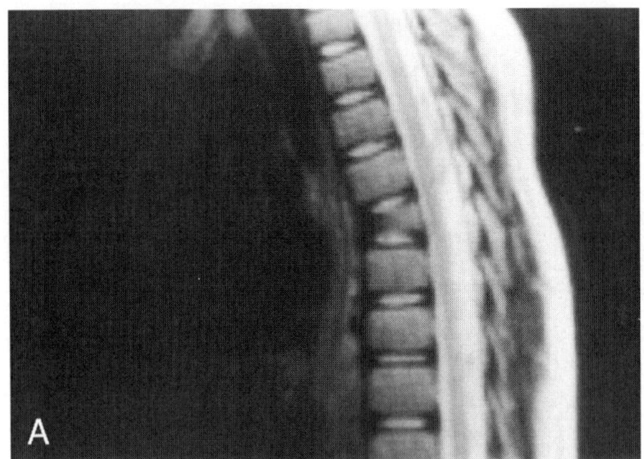

Figure 4.1 A

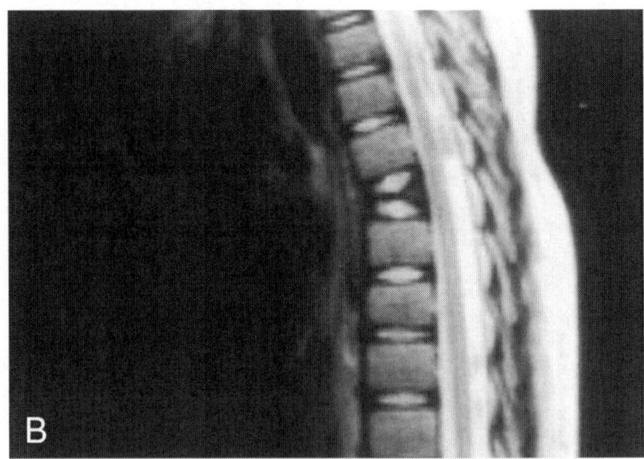

Figure 4.1 B

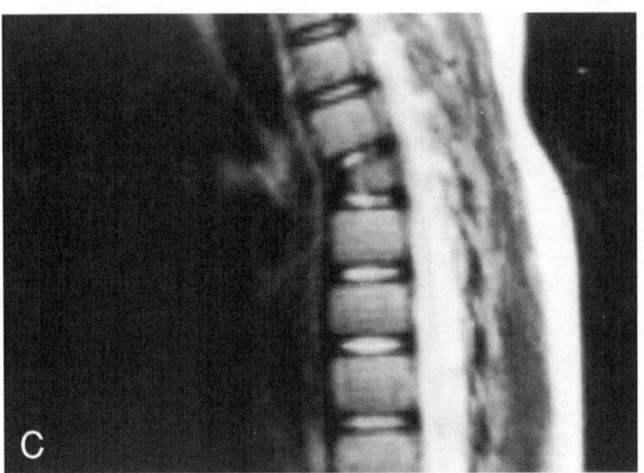

Figure 4.1 C

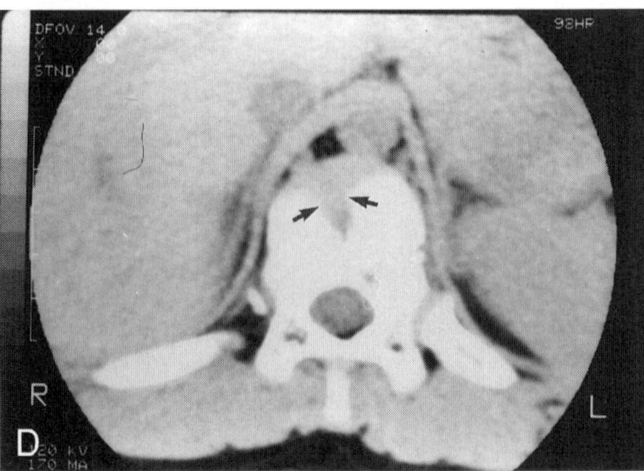

Figure 4.1 D

Findings: Fig. A is a right parasagittal MR T2-weighted image showing a wedge deformity involving a midthoracic vertebral body. In the same patient (Fig. B), the midsagittal MR T2-weighted image shows marked diminution of the height of that vertebra. A left parasagittal MR T2-weighted image (Fig. C) shows less deformity. Note that in both parasagittal images, the signal intensity from the vertebral bone marrow is normal, making a metastasis unlikely. In a different patient, axial CT (Fig. D) shows a cleft (arrows) in the midportion of a lower thoracic vertebral body.

Diagnosis: Butterfly vertebrae.

Discussion: During embryologic development, paired somites form along the sides of the centrally located notochord. These somites differentiate into cell masses that give origin to the skin and subcutaneous tissues (dermatome), paraspinal muscles (myotome), and vertebrae (sclerotome). Sclerotome segmentation and differentiation are probably under the control of the notochord and the neural tube. Fusion of one superior and one inferior sclerotome leads to "condensation" and formation of one vertebral body. This primitive vertebral body contains several ossification centers grouped around the notochord. The notochord then involutes. The posterior vertebral arches are formed under influence of the neural crest. Thus, it is possible to have abnormalities isolated to the vertebral body, the posterior arch, or both. Failure of development of paired sclerotomas leads to an absent vertebra, whereas failure of development of one sclerotome leads to formation of the hemivertebra. Failure or delay notochordal involution results in absence of the midline condensation of the sclerotomes, resulting in a butterfly vertebra. Any of these anomalies may result in scoliosis. However, butterfly vertebrae are commonly asymptomatic and incidental findings, not to be confused with destructive lesions of the vertebrae.

CASE 2

Clinical History: You are shown two patients. The first (Fig. A) is a 5-year-old who was born with an open spinal dysraphism. The second (Figs. B–D) was born with an open dysraphism at the upper lumbar level.

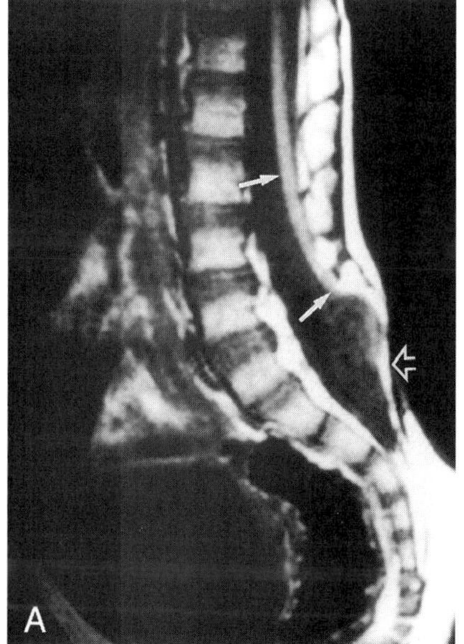

Figure 4.2 A

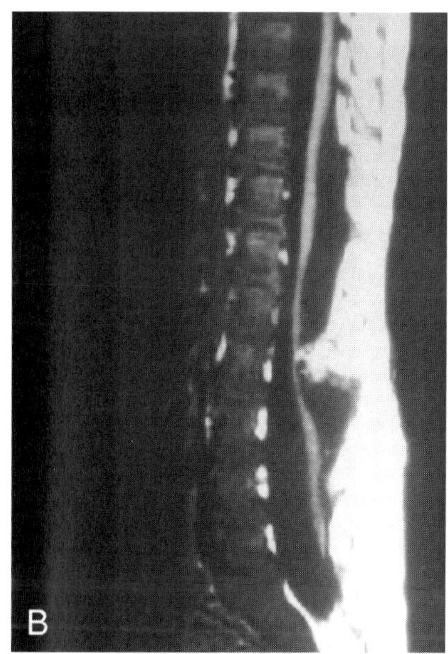

Figure 4.2 B

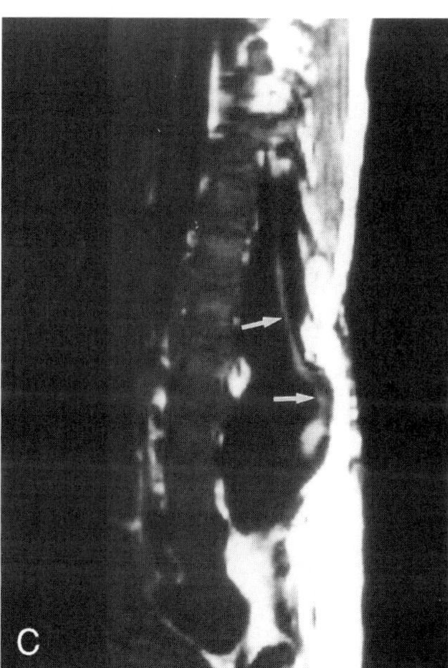

Figure 4.2 C

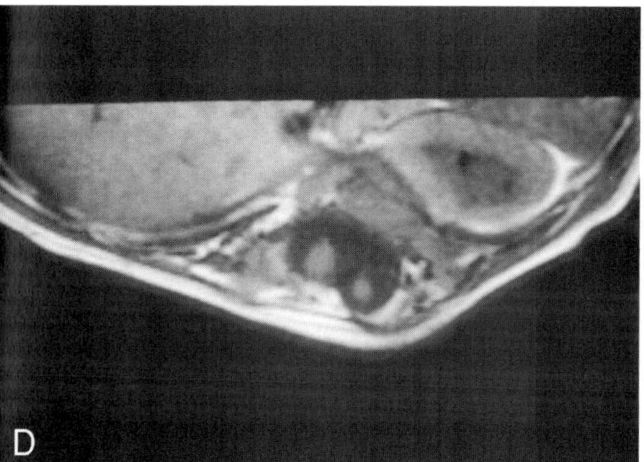

Figure 4.2 D

(continued)

Findings: Midsagittal MR T1-weighted image (Fig. A) shows that the spinal cord (solid arrows) extends into the site of a surgically closed myelomeningocele (open arrow). This is the expected appearance of a repaired myelomeningocele, and the spinal cord is likely tethered at the site of repair. In the second patient, a right parasagittal MR T1-weighted image (Fig. B) shows a dysplatic, thin spinal hemicord extending down to the level of L5-S1. A left parasagittal MR T1-weighted image (Fig. C) shows a thin hemicord (arrows) herniating into the previously repaired open defect. Axial MR T1-weighted image (Fig. D) shows two hemicords, the right one contained in the canal and the left one herniating into the repaired defect.

Diagnosis: Myelomeningocele (first case) and hemimyelocele (second case).

Discussion: Both myelocele and myelomeningocele are considered open spinal defects. The neural tube fails to close completely and allows for direct visualization of an unfolded spinal cord (placode). If the placode is at the level of the skin, a myelocele is present. Most commonly, a ventral and enlarged fluid-containing space displaces the placode, outwardly forming a myelomeningocele. Rare types of open dysraphisms include a myelocystocele and a hemimyelocele. In the heminyelocele, a hemicord is herniated through an open defect while the other remains within the spinal canal. Open dysraphisms occur in 1–3 of 1,000 newborns and are more common in females. It occurs in 4–8% of subsequent siblings. Elevated alpha feto protein is found in serum (80% sensitivity) and in aminiotic fluid (98% sensitivity) in cases of open spinal dysraphism. Hydrocephalus is present in more than 75% of these patients, and evaluation of the head is therefore mandatory. Without treatment, mortality is between 50–80%. Most open defects are found in the lower lumbar and upper sacral spine, followed by the craniocervical junction. Most defects are closed before any imaging is attempted. Imaging is used to follow patients who develop new and/or progressive symptoms. In all of the postoperative patients, the cord may be considered as tethered; therefore, imaging is used to determine other potentially correctable abnormalities. Such abnormalities include syringohydromyelia, arachnoid cysts, diastematomyelia, and epidermoid and dermoid tumors. Imaging of postoperative patients should include the entire spine.

Clinical History: You are shown two patients. The first (Figs. A–C) presented at birth with a large skin-covered mass in the lower back. The second (Figs. D and E) presented with fatty mass in the lower back, bladder retention, and varus deformity of the feet.

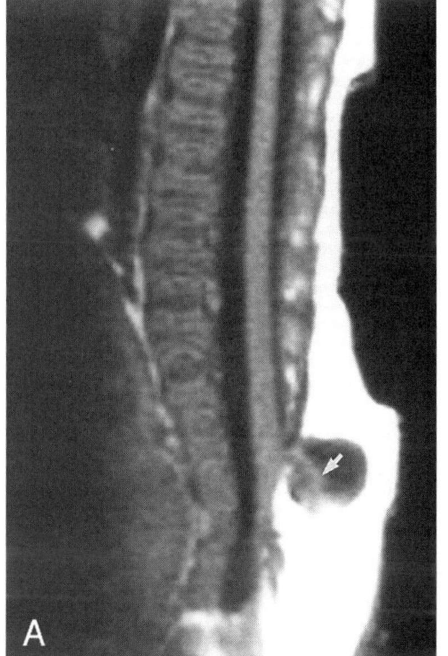

Figure 4.3 A

Figure 4.3 B

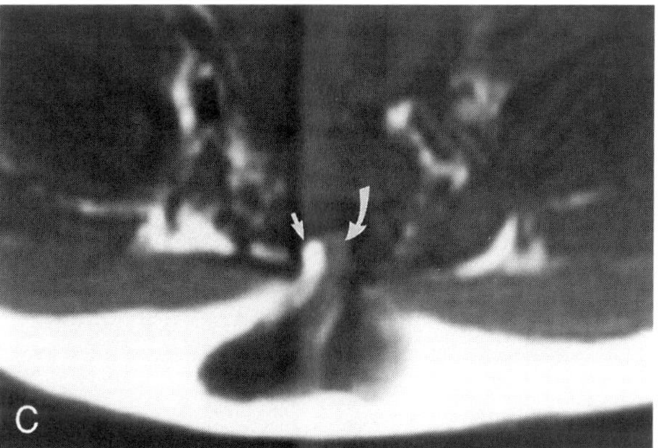

Figure 4.3 C

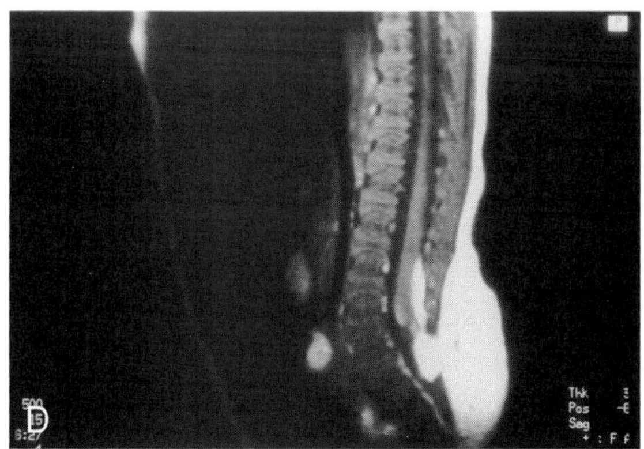

Figure 4.3 D

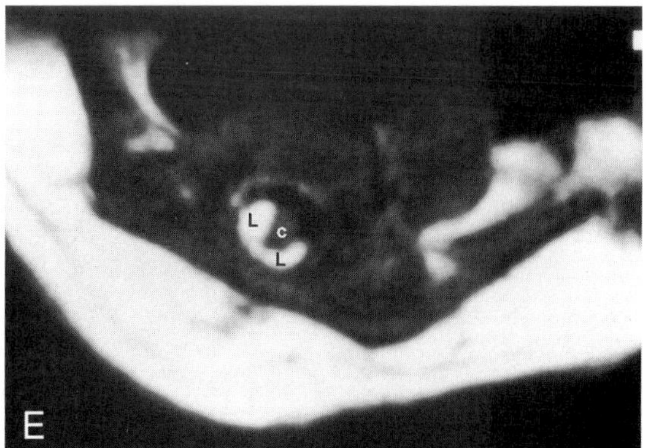

Figure 4.3 E

(continued)

Findings: In the first patient, a midline sagittal T1 weighted image (Fig. A) shows a fluid-filled cavity protruding into the subcutaneous fat at the S2 level. The meningocele contains neural elements (arrow) is covered by fat. On a slightly parasagittal image (Fig. B), there is extension of the subcutaneous fat into the meningocele and into the spinal canal. Axial T1 weighted image (Fig. C) shows that the intraspinal lipoma (small arrow) abuts the dysplastic (unfolded) and low-positioned spinal cord (curved arrow), which also herniates posteriorly into the defect. In the second patient, a midsagittal MR T1-weighted image (Fig. D) shows subcutaneous lipoma with continuation into the spinal canal through a bone defect in the lumbosacral region. The lipoma is in apposition with the dorsal spinal cord, which is dysplatic and low-lying but entirely located within the canal. Axial MR T1-weighted image (Fig. E) shows the lipoma (L) insinuating itself into an incompletely folded spinal cord (c).

Diagnosis: Lipomyelomeningocele (first case) and lipomyelocele (second case).

Discussion: Lipomyeloceles and lipomyelomeningoceles are considered "closed" dysraphisms because skin overlies the defect, preventing direct inspection. These disorders arise from incomplete and premature separation of the surface ectoderm from the folding neural tube. There is inclusion of ectodermal elements that later differentiate and grow into lipomas. Lipomas may be entirely intradural. In the lipomyeloceles and lipomyelomeningoceles, there is continuation of the subcutaneous fat into the canal and cord via spinal bifida. If the unfolded neural tube (placode) remains deep or at the level of the bone defect, the result is a lipomyelocele. If the placode is displaced outwardly from the spina bifida, a lipomyelomeningocele is formed. The most common of these defects is the lipomyelomeningocele. Associated syringohydromyelia is found in 2% of these patients. Concomittant anomalies of vertebral segmentation occur in up to 50% of cases. These defects are more commonly found in the lumbosacral region. Clinically, most of these patients have a soft fatty mass in the lower back. At this level, the skin is abnormal (hemangioma, atrophy, hairy patches). Common symptoms are weakness or flaccid paralysis of the lower extremities and bowel and bladder dysfunction. These defects are more common in females.

CASE 4

Clinical History: This patient presents with low back pain, lower extremity weakness, and bilateral varus deformity of the feet.

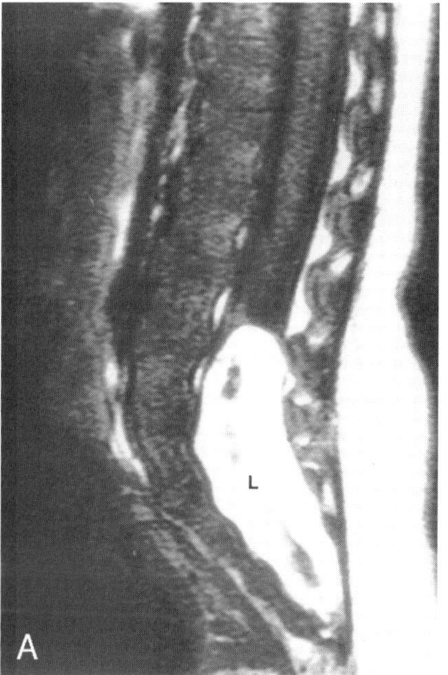

Figure 4.4 A

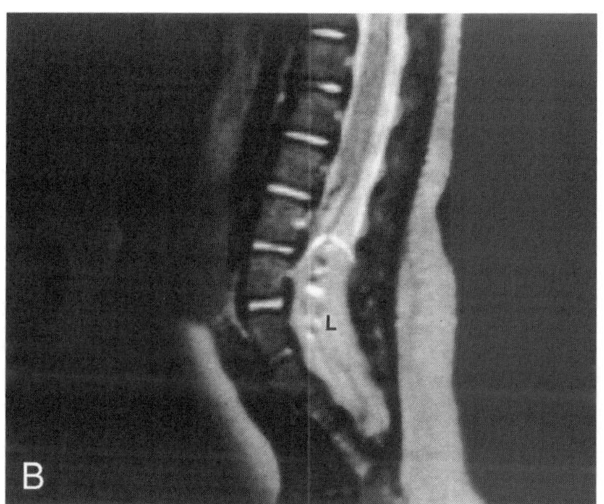

Figure 4.4 B

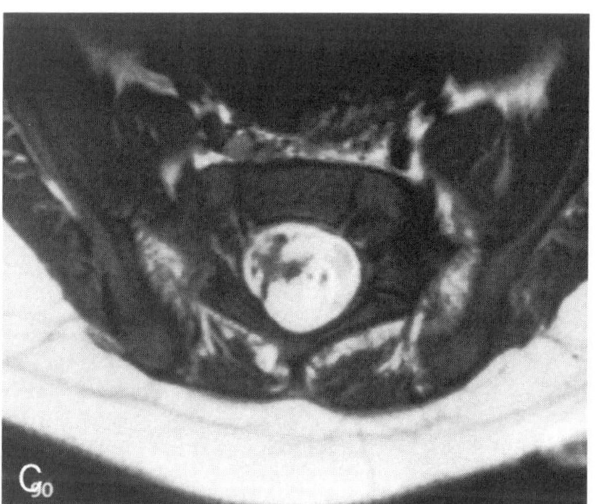

Figure 4.4 C

Findings: Midsagittal MR T1-weighted image (Fig. A) shows an intraspinal lipoma (L) expanding the canal. The spinal cord is low-lying. On a corresponding T2-weighted image (Fig. B), the lipoma (L) is of lower signal intensity (similar to that of the subcutaneous fat). Axial MR T1-weighted image (Fig. C) shows the lipoma has diffusely encased the distal dysplastic spinal cord and nerve roots.

(continued)

Differential Diagnosis: Dermoid, intraspinal lipoma.

Diagnosis: Intraspinal lipoma.

Discussion: Intradural lipomas represent only 1–4% of all spinal lipomas. They are believed to arise from pluripotential ectodermal cell rests trapped within the folding neural tube as a result of premature and incomplete separation of the neural tube from the cutaneous ectoderm. They are more common in females. The cervical region is affected the most often. Most intraspinal lipomas become symptomatic during the first 5 years of life. These masses compress the neural elements, and common symptoms include ascending paresis, spasticity, sensory loss, abnormal development, lower extremity weakness, and bowel and bladder dysfunction. MR is the imaging method of choice. Lipomas are generally located in the dorsal aspect of the spinal canal but may be found anywhere. They insinuate themselves into the spinal cord, which appears incompletely closed at that level. The spinal cord may be compressed by the lipoma. The lipoma may be contiguous with the fat in the epidural space. A fibrous band or a sinus tract may join it to a dermal ostium. Lipomas have the signal intensity of fat on all MR sequences. They may, however, appear somewhat inhomogenous because they may contain abundant fibrous tissues. Intraspinal lipomas may result in remodelling of the neighboring bones.

CASE 5

Clinical History: You are shown MR imaging studies of three different patients who presented with bladder and bowel retention and bilateral dislocated hips.

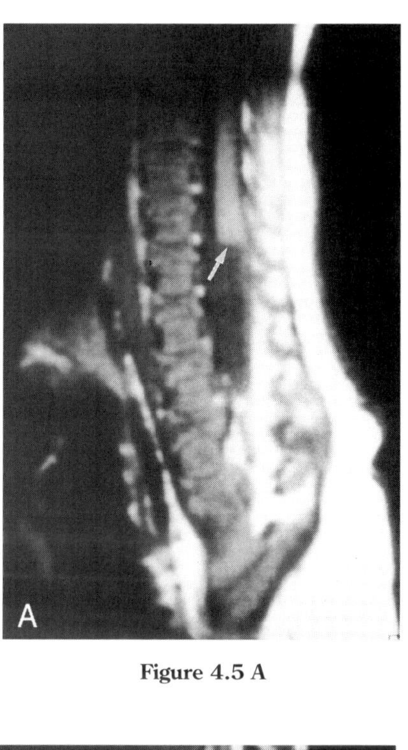

Figure 4.5 A

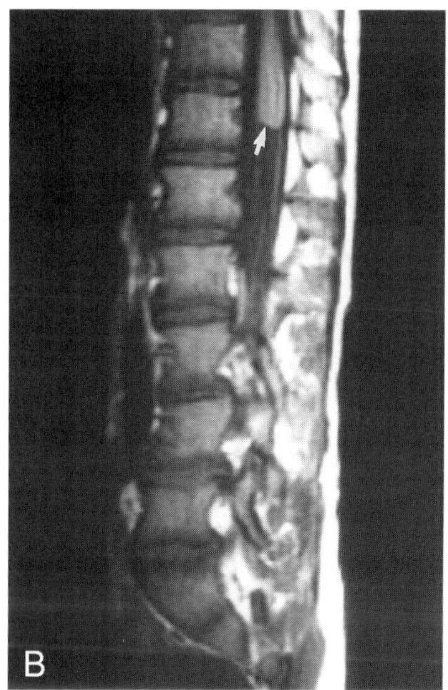

Figure 4.5 B

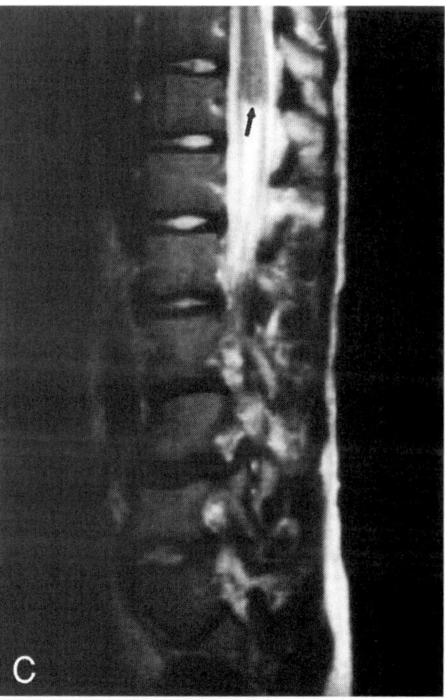

Figure 4.5 C

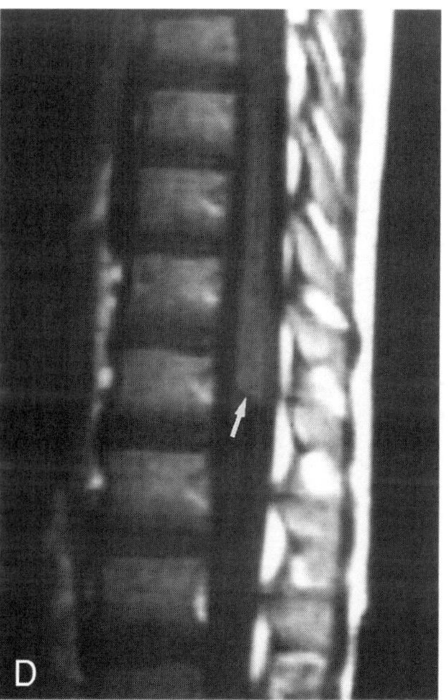

Figure 4.5 D

Findings: In the first patient, a midsagittal MR T1-weighted image (Fig. A) shows a truncated conus medullaris (arrow) with sparse roots in the cauda equina. There is absence of the mid- and lower sacral segments. In the second patient, midsagittal MR T1- (Fig. B) and T2- (Fig. C) weighted images show a truncated ("wedge-shaped") tip of the conus medullaris (arrows) and absence of the sacrum below the S2 segment. Note the sparse appearance of the cauda equina. In the third patient, a midsagittal MR T1 weighted (Fig. D) again shows a wedge-shaped tip (arrow) of the conus medullaris.

(continued)

Diagnosis: Caudal regression syndrome.

Discussion: The lower lumbar and sacral regions form by canalization and retrogressive differentiation. Early in life, the distal spine is formed by the caudal cell mass. This mass canalizes and joins the central spinal canal of the folded neural tube. The mass undergoes upward necrosis (retrogressive differentiation), leaving behind the filum terminale, distal conus medullaris, lumbar and sacral nerve roots, and ventriculus terminalis. Because the caudal cell mass is separated from the cloaca only by the notochord, anorectal and genitourinary anomalies are common with malformations of the distal spine. An insult to the caudal cell mass resulting in partial absence or exaggerated retrogressive differentiation may lead to the syndrome of caudal regression. This is a rare syndrome found in one of 7,500–25,000 newborns and is more common in the offspring of diabetic mothers. It varies in severity from a partially malformed sacrum (scimitar sacrum) to fusion of the lower extremities (mermaid). Most commonly, the sacrum is partially or completely absent. The tip of conus medullaris is not formed. Many lumbar and sacral nerve roots are also absent. Occasionally, the spinal cord is located low and displastic and tethered inferiorly by an intraspinal lipoma. Congenital dislocation of the hips is also common. MR is the imaging method of choice. Common symptoms include club feet, scoliosis, associated open spinal dysraphism, and Klippel-Feil syndrome. Motor deficits are more severe than the sensory abnormalities. Intelligence is usually normal.

CASE 6

Clinical History: You are shown two patients. The first (Fig. A) has low back pain and is being studied to rule out degenerative disease. The second (Fig. B) is being studied for mild bilateral lower extremity pain.

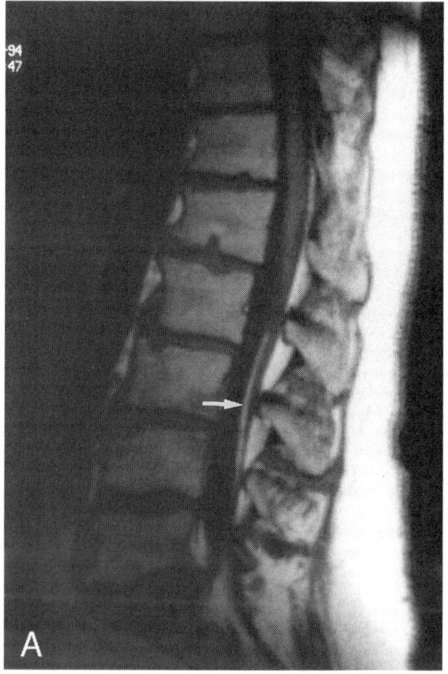

Figure 4.6 A

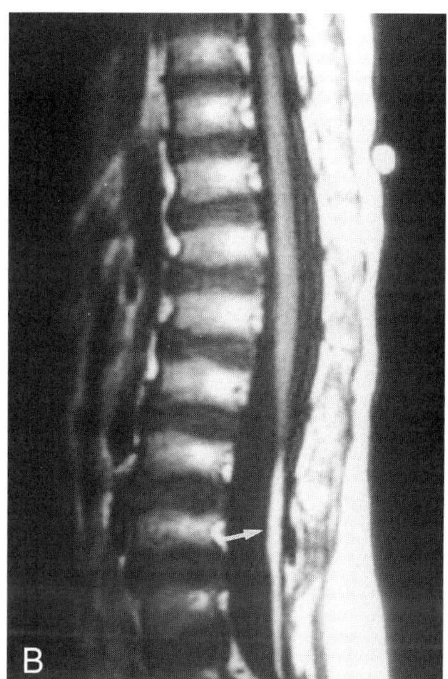

Figure 4.6 B

Findings: In the first patient, a midsgittal MR T1-weighted image (Fig. A) shows thin filar lipoma (arrow). Note that the level of the conus medullaris is normal at L1. In the second patient, a midsagittal MR T1-weighted image shows a thick filar lipoma (arrow). The conus medullaris is at L2, making it suspicious for tethering by the lipoma.

Diagnosis: Filar lipomas.

Discussion: Lipomas of the filum terminale are a common malformation found in approximately 1–6% of the population. They arise from an abnormality in retrogressive differentiation (see Case #5), although their exact etiology is not certain. There is fat infiltration of the ependyma/pia that forms the normal filum terminale. Fat may be found in the intra- and extradural portions of the filum. Commonly, the filum terminale remains of normal thickness, and these lipomas are incidental findings in asymptomatic individuals. The amount of fat present may correlate with the patient's symptoms. MR imaging shows these lipomas to have similar signal characteristics to normal fat. They do not enhance. The conus medullaris is usually at its normal position. In the presence of a low conus medullaris and symptoms, the diagnosis of tight filum terminale syndrome should be considered (see Case #7).

CASE 7

Clinical History: This patient is a 40-year-old male with spina bifida occulta and presents with problems emptying his bladder.

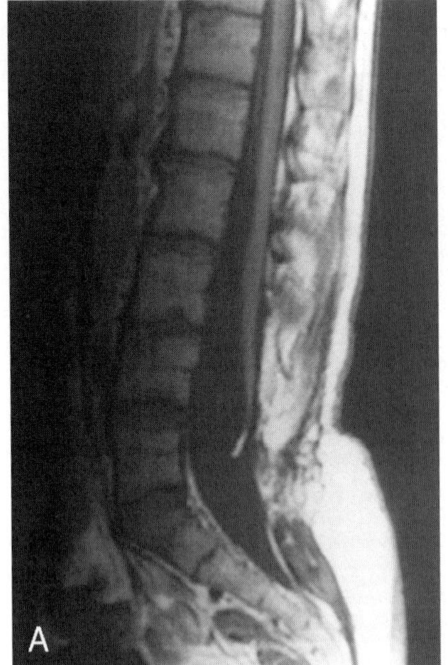

Figure 4.7 A

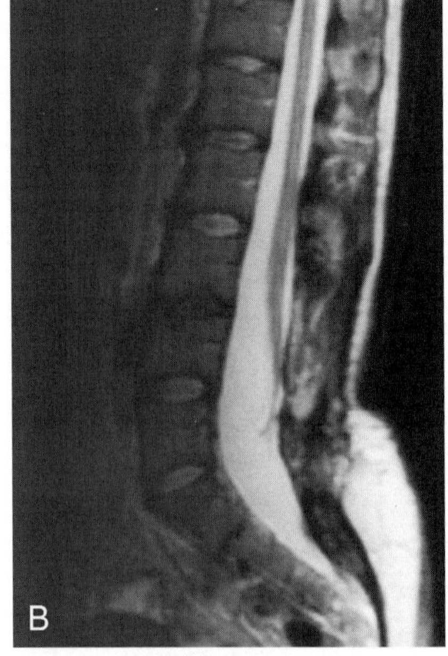

Figure 4.7 B

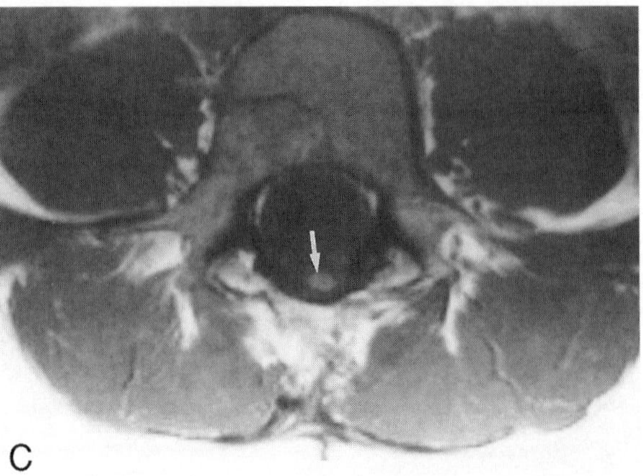

Figure 4.7 C

Findings: Midsagittal MR T1-weighted image (Fig. A) shows that the conus medullaris extends down to the level of L4. The proximal filum terminale is thick and contains a small focal lipoma. Corresponding MR T2-weighted image (Fig. B) clearly shows the low and abnormal position of the conus medullaris. Axial MR T1-weighted image (Fig. C) shows the thickenned proximal filum terminale (arrow).

(continued)

Diagnosis: Tight filum terminale syndrome.

Discussion: This syndrome ensues secondary to abnormal thickenning of the filum terminale and a conus medullaris in a low position. There is no specific age for it and no gender predilection. Patients report lower extremity weakness and/or muscle stiffness as well as bowel and bladder dysfunction. In severe cases, club feet may be present. These patients may also be scoliotic. The symptoms are increased by exercise, and therefore many patients present in late childhood and adolescence when involvement in sports is prominent. Some patients, however, remain asymptomatic during their lifetime. The underlying etiology is probably incomplete retrogressive differentiation (see Case #5) leading to a short filum terminale. Constant traction on the lumbar and sacral nerve roots and the conus medullaris may lead to ischemic myelopathy and neuropathy, resulting in symptoms. MR is the imaging method of choice to evaluate these patients. The conus medullaris is considered abnormally low if its tip is below the L2-L3 disk. The normal position of the conus medullaris is between T11 and L2. In patients with the tight filum terminale syndrome, the filum measures more than 2 mm in diameter and may be of normal signal intensity or infiltrated by fat. A spinal bifida occulta is present in 20% of these patients. Syringohydromyelia and evidence of myelomalacia are not uncommon.

CASE 8

Clinical History: This newborn is being imaged because of a spina bifida occulta.

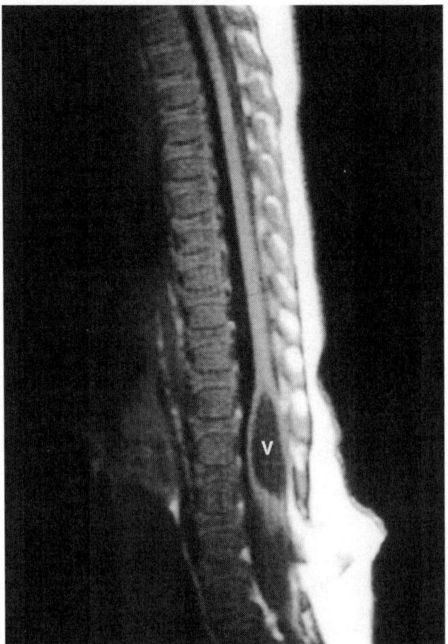

Figure 4.8

Findings: Midsagittal MR T1-weighted image (Fig. A) shows a cystic cavity (V) involving the distal conus medullaris. The position of the conus is at L1-L2. Therefore, the position of the conus medullaris is normal.

Differential Diagnosis: Syringohydromyelia, persistent ventriculus terminalis.

Diagnosis: Persistent ventriculus terminalis.

Discussion: The ventriculus terminalis is a small, fluid-filled cyst located in the distal-most conus medullaris. The cyst is lined by ependyma. It is not uncommon, is most often found in premature babies, and is more prominent in girls. It is also more common in patients with a Chiari 1 malformation. The cyst is probably related to persistent vacuoles related to the mechanism of canalization and retrogressive differentiation (see Case #5), and accesory spinal canal, or dilatation of the distal central spinal canal. Most patients are asymptomatic, but occasionally they may present with nonspecific problems, such as recurrent low back pain, sciatica, and bladder dysfunction. This abnormality is almost always found by MR imaging. The cavity is filled with fluid and measures 2–4 cm in length and 1–2.5 cm in diameter. They have no internal septations and do not enhance after contrast administration. In symptomatic patients, fenestration and/or shunting of this cyst may be indicated.

CASE 9

Clinical History: This patient, born by cesarean section, has a large, soft, skin-covered mass in the low back.

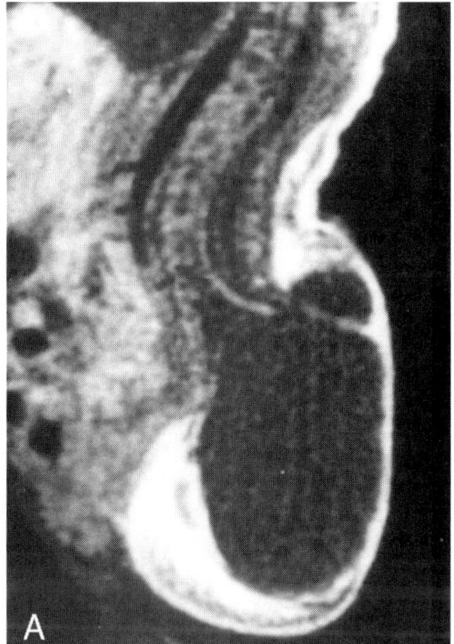

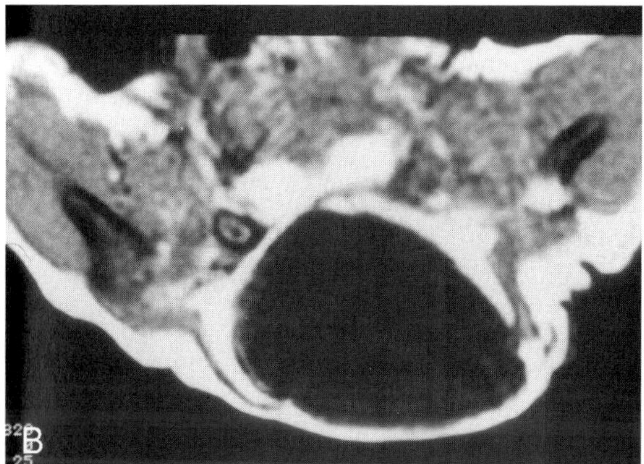

Figure 4.9 A   Figure 4.9 B

Findings: Midsagittal MR T1-weighted image (Fig. A) shows a large cystic structure protruding through the distal spine. Note that it is covered by subcutaenous fat and skin (therefore not a myelomeningocele). Axial MR T1-weighted image (Fig. B) confirms the cystic structure of the mass, whose walls are composed of thin and gliotic spinal cord.

Differential Diagnosis: Myelomeningocele and cystic spinal teratoma, terminal myelocystocele.

Diagnosis: Terminal myelocystocele.

Discussion: Terminal myelocystocele and myelocystocele (syringomyelocele) are rare types of occult spinal dysraphism (i.e., covered by skin) in which a fluid-filled spinal cord cyst herniates through a defect in the vertebrae, generally posterior in location. In the lower lumbar spine, covering skin may be absent. Although it may involve any portion of the spine, it is more commonly found in the lumbosacral region (terminal). In this location, it is most likely an anomaly of canalization and retrogressive differentiation (see Case #5) in which there is persistence and dilatation of distal vacuoles. As such, a terminal myelocystocele is generally accompanied by anorectal and genitourinary abnormalities. The mechanism responsible for myelocystoceles elsewhere in the spine is unknown. Most myelocystoceles present as skin-covered, soft, posterior spinal masses (similar to lipomyeloceles and lipomyelomeningoceles, see Case #3). MR is the imaging method of choice for these patients. The spinal cord terminates low and there is large, fluid-filled cyst herniating through a spina bifida. This cyst generally communicates superiorly with a syringohydromyelia. The cyst has no internal septations and does not communicate with the subarachnoid space. The cyst adheres to the surrounding tissues and tethers the spinal cord inferiorly.

CASE 10

Clinical History: You are shown two cases of the same anomaly in varying degrees of severity. The first case (Figs. A–C) involves a patient who has a weak right lower extremity. The second patient (Fig. D) is 10 years old and presents with bladder and bowel difficulties.

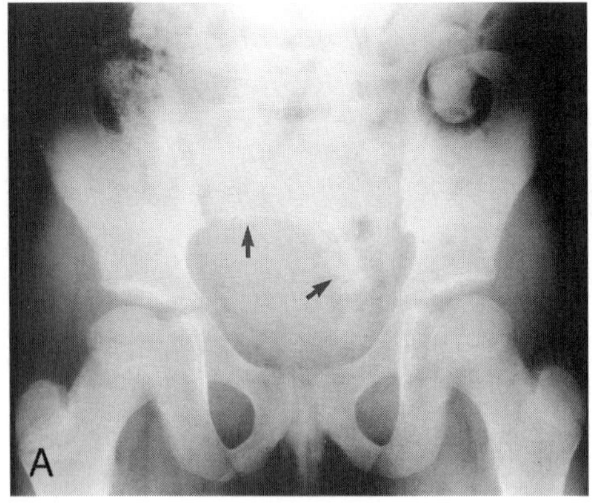

Figure 4.10 A

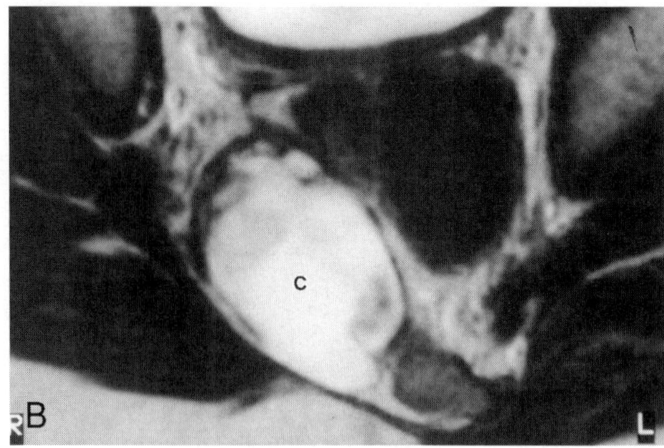

Figure 4.10 B

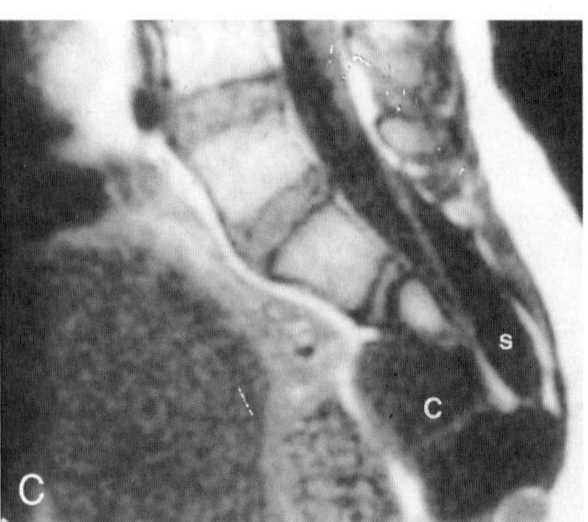

Figure 4.10 C

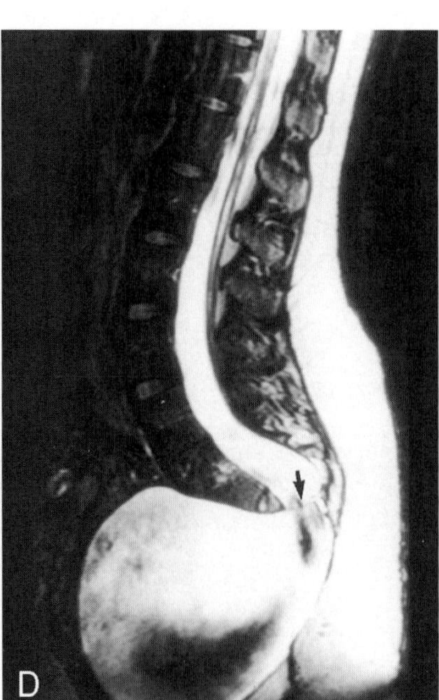

Figure 4.10 D

Findings: Frontal radiograph (Fig. A) shows a scimitar-shaped sacrum with excavation of its right side (arrows). Axial MR T2-weighted image shows that there is a cystic mass (C) involving the right side of the sacrum. Slightly parasagittal MR T1-weighted image (Fig. C) shows a septated cystic lesion (C) anterior to the sacrum communicating with spinal canal (s). In the second patient, midsagittal MR T1-weighted image (Fig. D) shows a large cystic mass anterior to the sacrum and a wide communication (arrow) with the spinal canal. The sacrum is almost absent. The spinal cord is dysplastic, thin, and tethered inferiorly. It also contains a linear area of high signal intensity, which may be a syrinx or myelomalacia.

(continued)

Differential Diagnosis: Cystic sacral teratoma, large perineurial cyst, duplication cyst, cloacal abnormalities (diverticulum), anterior sacral meningoceles.

Diagnosis: Anterior sacral meningoceles.

Discussion: A meningocele is a dural sac filled with cerebrospinal fluid (CSF) that projects outside the spine through a bone defect. Meningoceles do not contain neural structures. Anterior sacral meningoceles herniate through eroded or congenitally absent sacral segments. They are more commonly found in individuals age 10 to 30 years, and there is no gender predilection. The most common symptoms are related to mass effect upon pelvic viscera (rectum and bladder), pressure on nerve roots, resulting in radiculopathies, and abnormal flow of CSF, resulting in headaches. Overall, meningoceles are more common in patients with neurofibromatosis type 1 (particularly lateral thoracic ones) and Marfan and Ehler-Danlos syndromes. The etiology of these lesions is not certain. MR is the imaging method of choice for the evaluation of suspected anterior sacral meningoceles. These fluid-filled masses are anterior to the sacrum. The sacrum may be absent, partially missing (scimitar-like), or nearly intact. The masses may be large or small and may communicate with the remaining subarachnoid space via a narrow neck. The fluid within them may be pulsatile and proteinaceous, leading to a signal intensity that is different from that of CSF. The identification of nerves within the meningocele is paramount because it precludes simple ligation and resection of the mass.

CASE 11

Clinical History: A 35-year-old male presents with chronic pain in the sacrum.

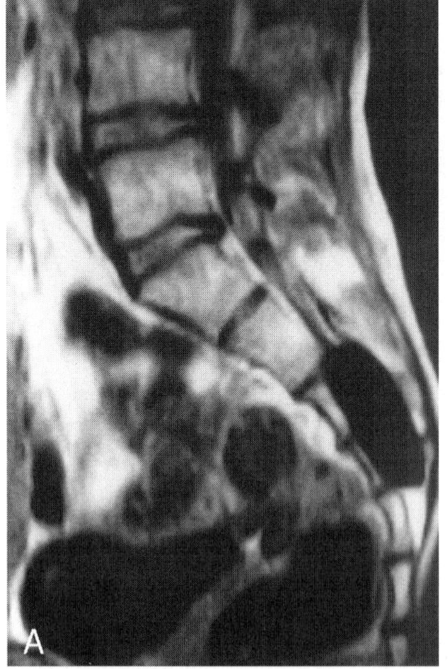

Figure 4.11 A

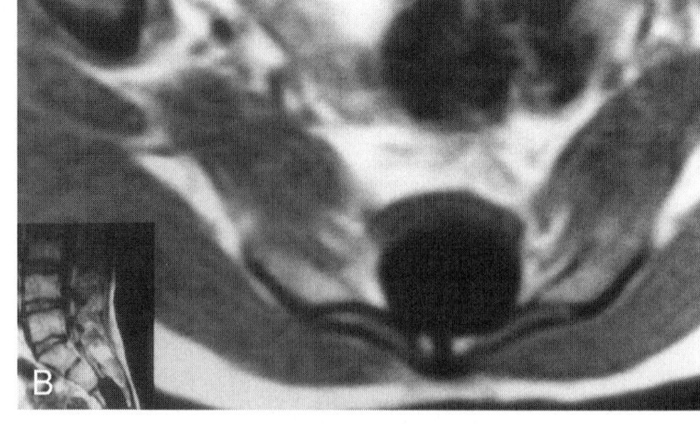

Figure 4.11 B

Findings: Midsagittal MR T1-weighted image (Fig. A) shows a cystic lesion in the sacral canal producing erosion. Axial MR T1-weighted image (Fig. B) shows the cystic lesion involving the distal sacrum.

Differential Diagnosis: Perineurial cyst, arachnoid cyst, epidermoid, cystic teratoma, parasitic disorders (echinococcus, cysticercosis), intrasacral (occult) meningocele.

Diagnosis: Intrasacral (occult) meningocele.

Discussion: The term occult intrasacral meningocele is a misnomer because meningoceles usually protrude outside the spine through a bone defect. However, the term is commonly used to denote a fluid-filled sac contained within an expanded sacrum. The walls of this lesion are composed of fibrous tissues and arachnoid. It communicates with the remaining subarachnoid space via a wide passage that generally allows for free flow of cerebrospinal fluid. Growth of these lesions is very slow and probably occurs secondary to the hydrostatic pressure exerted by the fluid. Their etiology is uncertain but they are probably related to a congenital malformation of the dura and subarachnoid space (meninx primitiva). They are generally asymptomatic. They displace the nerve roots and may occasionally compress them, producing radiculopathies and local pain. When these lesions require surgical treatment, interruption of the connection with the subarachnoid space and deflation of the meningocele generally suffice. In general, extramedullary cystic cavities involving the meninges may be classified as: 1) those containing no nerve roots (diverticula and intrasacral meningoceles); 2) those containing nerve roots (perineurial or Tarlov cysts); and 3) intradural cysts, particularly involving the posterior subarachnoid space (arachnoid and subarachnoid cysts, and cysts of the septum posticum in the thoracic region).

CASE 12

Clinical History: You are shown two patients. The first (Figs. A–C) presents with mild bilateral lower extremity weakness and hyperreflexia. The second (Figs. D and E) is a newborn being studied because of the palpable spinal deformity in the upper lumbar region.

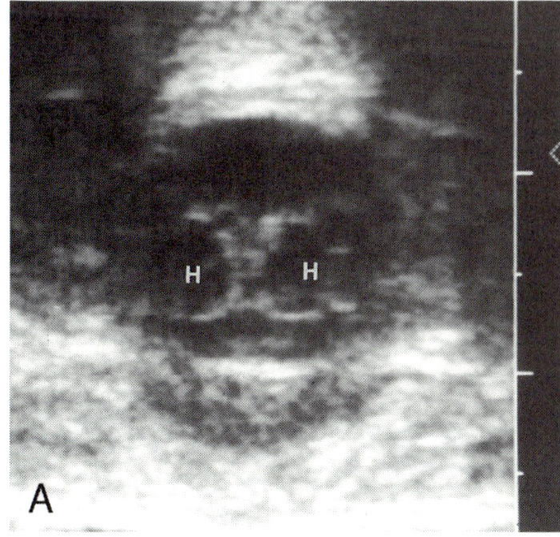

Figure 4.12 A

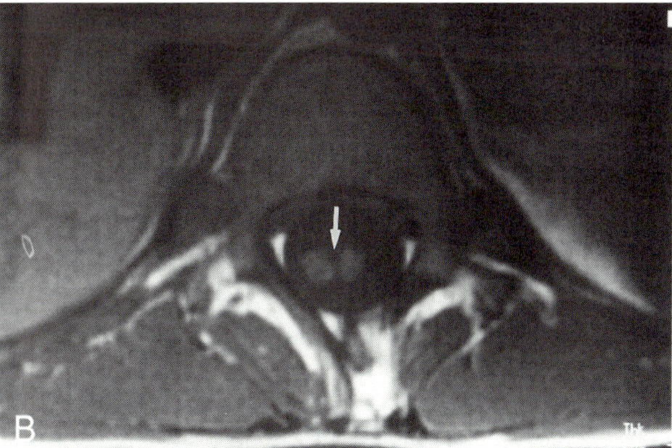

Figure 4.12 B

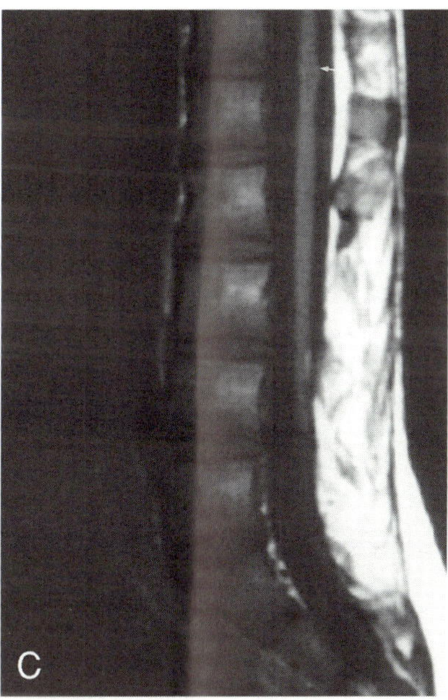

Figure 4.12 C

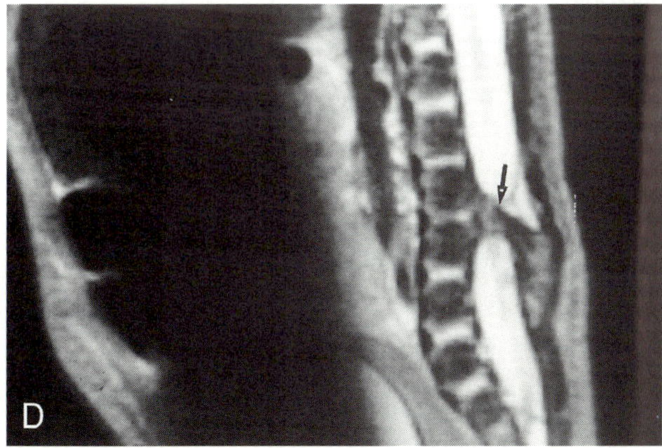

Figure 4.12 D

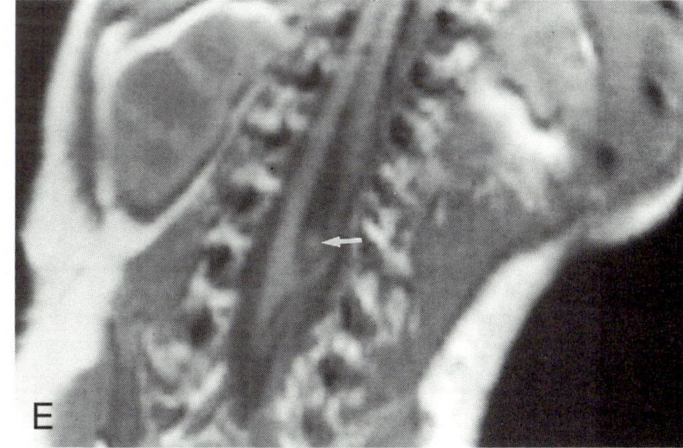

Figure 4.12 E

(continued)

Findings: Axial sonogram (Fig. A) shows two hemicords (H). Corresponding MR T1-weighted image (Fig. B) shows the hemicords divided by a cleft (arrow) and no spur. Midsagittal MR T1-weighted image (Fig. C) shows a minimal deformity of the spinal cord (arrow) at the level of the splitting. The conus is abnormally low, terminating at L4. In the second patient, a midsagittal MR T2-weighted image (Fig. D) shows a thick bone bar (arrow) traversing the center of the spinal canal. The posterior elements at this level are prominent. Coronal MR T1-weighted image (Fig. E) shows the assymetric hemicords traversed by the spur (arrow).

Diagnosis: Diastematomyelia.

Discussion: Diastematomyelia refers to a midline splitting of the spinal cord. This anomaly is found mostly in females. It occurs in 1–5% of patients with scoliosis and in 20–30% of patients with open spinal dysraphism. Clinically, these patients present with muscle atrophy, decreased or absent deep tendon reflexes, weakness of the lower extremities, deformities of the feet, and urinary dysfunction. The skin overlying the site of diastematomyelia is abnormal in 50–75% of patients. This abnormality may be in the form a hemangioma, dermal sinus, lipoma, and pigmented or hairy patches. Histologically, the hemicords may reside in one dural sheath with no true physical separation between them (internal diastematomyelia). However, approximately 50% of patients harbor a true spur separating the hemicords (external diastematomyelia). This spur may be composed by bone, cartilage, fat, fibrous tissues, or any combination of these. Segmentation anomalies of the vertebrae in the region of the diastematomyelia are found in more than 95% of patients. Kyphoscoliosis is present in 50% of patients. MR is the imaging method of choice for evaluation of these patients. In most instances, the hemicords are asymmetrical and unite inferiorly into a single spinal cord. Approximately 50% of patients harbor a syringohydromeylia within one or both hemicords, or in the spinal cord superior or inferior to the diastematomyelia. The spurs are multiple in 6% of patients. Imaging requires T2-weighted gradient echo sequences through the level of the hemicords to exclude a spur reliably. Spurs need to be surgically resected because they tether the spinal cord.

CASE 13

Clinical History: You are shown two patients. The first (Figs. A–C) presents with a myelopathy, and radiographs demonstrate segmentation anomalies at T1-T3. The second (Figs. D and E) also presents with myelopathy.

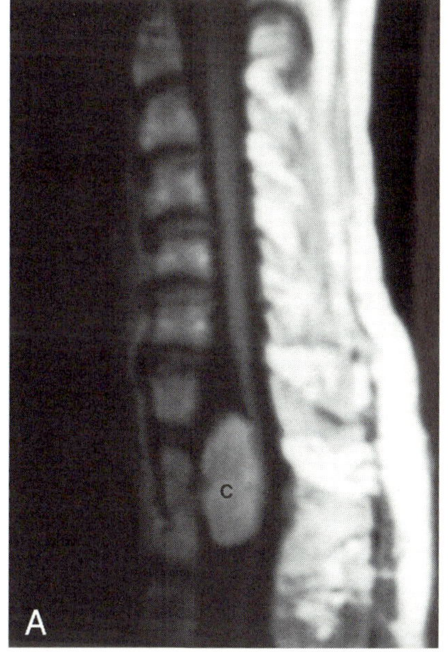

Figure 4.13 A

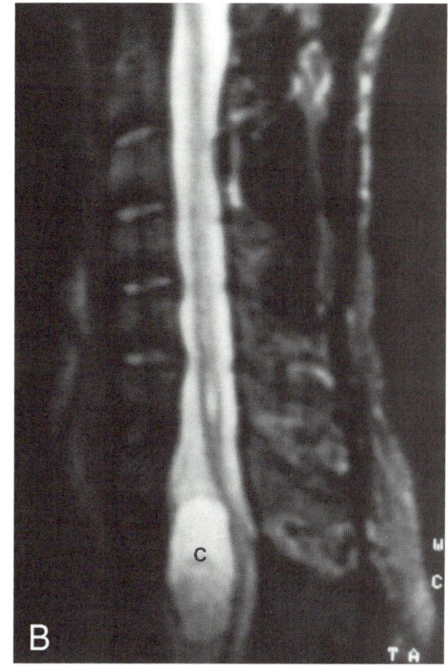

Figure 4.13 B

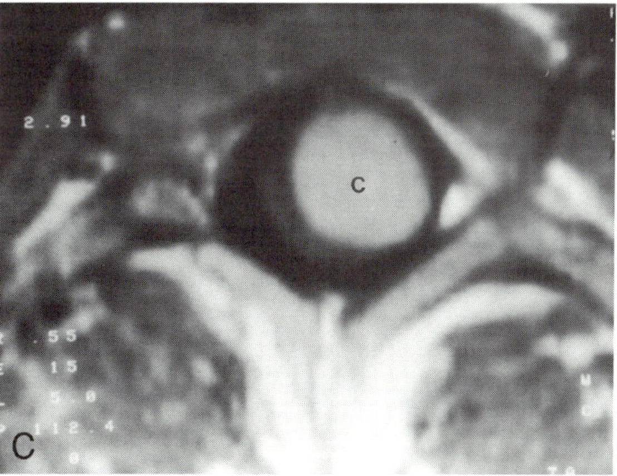

Figure 4.13 C

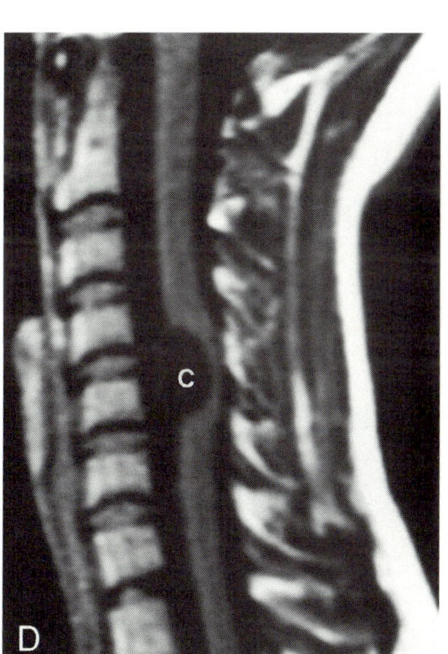

Figure 4.13 D

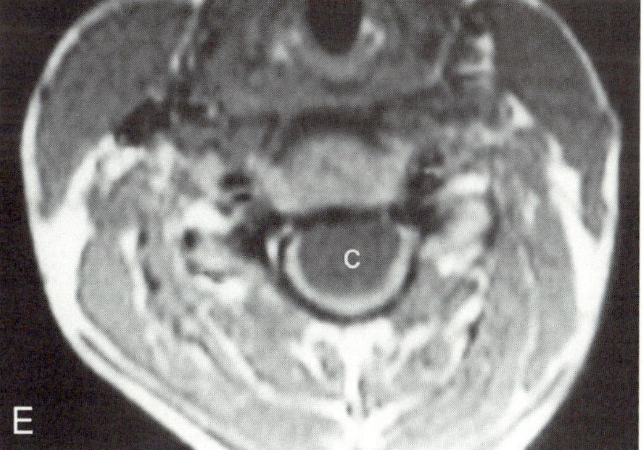

Figure 4.13 E

(continued)

Findings: In the first patient, a midsagittal MR T1-weighted image (Fig. A) shows an intraspinal bright mass (C) with compression of the spinal cord (which is thin). The spinal canal is wide at this level and the vertebrae anterior to the mass are dysplastic. Corresponding MR T2-weighted image (Fig. B) shows the mass (C) to be hyperintense. Note a linear area of high signal intensity in the spinal cord at the C6 level. Because this latter finding was not present on Fig. A, it is most likely myelomalacia. Axial MR T1-weighted image (Fig. C) shows the hyperintense lesion (C) compressing the spinal cord. Note the deformed vertebra. In the second patient, a midline sagittal MR T1-weighted image (Fig. D) shows an extramedullary cystic mass (C) indenting the anterior aspect of the spinal cord at the C4–5 levels. An axial T1-weighted image (Fig. E) again shows the cyst (C) compressing the spinal cord. (Case courtesy R. Quencer, M.D., Miami, Fl.)

Diagnosis: The first case is a surgically proven intraspinal duplication cyst (split notochord syndrome). The second case is a presumed intraspinal duplication cyst.

Discussion: The split notochord syndrome refers to a group of anomalies in which the notochord is divided and allows for communication of the surface ectoderm (skin) with the endoderm (gastrointestinal tract). The most severe variation is the dorsal enteric fistula in which the bowel communicates or is extruded through a defect in the spine. The intermediate form is the dorsal enteric sinus in which there is a blind ending pouch projecting through the spinal defect. The least severe abnormalities are the dorsal enteric cyst and diverticula. These cysts are generally found ventral to the spinal cord but may be lateral or even posterior to it. The most severe abnormalities are obvious at birth. The intraspinal enteric cysts present with radicular pain in adolescents. Chronic compression of the spinal cord may lead to a myelopathy. These unilocular cysts are generally found in the low cervical and high thoracic regions. They are generally accompanied by vertebral segmentation anomalies and occasionally by a diastematomyelia. MR is the imaging method of choice for these patients. The cyst may have a signal intensity similar to that of cerebrospinal fluid or be hyperintense on T1-weighted images because of proteinaceous contents. It is important to clearly define the location of the cyst with relation to the spinal cord before surgery.

CASE 14

Clinical History: A 20-year-old man presents with mild bilateral pain and weakness. Since birth, he has had a small opening in the skin above the interglutteal fold.

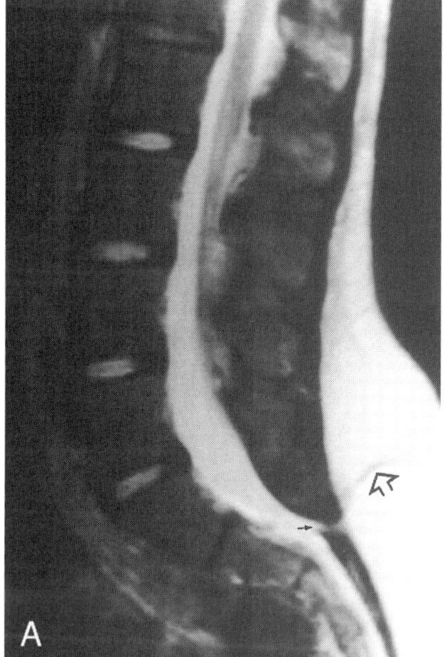
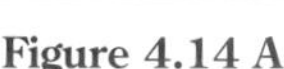

Figure 4.14 A

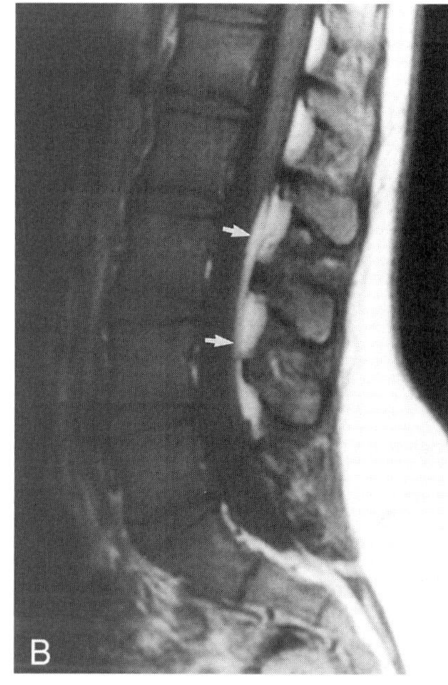

Figure 4.14 B

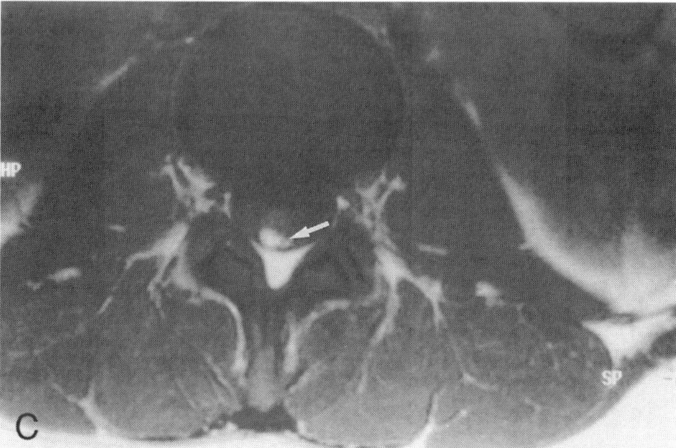

Figure 4.14 C

Findings: Midsagittal MR T2-weighted image (Fig. A) shows a sinus tract (open arrow) extending through the subcutaneous fat into the spine (tiny arrow) through an occult defect. Corresponding T1-weighted image (Fig. B) shows that there is an intradural lipoma (arrows) posteriorly in the thecal sac following the course of the filum terminale. Axial MR T1-weighted image (Fig. C) at the level of the distal conus medullaris confirms the lipoma (arrow) in the dorsal aspect of the thecal sac.

(continued)

Diagnosis: Dorsal dermal sinus tract with intraspinal lipoma.

Discussion: A dorsal dermal sinus is a tract lined with squamous epithelium that connects the skin with neural tube or the meninges. This anomaly occurs in approximately 1 of 2500–3000 newborns. These sinuses are caused by incomplete or delayed separation of the cutaneous ectoderm from the closing neural tube. Dermal sinuses are more commonly found in the lumbar region but may also occur in the cervical spine, occiput, and nasion. These sinuses are different from the simple sacral or coccygeal dimple, which occurs in 2–4% of children. The skin surrounding the dimples is usually normal, whereas that surrounding a true sinus tract contains anomalous pigmentation, tags, lipomas, and hypertrichosis. Patients with dermal sinus tract may present with neurologic symptoms caused by tethering of the spinal cord, local infection, or meningitis, which may be bacterial or chemical in origin. The tract terminates in an intraspinal dermoid or epidermoid in 50% of patients. The sinus tracts may also terminate in the filum terminale, conus medullaris, or the nerve roots. The tract courses upwardly in all patients. Bone abnormalities are common and many patients have a spinal bifida occulta. MR is the imaging method of choice to evaluate these patients.

CASE 15

Clinical History: You are shown three patients. The first (Figs. A–C) is a boy with bilateral and progressive lower extremity weakness. The second (Fig. D) has had surgery for closure of a myelocele and now presents with new onset of urinary retention and lower extremity weakness. The third (Figs. E and F) is a 34-year-old female with a skin defect in her lower back since birth. This patient was asymptomatic until 2 months before this study when she began having problems urinating.

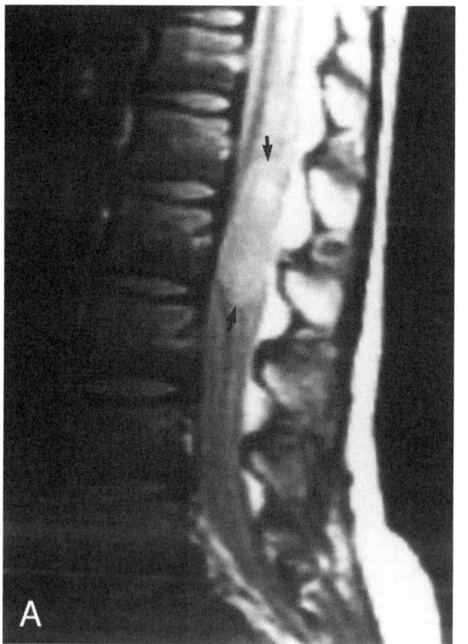

Figure 4.15 A

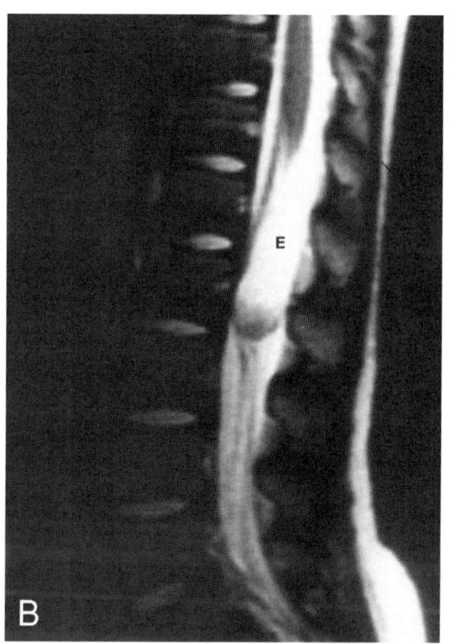

Figure 4.15 B

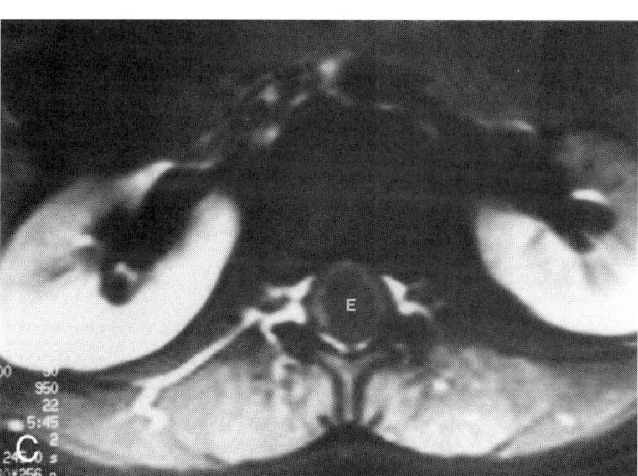

Figure 4.15 C

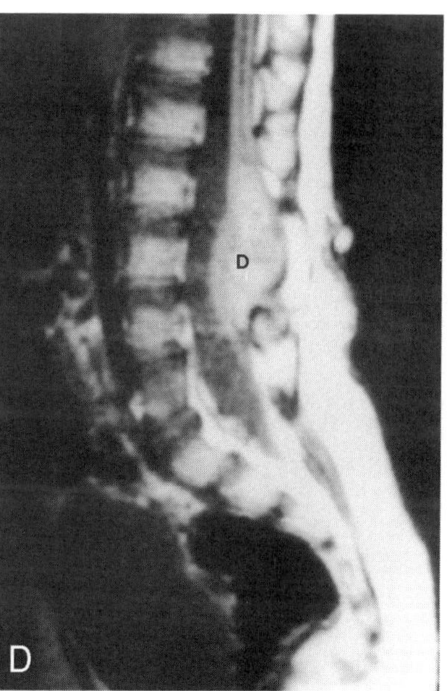

Figure 4.15 D

(continued)

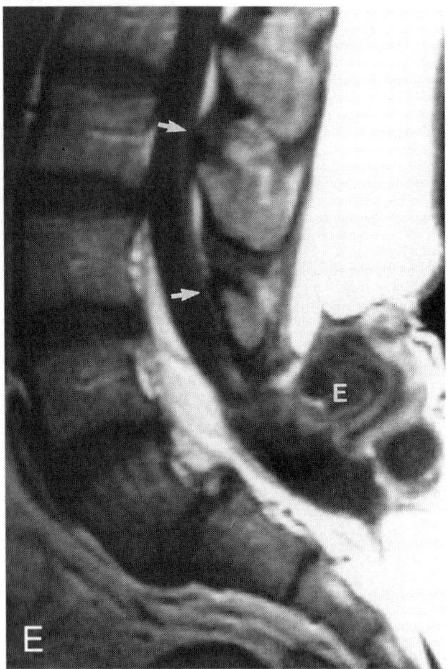

Figure 4.15 E

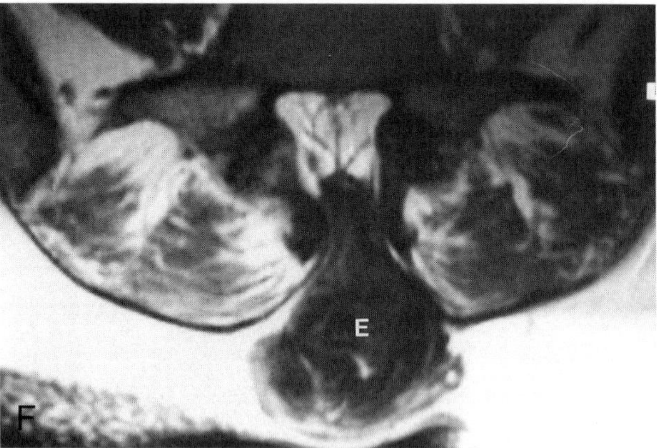

Figure 4.15 F

Findings: In the first patient, a midsagittal MR proton density image (Fig. A) shows an intradural mass (arrows) at the L1-L2 level. The mass is slightly hyperintense when compared with CSF. Corresponding MR T2-weighted image (Fig. B) shows the mass (E) to be mostly bright. On an axial MR T1-weighted image (Fig. C), the lesion (E) is of low signal intensity and insinuates itself into the spinal cord (note thin circumferential rim of spinal cord surrounding the lesion). In the second patient, midsagittal MR T1-weighted image (Fig. D) shows a hyperintense mass (D) at the L3-L4 level. The mass merges with low-lying spinal cord at the level of a repaired open dysraphism. The distal spinal cord contains a linear area of decreased signal intensity, suggesting the presence of a syrinx. In the third patient, a midsagittal MR T1-weighted image (Fig. E) shows a mostly hypointense mass (E) in the subcutaneous tissues extending anteriorly into the spinal canal. Note that the mass contains serpiginous areas of intermediate signal intensity. The spinal cord (arrows) is thin, dysplastic, and tethered inferiorly by the mass. Axial T1-weighted image (Fig. F) shows the mass (E) extending into the spinal canal via a spina bifida.

Differential Diagnosis: For epidermoid: arachnoid cyst, cystic teratoma, dermoid, congenital intraspinal epidermoid; for dermoid; lipoma, epidermoid, postoperative inclusion dermoid.

Diagnosis: Congenital intraspinal epidermoid (first and third cases) and postoperative inclusion dermoid (second case).

Discussion: Epidermoids and dermoids account for 3–17% of spinal tumors in children. Approximately 20–30% of them are associated with dermal sinus tract (see Case #14). The epidermoid is a cystic mass whose wall is composed by fibrous tissue lined with squamous epithelium. The wall of a dermoid has, in addition to the above, cutaneous appendages (such as hair follicles and sebaceous and sweat glands). Both contain cholesterol and keratinized elements but a dermoid also contains glandular secretions. In an epidermoid, the cholesterol tends to be in a liquid form, whereas in a dermoid it tends to be solid. If these tumors rupture into the subarachnoid space, their fatty acids induce a chronic chemical meningitis. Most patients with these lesions present during the first two decades of life. Epidermoids are slightly more common in males, whereas dermoids occur equally in both genders. Most are found in the lumbosacral junction and are intradural. However, epidermoids and dermoids may also be intramedullary. They may tether the spinal cord inferiorly, particularly if they occur along a dermal sinus tract. These tumors grow slowly and produce back pain, weakness of the lower extremites, or bladder dysfunction. Scoliosis may also be present. MR is the imaging method of choice for the evaluation of these patients. Epidermoids are difficult to visualize because their signal characteristics are very similar to those of cerebrospinal fluid. Dermoids are bright on T1- and T2-weighted images. Administration of contrast is not indicated unless infection is suspected. Once an epidermoid or dermoid has ruptured, it becomes difficult to visualize the remaining capsule.

CASE 16

Clinical History: Toddler who presents with a history of delayed walking. At physical examination there was bilateral lower extremity spasticity.

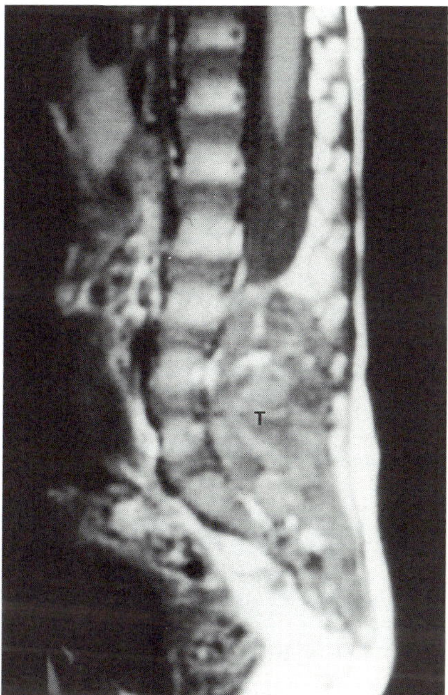

Figure 4.16

Findings: Midsagittal postcontrast MR T1-weighted image shows a complex and partially enhancing mass (T) in the lumbosacral spinal canal. Note significant widening of the canal and posterior scalloping of the lower lumbar vertebrae and sacrum.

Diagnosis: Intraspinal teratoma.

Discussion: Sacrococcygeal teratoma is the most common spinal tumor in newborns. It occurs in 1 in 35,000 newborns. Although most fetuses are asymptomatic, most teratomas are diagnosed by prenatal sonography. Polyhydramnios may be present. Prenatal diskovery of spinal teratoma is important because, if vaginally delivered, 11% of these babies will sustain significant trauma. Thus, cesarean section is done for babies with large sacrococcygeal teratomas. Prognosis is better if the presentation is after 30 weeks of gestation. Approximately 5–25% of these children harbor other unrelated congenital anomalies. Most patients are female. More than 90% of these teratomas are histologically benign. Teratomas produce alpha-fetoprotein and human chorionic gonadotropin. Resection is indicated because anemia, hemorrhage, ulceration and infection, and high output cardiac failure lead to death in most of these babies. Sacrococcygeal teratomas may be classified as totally external, mostly external, mostly internal, and completely internal. At birth, 5% of patients have distant metastases. Both CT and MR may be used to image teratomas. Most tumors originate in the sacrum and may destroy or remodel it. Calcifications are seen in 50% of cases. These tumors are heterogeneous in appearance. Their solid portions enhance after contrast administration. Malignant teratomas tend to be homogeneous and enhance uniformly after contrast administration. They tend to invade the surrounding structures. Surgical resection, followed by chemotherapy, is generally employed for the treatment of these tumors.

Clinical History: This boy presents with occipital headaches.

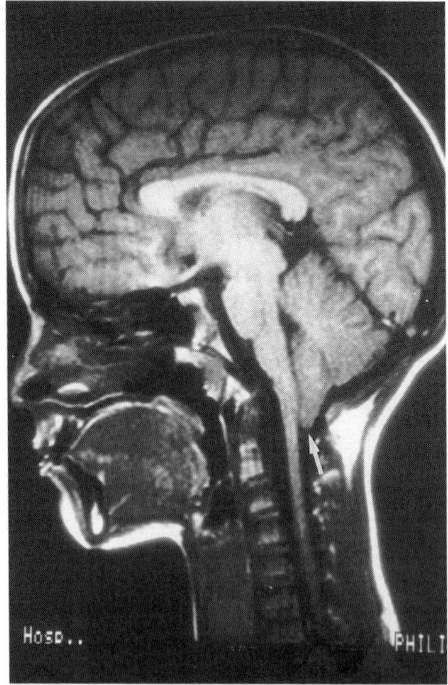

Figure 4.17

Findings: Midsagittal MR T1-weighted image (Fig. A) shows that the cerebellar tonsils project inferiorly to the level of the foramen magnum. Also note that the tonsils are "pointing" down.

Diagnosis: Chiari type 1 malformation.

Discussion: The Chiari type 1 malformation is characterized by displacement of the cerebellar tonsils inferior to the foramen magnum. Its true incidence is uncertain but it is found in approximately 1% of brain MR imaging studies. It is more common in females. Thirty percent of patients in which the cerebellar tonsils are herniated between 6 and 10 mm have symptoms. Most patients with herniations exceeding 12 mm are symptomatic. The symptoms generally consist of neck pain, abnormal gait, ataxia, nystagmus, and lower cranial nerve dysfunction. Myelopathy and hydrocephalus may develop. Approximately 20–40% of these patients develop a syringohydromyelia.

CASE 18

Clinical History: This 5-year-old patient has a progressive myelopathy. He had a myelomeningocele repaired at birth and has had a shunt placed for hydrocephalus.

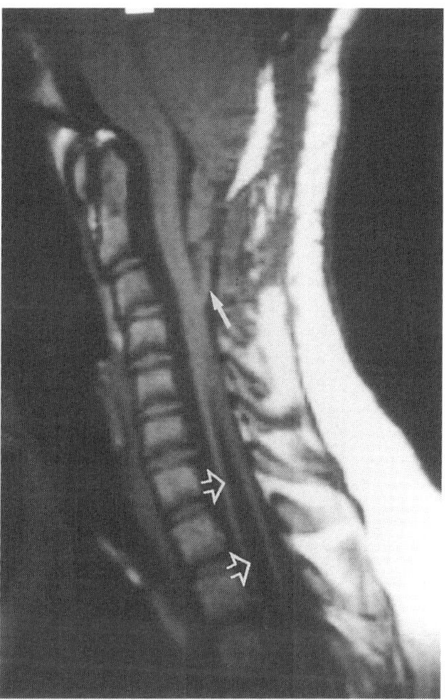

Figure 4.18

Findings: Midsagittal MR T1-weighted image (Fig. A) shows inferior herniation of the cerebellar vermis (solid arrow) down to the level of C3-C4. A syrinx (open arrows) is present in the lower cervical and upper thoracic regions. The fourth ventricle is small.

Diagnosis: Chiari type 2 malformation.

Discussion: The Chiari type 2 malformation is a complex anomaly involving the spine and brain. For practical purposes, all of these patients have an open spinal dysraphism (myelocele or myelomeningocele, see Case #2). It occurs in approximately 2–3 in 1000 newborns and repeats itself in 4–8% of subsequent siblings. The intracranial abnormalities seen in patients with Chiari 2 malformation are not addressed here. MR is the imaging method of choice to evaluate these patients. The cerebellar vermis extends downward and posterior to the cervical spinal cord generally to the level of C3. Fourth ventricular choroid plexus may also be displaced into the cervical spinal canal and simulate an enhancing mass in studies obtained after contrast administration. The medulla is also displaced inferiorly and in 70% of patients it "kinks" where it joins the dentate ligaments. Syringohydromyelia develops in 40–80% of cases. Segmentation anomalies of the high cervical spine, particularly the posterior arch of C1, are present in 10% of patients. Diastematomyelia (see Case #12) may be present in up to 30% of these patients.

CASE 19

Clinical History: A 20-year-old male presents with chronic and progressive weakness and decreased pain sensation in both upper extremities.

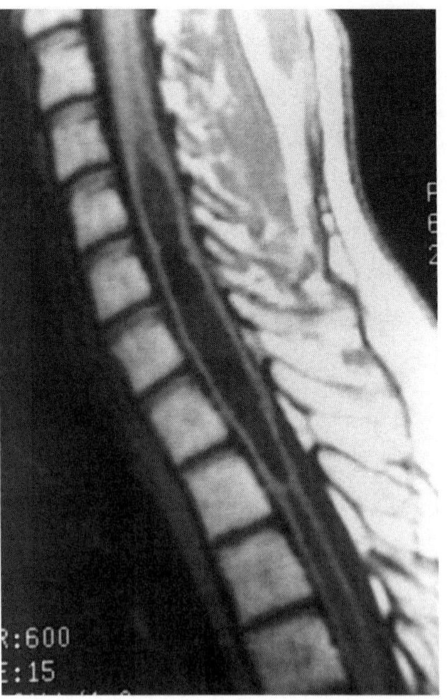

Figure 4.19

Findings: Midsagittal MR T1-weighted image (Fig. A) shows a septated fluid-filled cavity within the cervical spinal cord extending inferiorly into the thoracic region. The cord is expanded. After contrast administration, no abnormal enhancement was present. The structures at the level of the foramen magnum were normal.

Differential Diagnosis: Primary spinal cord tumor, cysticercosis, syringohydromyelia (idiopathic).

Diagnosis: Syringohydromyelia (idiopathic).

Discussion: Syringohydromyelia is a term used to describe the presence of fluid-filled cyst(s) in the spinal cord. These cysts are generally surrounded by gliosis. Hydromyelia is an expansion of the central spinal canal; therefore, its walls are lined by ependyma. A syringomyelia occurs outside the central spinal canal and its walls are composed of gliosis. Because the differentiation between is difficult even at histology, the term syringohydromyelia is commonly employed. This disease predominantly affects adults and is generally found after spinal trauma. A long latent period between the trauma and the onset of symptoms arising from the cyst is the general rule. In children, it is almost always associated with congenital anomalies of the spine, such as the Chiari malformations, scoliosis, open dysraphism, diastematomyelia, and other causes of spinal cord tethering. The most common symptoms at presentation are a tethered spinal cord, muscle atrophy and weakness, loss of pain and temperture, and pain occuring in any of the extremities. The etiology of these cysts is uncertain but most of these patients have abnormal flow of cerebrospinal fluid (CSF). If symptomatic, the cyst(s) may need to be decompressed by shunting into the subarachnoid space or to the peritoneal cavity. In some patients, decompression of hydrocephalus may lead to disappearance of the syrinx. MR is the imaging method of choice for the evaluation of patients suspected of harboring a spinal cord cyst. The cysts are isointense to CSF in most sequences and should not demonstrate any enhancement after contrast administration. Areas of increased T2 signal in the adjacent spinal cord may be related to gliosis. The cysts may be multiseptated. The entire spinal cord, including the foramen magnum, needs to be imaged. Extension of the cyst into the brainstem is termed "syringobulbia."

Clinical History: You are shown two patients. The first (Figs. A–D) is a male with chronic thoracic back pain and a myelopathy. The second (Fig. E) is a 40-year-old female with chronic upper lumbar pain.

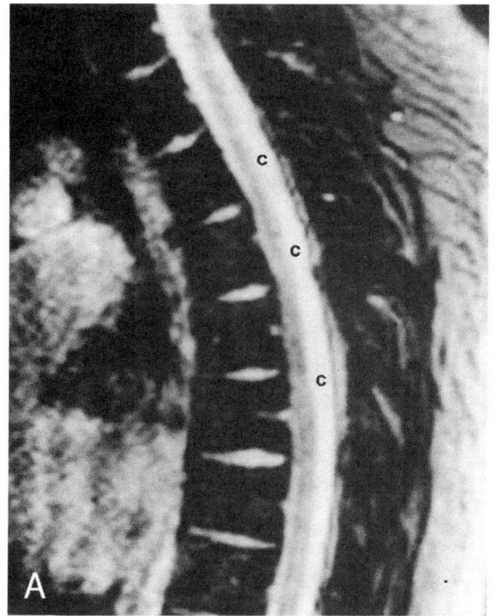

Figure 4.20 A

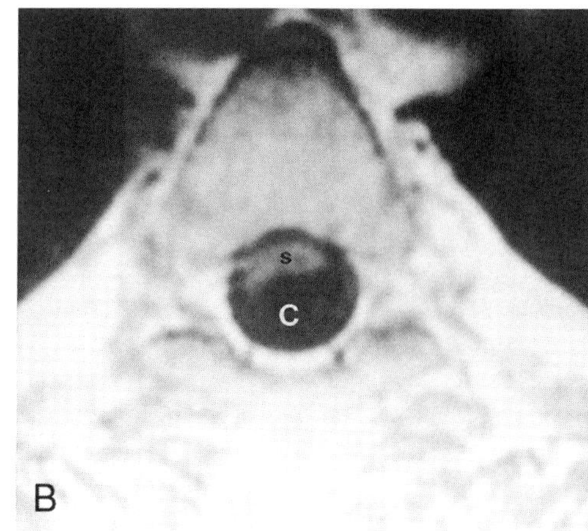

Figure 4.20 B

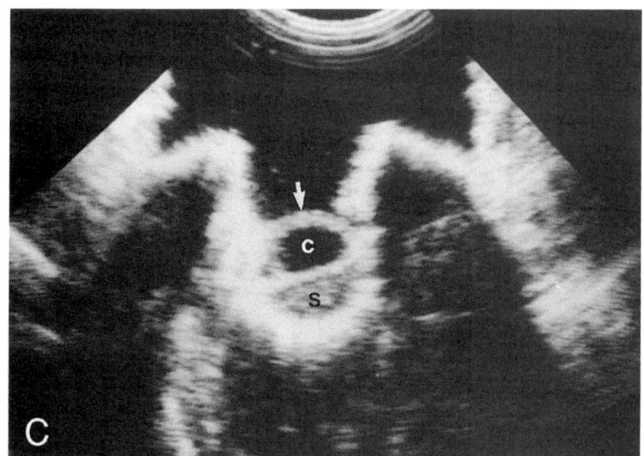

Figure 4.20 C

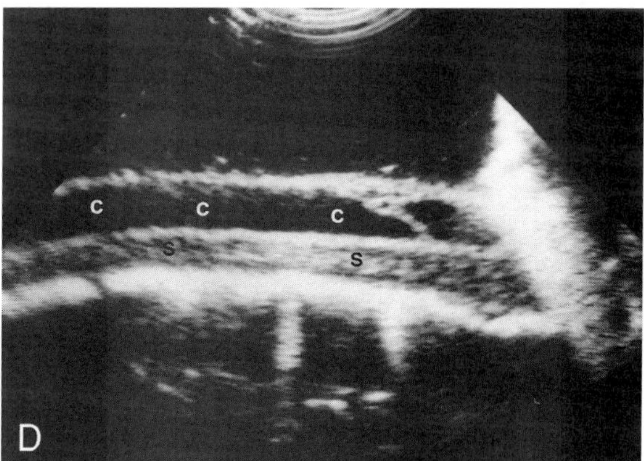

Figure 4.20 D

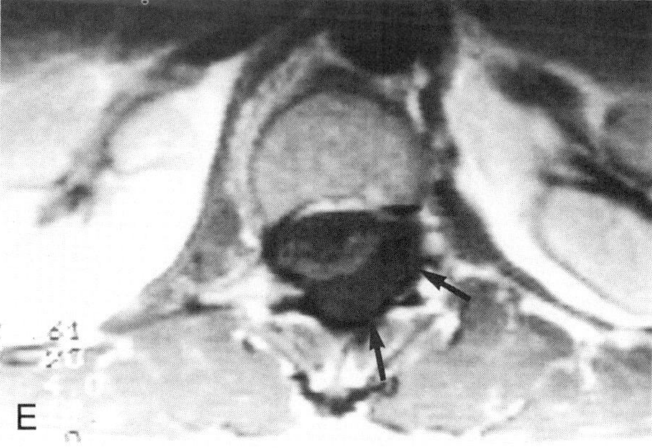

Figure 4.20 E

(continued)

Findings: In the first patient, a midsagittal MR T2-weighted image (Fig. A) shows the presence of a hyperintense cyst (c) posterior to the thoracic spinal cord. Axial MR T1-weighted image (Fig. B) shows the cyst (C) posterior to the spinal cord (s). Note the compression and ventral displacement of the spinal cord. Transverse view (Fig. C) during intraoperative sonography shows the cyst (C) posterior to the displaced spinal cord (s) but deep to the dura (arrow) confirming its subarachnoid location. Sagittal intraoperative sonogram (Fig. D) shows the cyst (C) and the spinal cord (S). Note a septation within the cyst. (Case courtesy of R. M. Quencer, M.D., Miami, FL.) In the second patient, an axial MR T1-weighted image (Fig. E) shows a cyst (arrows) located dorsolaterally to the cauda equina which has eroded the posterior vertebral elements.

Differential Diagnosis: In the first patient, consider the following: exophytic syringohydromyelia, cysticercosis, epidermoid, echinococcus, arachnoid cysts. In the second patient, erosive changes from ankylosing spondylitis or dural ectasia secondary to neurofibromatosis or collagen disorders may have a similar appearance. Consider arachnoid cysts.

Diagnosis: Arachnoid cysts.

Discussion: Arachnoid cysts are encapsulated collections of cerebrospinal fluid (CSF) within the arachnoid membrane. Approximately 50% are extradural and the rest are intradural. Intradural arachnoid cysts are probably the result of incomplete trabeculation of the membrane. Extradural cysts result from a deficiency in the dura that allows the arachnoid and CSF to herniate and form a fluid collection. They grow slowly over time and produce symptoms by virtue of compression of the neural elements. These cysts are commonly idiopathic and are associated with congenital spinal anomalies, such as closed and open dysraphisms. They may also occur secondary to previous inflammatory processes and have been seen after inadvertent intradural administration of spinal anesthetics. The treatment involves decompression of these cysts via a fenestration. The walls of these cysts are generally not resected. If needed, the cyst may be shunted to the subarachnoid space, peritoneal cavity, or pleura. MR is the imaging method of choice. The cysts are of signal intensity equivalent to CSF in all sequences and do not enhance after contrast administration. They are more common in the thoracic region and are generally dorsal to the spinal cord. The spinal cord is displaced ventrally and compressed by the cyst.

CASE 21

Clinical History: Adolescent female with progressive scoliosis.

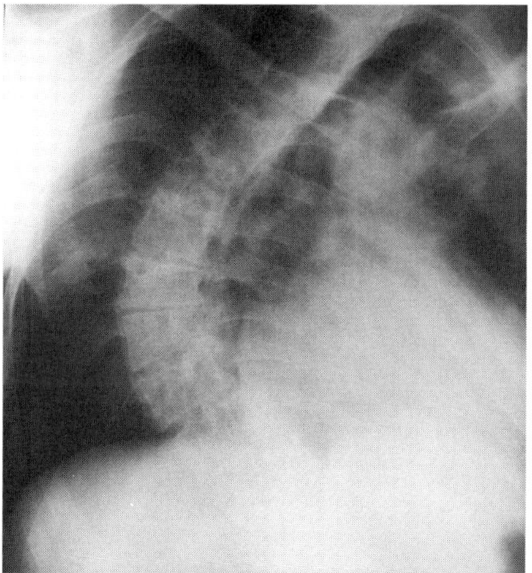

Figure 4.21

Findings: Frontal radiograph (Fig. A) shows a midthoracic dextro scoliosis. Note the absence of segmentation or fusion anomalies at the apex of the curve.

Diagnosis: Adolescent idiopathic scoliosis.

Discussion: The overall incidence of idiopathic scoliosis is approximately 5%. It is divided into the following types: infantile (0–3 years of age), juvenile (4–9 years of age), and adolescent (more than 10 years of age). The juvenile type accounts for more than 20% of scoliosis cases and is more common in females. There may be a family history in patients with juvenile scoliosis. Adolescent scoliosis is also more common in girls. Boys are more commonly affected during the infantile period. Patients with early-onset scoliosis may develop pulmonary and cardiac complications. Back pain is probably the most common symptom in all patients with scoliosis. In patients with juvenile scoliosis, progression occurs in about 70%. Patients with progressive curves will require therapy. The initial diagnosis is made on radiographs. In the infantile type, the curves are convex to the left and centered in the thoracic region. In the juvenile type, there is no particular segment or side affected more than others. In adolescents, most curves are to the right and centered in the thoracic region. CT may be done to evaluate underlying congenital deformities of the vertebrae, such as hemivertebrae, fusions, and butterfly vertebrae (see Case #1). MR imaging is generally obtained before surgical treatment to exclude tumors, synringohydromyelia (see Case #19), or a tethered spinal cord. In adults, kyphoscoliosis may be sequela of prior spinal infection. Patients with curves greater than 40° as measured by the Cobb method are generally treated surgically.

Clinical History: You are shown the spine imaging studies in four different patients, all suffering from the same systemic and congenital disorder.

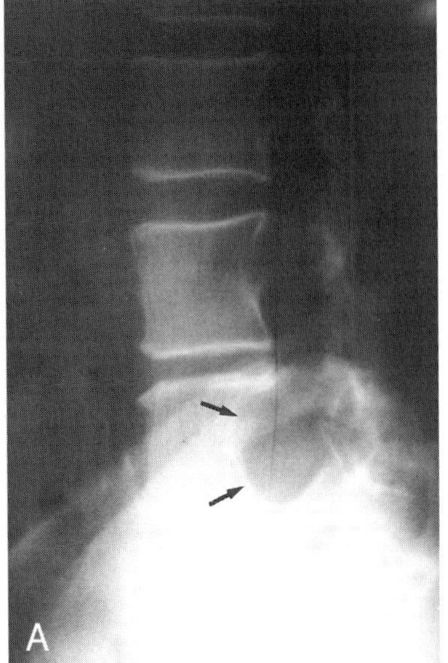

Figure 4.22 A

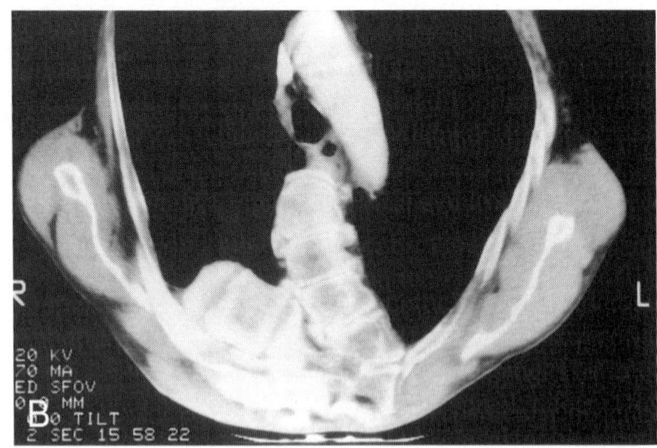

Figure 4.22 B

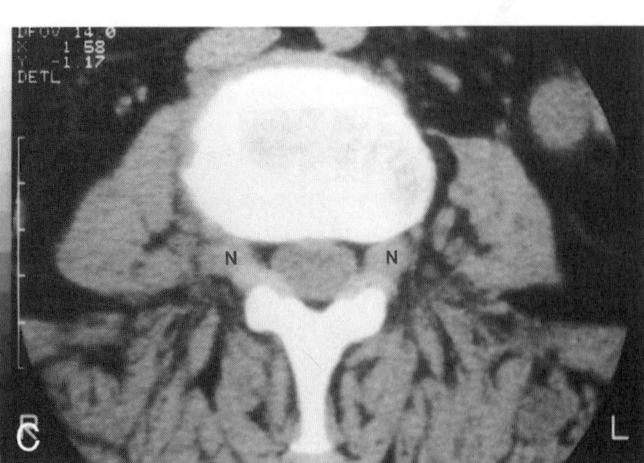

Figure 4.22 C

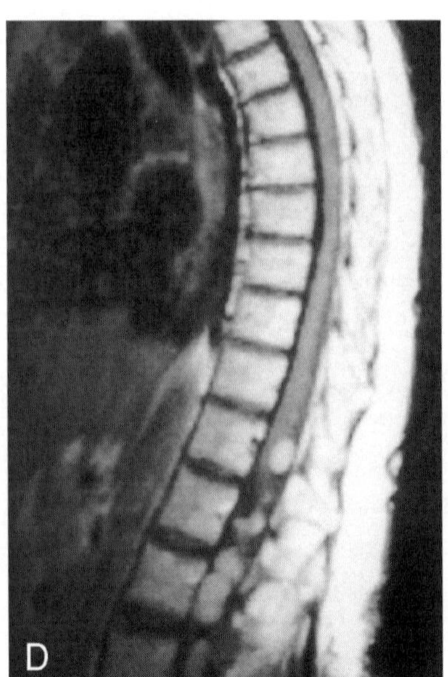

Figure 4.22 D

Findings: Lateral radiograph (Fig. A) of the lumbar region shows significant scalloping (arrows) of the posterior aspect of L5. In a different patient, axial CT (Fig. B) shows acute angle kyphoscoliosis at the midthoracic spine. Axial CT (Fig. C) in a different case shows masses (N) in the neural foramina at the L3-L4 level. In the last patient, midsagittal postcontrast MR T1-weighted image (Fig. D) shows multiple enhancing masses in the region of the conus medullaris and the cauda equina.

Diagnosis: Neurofibromatosis (type 1 in all patients).

(continued)

Discussion: Spinal abnormalities are present in 70% of patients with neurofibromatosis type 1 (NF1) and in 90% of patients with neurofibromatosis type 2 (NF2). In patients with NF1, neurofibromas are common, particularly in the cervical and thoracic regions. Approximately 5% of these tumors eventually undergo malignant degeneration. Astrocytomas of the spinal cord are relatively unusual. Mesodermal abnormalities include dural ectasia with formation of meningoceles and scalloping of the vertebrae. In these patients, lateral thoracic meningoceles are believed to be the most common paraspinal mass. Thoracic scoliosis is relatively common in patients with NF1. Acute angle kyphoscoliosis is typical but less common than just mild-to-moderate scoliosis. Spinal dislocations and pseudoarthroses also may be found. In patients with NF2, spinal schwannomas and meningiomas are relatively common. These patients have an increased incidence of intramedullary masses and most are ependymomas, but astrocytomas may also be present. Syringohydromyelia may be present as well. In patients with NF2, the spinal bone abnormalities are usually the result of remodeling by tumors. MR is the imaging method of choice for these patients. Meningiomas, schwannomas, and neurofibromas all enhance after contrast administration. Lateral thoracic meningoceles are of signal intensity equivalent to cerebrospinal fluid in all imaging sequences and do not enhance after contrast administration (see Case #31).

Clinical History: You are shown images from three different patients suffering from the same systemic disorder. Physical examination of all individuals shows ectopia lentis and tall stature.

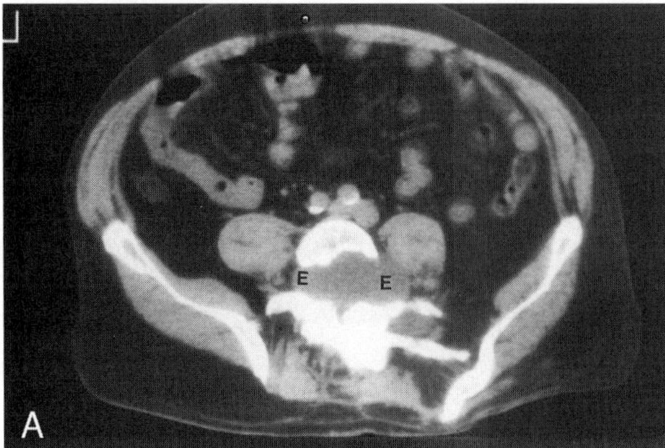

Figure 4.23 A

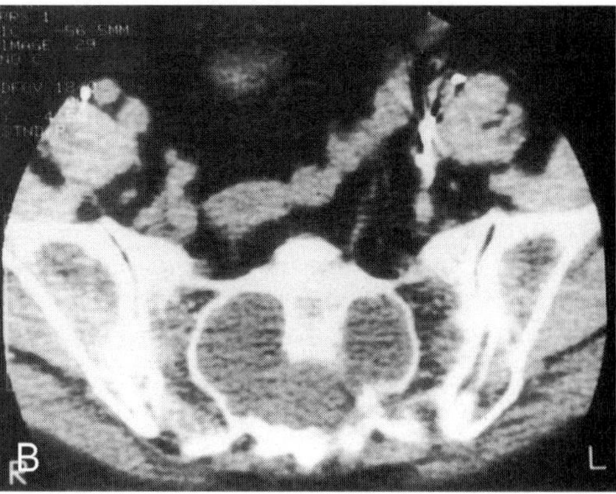

Figure 4.23 B

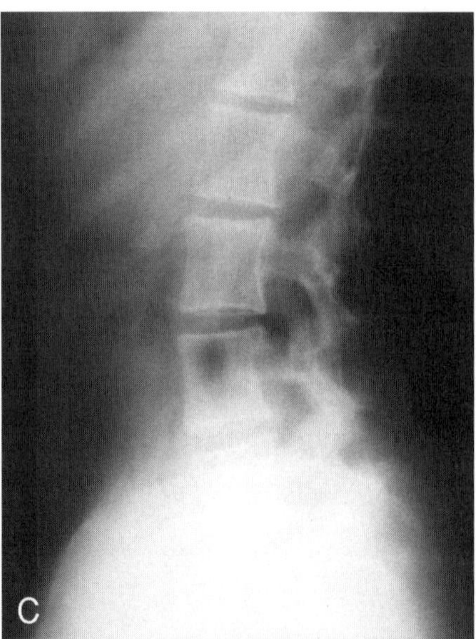

Figure 4.23 C

Findings: In the first patient, an axial CT (Fig. A) shows dural ectasia with a patulous thecal sac projecting through both neural foramina (E). There is scalloping of the posterior aspect of the vertebral body. The bony abnormality of the posterior elements is of uncertain etiology. Axial CT of the second patient (Fig. B) shows marked expansion of the sacral canal and foramina by a patulous thecal sac and nerve root sleeves. Lateral spine radiograph (Fig. C) in the third patient shows mild posterior scalloping of all lumbar vertebrae.

(continued)

Differential Diagnosis (For Vertebral Scalloping): Ehlers-Danlos syndrome, homocystinuria, neurofibromatosis, acromegaly, uncontrolled and long-standing hydrocephalus, dural ectasia secondary to Marfan syndrome.

Diagnosis: Dural ectasia secondary to Marfan syndrome.

Discussion: Marfan syndrome is an autosomal dominant disorder with variable expression. It affects all connective tissue in the body, but particularly the musculoskeletal system. Patients may either have the full syndrome or just a Marfanoid habitus. It occurs in approximately 4–5 of 100,000 individuals, and 25% of cases are new mutations. The average lifespan for these patients is 40 years. The abnormality resides in chromosome 15q, which encodes for fibrillin. Clinically, the cardiovascular, musculoskeletal, and ocular systems are affected. The most common abnormalities include ectopia (superolateral subluxation) lentis (80% of patients), dissecting aortic aneurysm, and kyphoscoliosis. Musculoskeletal abnormalities are present in more than 50% of patients and include: ligamentous laxity, dolichocephaly, pectus excavatum and carinatum, increased length of the long bones, and increased length of the hands (arachnodactyly). The cervical spine is usually normal. The thoracic spine may show scoliosis, kyphosis, lordosis, scalloping of the vertebral bodies, other vertebral dysplasias, elongation of the vertebrae, and spondylolisthesis. Spinal abnormalities are found in approximately 75% of patients with Marfan syndrome. Scoliosis may be managed conservatively initially but becomes progressive on most patients. Once the curvature reaches 40°, surgical stabilization and fusion are necessary.

Clinical History: This patient has a history of a systemic inherited disorder. He now presents with neck pain and a history of episodic weakness of all extremities.

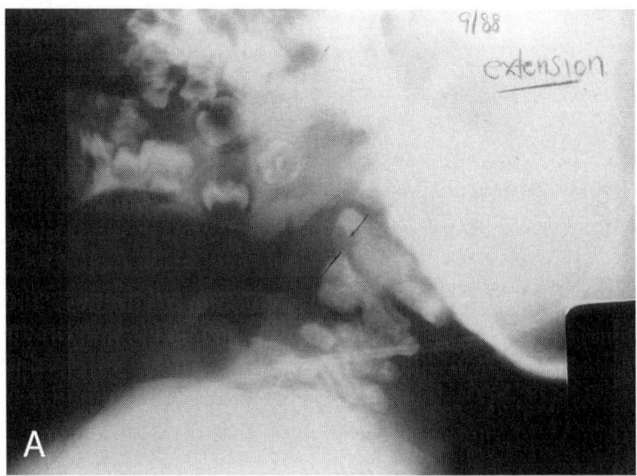

Figure 4.24 A

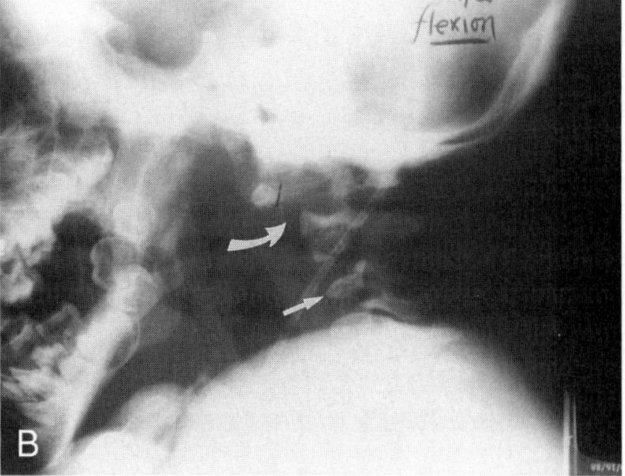

Figure 4.24 B

Findings: Lateral extension radiograph (Fig. A) shows a normal atlanto-dental distance (traced). Flexion lateral radiograph (Fig. B) shows increased (curved arrow) atlanto-dental distance; the dens is not well seen. There is beaking (straight arrow) of the cervical vertebrae.

Differential Diagnosis (for vertebral beaking): Central: Morquio syndrome, achondroplasia, spondyloepiphyseal dysplasia, and normal. Inferior: Hurler syndrome, cretinism, diastrophic dwarfism, Down syndrome, phenylketonuria, muscular hypotonia, trauma, normal (children who sit early). For atlanto-dental subluxation: trauma, pharyngeal infections (particularly in children), rheumatoid arthritis, ankylosing spondylitis, Down syndrome, mucopolysaccharidoses, and congenital anomalies of the dens.

Diagnosis: Atlanto-dental subluxation secondary to Hurler syndrome.

Discussion: The mucopolysaccharidoses are a group of genetic disorders characterized by enzymatic defects affecting the breakdown of heparan sulfate, dermatan sulfate, and keratan sulfate. The most common of these disorders are Hurler and Hunter diseases. Others include Sanfilippo, Morquio, Scheie, Maroteaux-Lamy, and Sly. Most of these patients have (at least initially) macrocephaly caused by deposition of mucopolysaccharides in the brain. This leads to mental retardation. Other clinical features include hearing loss, facial dysmorphism, corneal clouding, hepatosplenomegaly, and multiple areas of skeletal involvement. In the spine, the lumbar lordosis is accentuated and there is thoracic kyphosis. There is beaking of the anterior surface of the vertebral bodies. The exact location of these beaks varies according to the type of mucopolysaccharidosis. In Morquio disease, the beaks tend to arise in the middle and anterior of the vertebral bodies, whereas in others they usually arise in the anterior and inferior aspect of the vertebral bodies. Thoracolumbar gibbus or kyphosis is common. Subluxations of C1 and C2 may result in serious complications, including compression of the spinal cord. This occurs because of laxity of the transverse ligaments, and flexion and extension radiographs and/or MR images are needed to document this abnormality.

CASE 25

Clinical History: You are shown the imaging studies in a boy with very short stature who now presents with symptoms of neurologic claudication in both lower extremities.

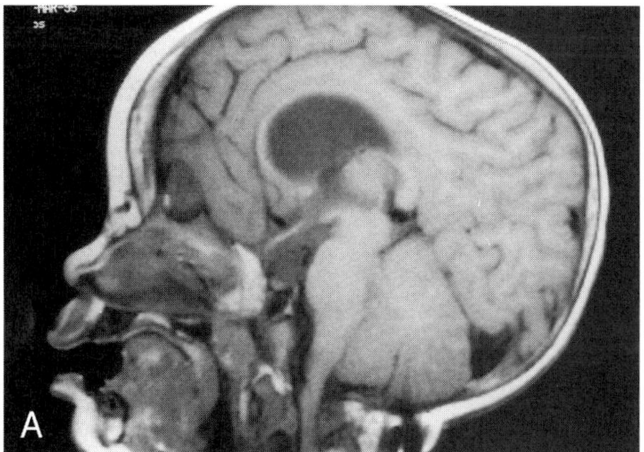

Figure 4.25 A

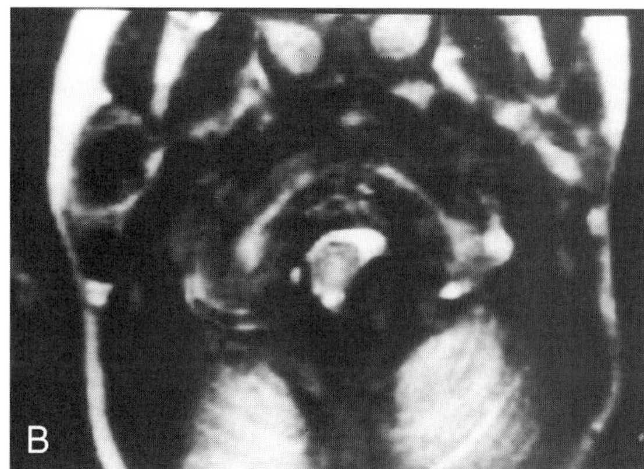

Figure 4.25 B

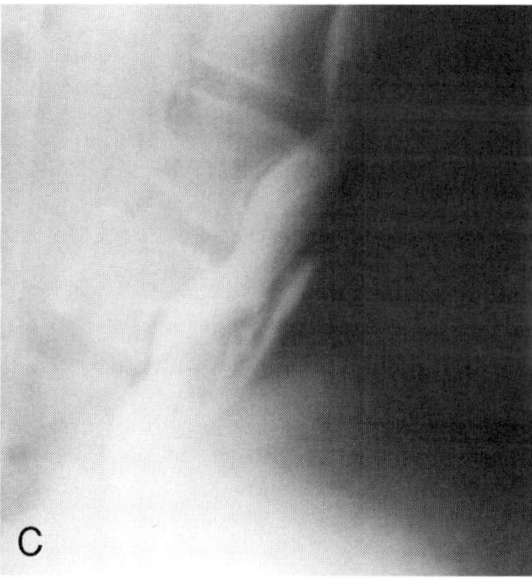

Figure 4.25 C

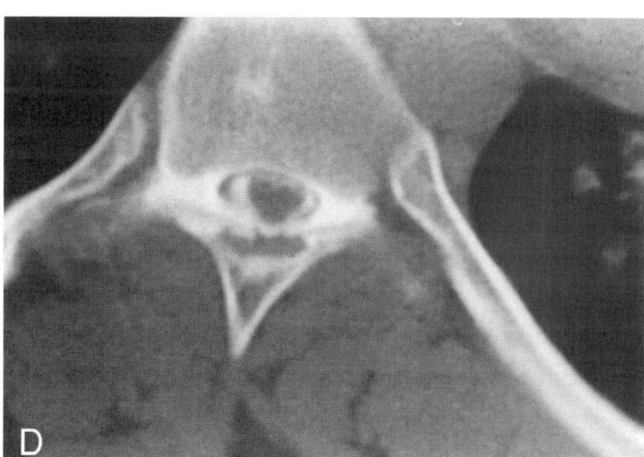

Figure 4.25 D

Findings: Midsagittal MR T1-weighted image (Fig. A) shows a very small foramen magnum and a vertical clivus. The lateral ventricles are prominent. Axial MR T2-weighted image (Fig. B) shows the severe narrowing of the foramen magnum. There is some questionably abnormal increased signal intensity in the medulla. Lateral radiograph from a myelogram (Fig. C) shows scalloping of the posterior lumbar vertebrae and spinal canal stenoses at the disk levels. Axial CT section after myelography (Fig. D) shows congenital spinal canal stenosis that was caused by short pedicles (not shown). The spinal cord is compressed and has a "triangular" thoracic appearance.

(continued)

Diagnosis: Achondroplasia.

Discussion: Achondroplasia is a defect of enchondral bone formation and is the most common type of dwarphism to affect the spine, particularly at the craniocervical junction. It occurs in approximately 1 of 25,000 individuals and has no gender predilection. It is autosomal dominant, although most new cases represent spontaneous mutations. Clinically, the most important features are short stature, dysmorphic facies, congenital skeletal abnormalities, and neurologic abnormalities. Hypotonia at birth suggests compression of the brainstem by craniocervical abnormalities. Spinal abnormalities resulting in symptoms before the age of 5 years generally require aggressive surgical treatment. Kyphoscoliosis is prominent but improves spontaneously in most patients. MR is the imaging method of choice in these patients. Narrowing of the foramen magnum to less than 10 mm in its anteroposterior dimension may indicate the need for decompression. Os odontoideum, dens hypoplasia, and congenital fusion of the occipital bone to C1 may result in C1-C2 instability and dictate the need for fusion. Stenosis of the cervical spinal canal is present in approximately 30% of these patients. Diffuse stenosis involving most of the spine is present in 10% of achondroplastic patients. In the lumbar spine, the interpedicular distance is shortened (diastrophic and thanotophoric dwarphisms may have similar findings). Bulging disks are common and, because of the accompanying congenital stenosis, lead to severe stenoses. Syringomyelia may be occasionally present.

Clinical History: Young male with a long-standing history of decreased neck mobility and bilateral upper extremity pain and weakness.

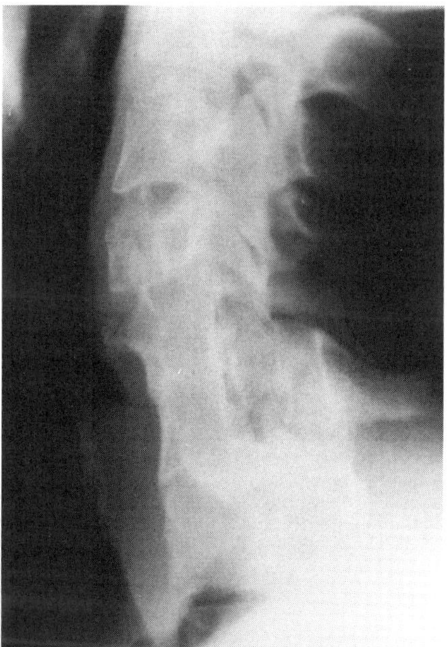

Figure 4.26

Findings: Lateral radiograph (Fig. A) shows congenital fusion of the C4-C6 vertebrae. A radiograph of the chest (not shown) demonstrated rotation and elevation of the scapulae (Sprengel's deformity).

Diagnosis: Klippel-Feil syndrome.

Discussion: Signs of Klippel-Feil syndrome include a short neck, low posterior hairline, and limitation of neck motion because of congenital fusion of several vertebral bodies. It probably occurs in approximately 1 of 42,000 individuals. Its etiology is uncertain, and primary vascular disruption, fetal insults, neural tube abnormalities, failure of spinal segmentation, and other genetic abnormalities have been implicated. It has both autosomal and dominant and recessive inheritance patterns. It is slightly more common in males. The age of presentation is variable and in accordance to the severity of the cervical spine fusion. Patients with fusions involving C1 and C2 present early in life. Approximately 20% of cases are discovered before the age of 5 years. The most common symptoms are neck pain and limited motion (50 to 75% of patients). Radiculopathies and slowly progressive or acute quadriparesis may also occur. The diagnosis is readily made by radiographs. Most patients have fusions involving only one disk space. In 35% of patients, the fusion involves multiple levels. The diameter of the spinal canal may be diminished because of degenerative changes immediately above and below the fusions. There may be C1-C2 (os odontoideum and occipitalization of the atlas) instability that requires evaluation with flexion and extension radiographs or MR imaging. Scoliosis and other anomalies involving the thoracic and lumbar regions are common.

CASE 27

Clinical History: Patient with known cleido-cranial dysostosis and increasing episodes of apnea.

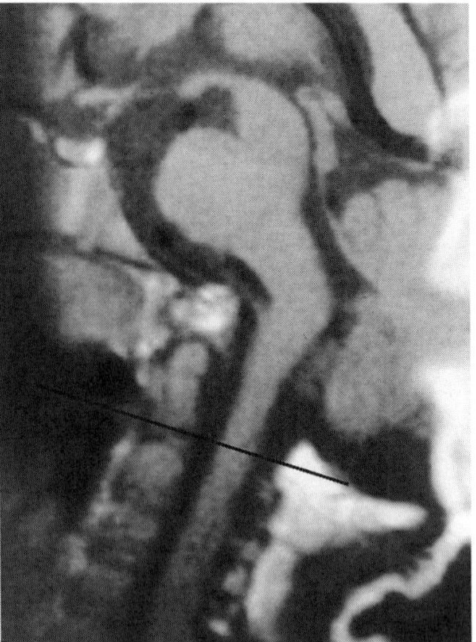

Figure 4.27

Findings: Midsagittal MR T1-weighted image (Fig. A) shows upward projection of the dens that compresses the pontomedullary junction of the brainstem. Note that most of C2 is superior to McGregor's line (black line).

Diagnosis: Basilar invagination.

Discussion: The term "basilar invagination" refers to a congenital dyplasia of the craniocervical junction in which there is upward displacement of C1 and C2 into the foramen magnum. The term "basilar impression" refers to a similar abnormality that is the result of acquired softening of bones forming the skull base. The etiology of basilar invagination is uncertain, but basilar impression is caused by fibrous dysplasia, Paget disease, hyperparathyroidism, multiple myeloma, mucopolysaccharidoses, osteogenesis imperfecta, rheumatoid arthritis, and osteomalacia. Basilar invagination may be associated with occipitalization of C1, hypoplasia of C1, absent posterior arch of C1, odontoid process abnormalities, Klippel-Feil syndrome (see Case #26), Down syndrome, Chiari malformations (see Cases #17 and 18), achondroplasia (see Case #25), and cleidocranial dysostosis. Treatment includes decompression and fusion of the upper cervical spine as well as enlargement of the foramen magnum. On frontal radiographs, the tip of the odontoid process should not project more than 10 mm above a bimastoid line. On lateral radiographs, the tip of the odontoid process should not lie more than 6 mm above Chamberlain's line (which extends from the posterior hard palate to the tip of posterior lip of the foramen magnum). The tip of the dens may project slightly superior to McGregor's line (from the posterior hard palate to the undersurface of the posterior lip of the foramen magnum) normally. On CT and MR imaging, the posterior fossa is small and margins of the foramen magnum are irregular. The high odontoid process may compress the medulla. Flexion and extension radiographs and/or MR images are needed to document C1-C2 instability.

Clinical History: You are shown two patients. The first (Fig. A) presents with neck pain. The second (Figs. B and C) presents with recent onset of episodic weakness in all extremities.

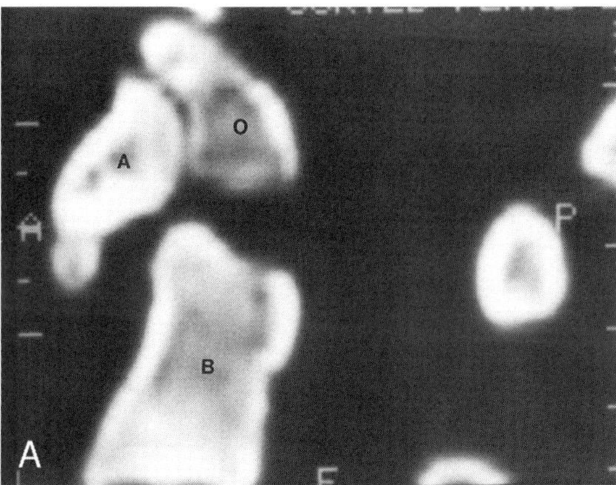

Figure 4.28 A

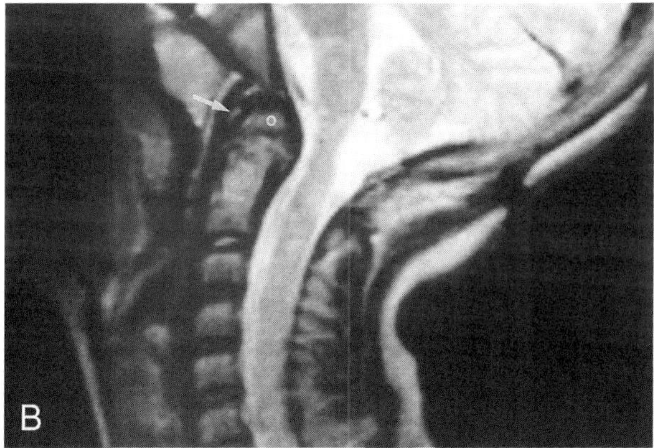

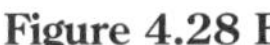

Figure 4.28 B

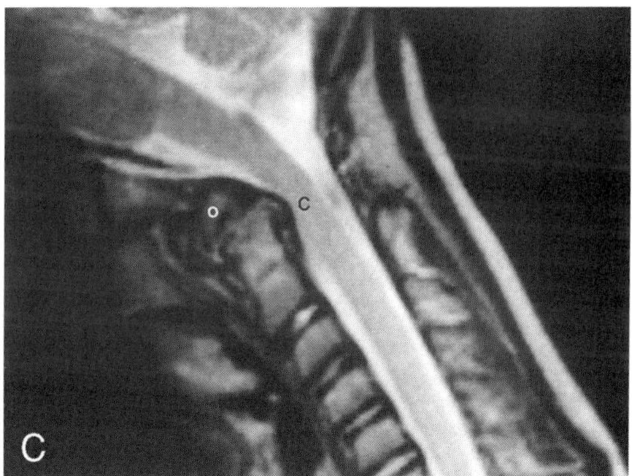

Figure 4.28 C

Findings: In the first patient, a midsagittal CT reformation (Fig. A) shows an os odontoideum (O) widely separated from the body (B) of C2. The atlanto-dental distance is normal and the anterior arch (A) of C1 is dysplastic. In the second patient, midsagittal extension MR T2-weighted image (Fig. B) shows an os odontoideum (o) which is aligned with the body of C2. Note the anterior arch (arrow) of C1 and the normal atlanto-dental distance. The perimedullary cistern is normal. On a corresponding flexion image (Fig. C), the os odontoideum (o) slides anteriorly while the atlanto-dental distance is preserved. The superior aspect of C2 now compresses the spinal cord (c) and effaces the perimedullary cistern.

(continued)

Differential Diagnosis: Type 2 fracture of the dens, os odontoideum.

Diagnosis: Os odontoideum.

Discussion: The most common abnormalities involving the dens are the os odontoideum and hypoplasia of the dens. The least common of these abnormalities is aplasia of the dens. There is no gender predilection. All of these abnormalities produce symptoms by virtue of C1-C1 instability and compression of the spinal cord. Compression of the vertebral arteries leading to vertebrobasilar insufficiency may also occur. The etiology for the os odontoideum is not clear, but trauma early in life may play an important role. Although it is generally an isolated anomaly, an os odontoideum may be associated with Down, Morquio, or Klippel Feil syndromes (see Cases #24 and 26). It may also be found in patients with spondyloepiphyseal dysplasia. On radiographs, the os odontoideum appears as a well-corticated, round ossicle, separated by a relatively wide radiolucent gap from the body of C2. In the orthotopic variety, the os odontoideum is located at the normal and expected position of the dens. In the dystopic variety, the os odontoideum lies under the anterior lip of the foramen magnum and may be fused to it. Both types may be accompanied by laxity of the transverse ligament and C1-C2 instability. Flexion and extension radiographs or MR images are needed to document instability. Coronal CT reformations help exclude a fracture of the dens.

Clinical History: This patient has a long-standing history of anemia, hepato-splenomegaly, and multiple cranial nerve palsies.

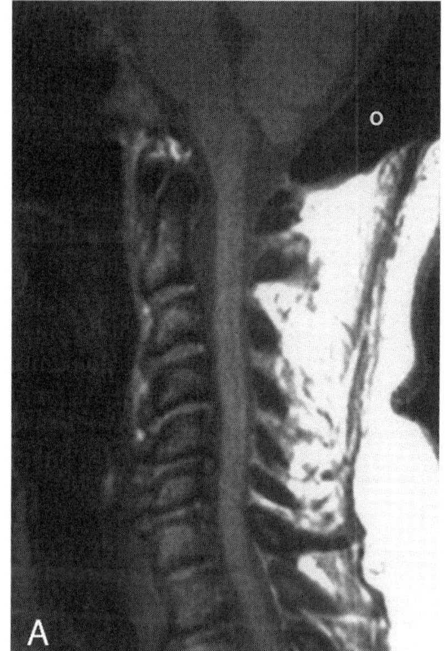

Figure 4.29 A

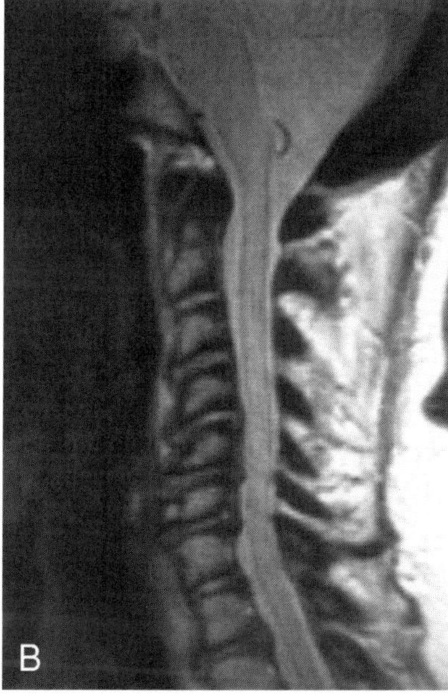

Figure 4.29 B

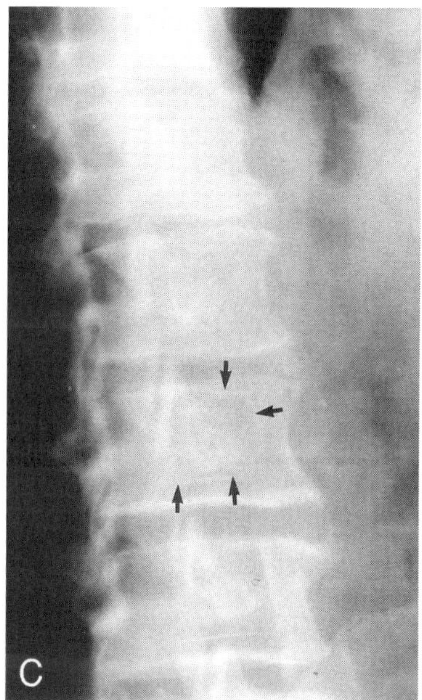

Figure 4.29 C

Findings: Midsagittal MR T1-weighted image (Fig. A) shows reduction in the size of the bone marrow cavities in the vertebrae. The cortical margins of the vertebrae appear more prominent than usual. Note the marked thickening of the occipital bone (O) and its low signal intensity. The spinous processes are also of low signal intensity. Corresponding proton density image (Fig. B) shows similar findings and some degenerative changes at C5-C6. Oblique radiograph of the lumbar spine (Fig. C) shows a "bone within bone" (arrows) appearance.

Differential Diagnosis (For "Bone Within Bone" Appearance): Normal, previous severe systemic illness, chronic intermittent disease, heavy metal intoxication, radiation therapy, osteopetrosis.

Diagnosis: Osteopetrosis (intermediate form).

Discussion: Osteopetrosis is a heterogeneous group of disorders that result in thick and sclerotic bones that fracture easily, hepatosplenomegaly, mental retardation, and reduced lifespan. The most severe form of the disease is the precocious type in which obliteration of all bone marrow cavities occurs, leading to anemia and infections. These patients have hepatosplenomegaly and suffer from compression of neural structures. These patients die young. Radiographically, the presence of "bone within bone" is unusual, and the most common findings are osteosclerosis and obliteration of the bone marrow cavities. The delayed type of osteopetrosis is also known as Albers-Schönberg disease and is autosomal dominant. Clinical features include anemia, fractures, and cranial nerve palsies. Some patients have only mild problems. Osteosclerosis and obliteration of the marrow cavities are common, and "bone within bone" appearance is sometimes seen.

The intermediate or recessive form is characterized by symptoms that are even more mild than those of the delayed form. There is diffuse increased bone density with obliteration of the marrow cavities, and the appearance of "bone within bone" is common. The prominent bone density is caused by an increase in the amount of bone and not from an increase in the percentage of mineralized bone per unit volume of tissue. Osteopetrosis with tubular acidosis and brain calcifications is an autosomal recessive disorder with a long survival time, and these patients tend to be mentally retarded. The most common imaging findings are osteosclerosis and obliteration of the marrow cavities. On MR imaging, the least severe forms of osteopetrosis show dense cortical bone and partial or complete obliteration of the normal high signal intensity of the bone marrow cavities.

CASE 30

Clinical History: This patient presents with nonspecific low back pain.

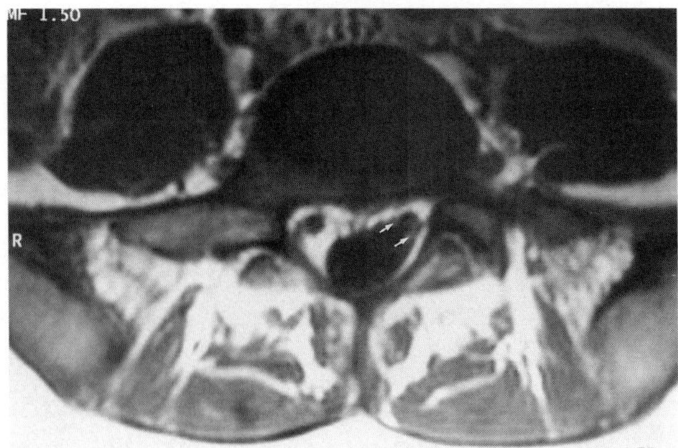

Figure 4.30

Findings: Axial MR T1-weighted image (Fig. A) shows widening of the left S1 nerve root sleeve. Note that this sleeve contains two nerve roots (arrows).

Diagnosis: Conjoined nerve roots.

Discussion: Conjoined or fused nerve roots are a relatively common anomaly of the lumbar spine in which two roots share a common dural sleeve. They run a parallel course and may emerge from a neural foramen as a fused root. Fused roots may emerge together at the appropriate level for the lower-most root or midway between the expected levels for both roots. A second (but rare) anomaly of the lumbar nerve roots is anastomosis. In these cases, a normal root bifurcates after it emerges from the dura and then anastomoses with the nerve root immediately inferior to it. Occasionally, a lumbar nerve root has a transverse course that may simulate conjoined roots. In these cases, the origin of the root is normal but its course is horizontal instead of oblique and caudal. Most conjoined nerve roots occur at the L4 through S1 levels. If a disk herniation occurs in patients with conjoined roots, the symptoms may be atypical and result in biradicular pain. It is important to report these anomalies to the surgeon if surgery is contemplated. After a laminectomy, the conjoined root sleeve may be mistaken for a herniation and inadvertently resected.

Clinical History: This patient's chest radiograph shows a right paraspinal mass. He is asymptomatic.

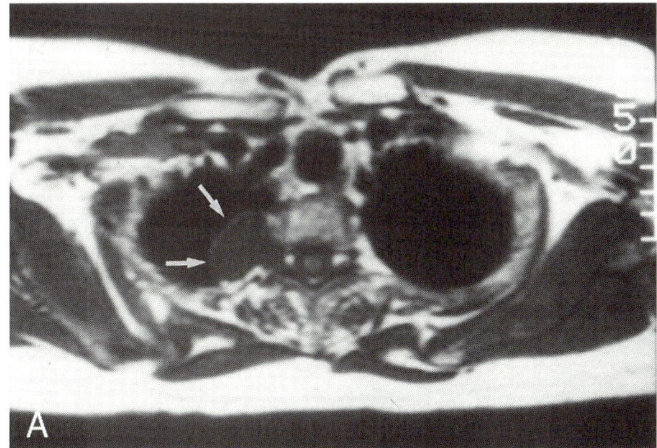

Figure 4.31 A

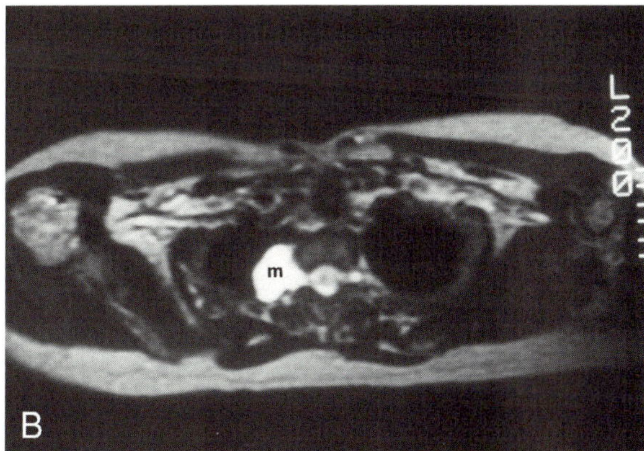

Figure 4.31 B

Findings: Axial MR T1-weighted image (Fig. A) shows a right paraspinal mass (arrows) of low signal intensity. Corresponding T2-weighted image (Fig. B) shows the mass (m) to be of high signal intensity and to communicate with the subarachnoid space in the spinal canal. The corresponding neural foramen is expanded. On a contrast study (not shown), the lesion did not enhance.

Diagnosis: Lateral thoracic meningocele.

Discussion: Lateral meningoceles are protrusions of dura and arachnoid through an enlarged neural foramen. They are filled with cerebrospinal fluid. The most commonly affected region is the thoracic spine, followed by the lumbar spine. Approximately 60–70% of patients with lateral thoracic meningoceles have neurofibromatosis type 1. In these patients, a lateral thoracic meningocele is a more than a neurofibroma. Contrary to true tumors from the nerve root, these meningoceles are generally asymptomatic. When symptoms occur, they result from compression of the nerve roots. They may be associated with kyphoscoliosis, particularly in patients with neurofibromatosis (see Case #22). They are easily diagnosed by MR imaging and, during myelography, they fill immediately after the instillation of intrathecal contrast material.

chapter 5

VASCULAR DISORDERS

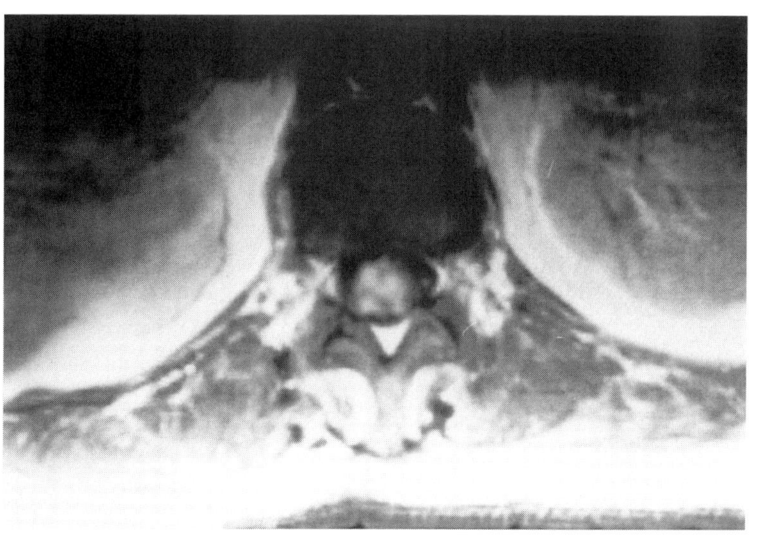

CASE 1

Clinical History: A 55-year-old male presents with progressive paraplegia of 2 years duration. This patient has a history of spine trauma from 10 years previously.

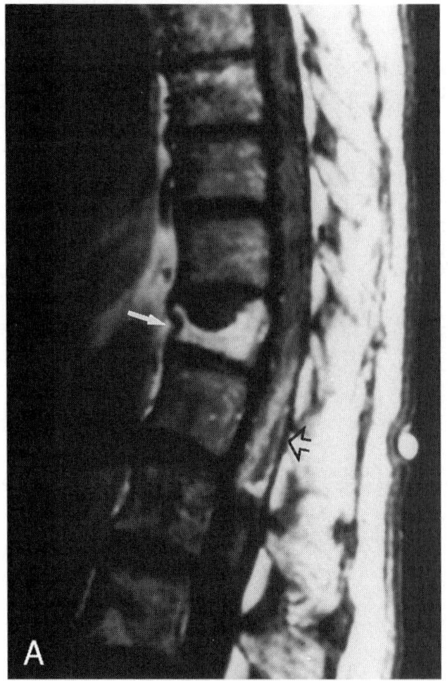

Figure 5.1 A

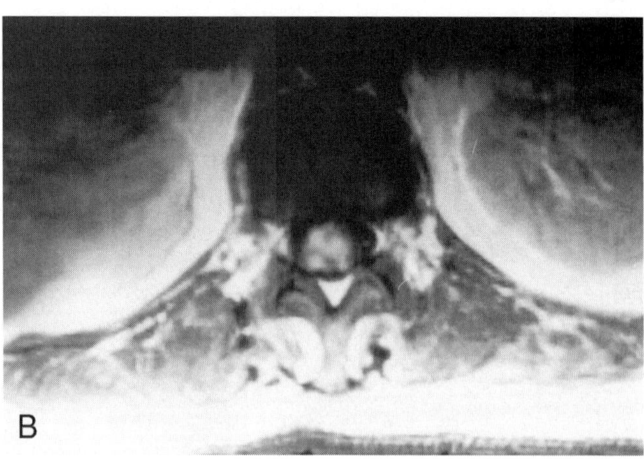

Figure 5.1 B

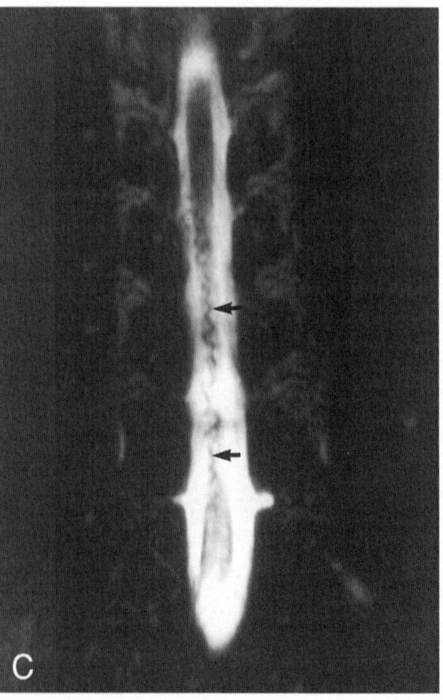

Figure 5.1 C

(continued)

Findings: Midsagittal postcontrast MR T1-weighted image (Fig. A) shows collapsed T11 vertebral body (solid arrow) and enhancement of the conus medullaris (open arrow). Axial postcontrast MR T1-weighted image (Fig. B) shows widening and diffuse enhancement of the conus medullaris. T2-weighted coronal partition (Fig. C) from an MR myelogram shows a large vessel (arrows) on the surface of the spinal cord.

Diagnosis: Spinal arteriovenous fistula (AVF).

Discussion: Spinal (or paraspinal) AVFs are characterized by arteriovenous blood shunting between one or more radiculomedullary arteries and a vein on the surface of the spinal cord. They occur more often in the conus medullaris but may also be found in the thoracic and cervical regions. They may be congenital or acquired. The patients generally present with long-standing and slowly progressive neurologic symptoms particularly involving the lower extremities. Their treatment consists of catheter embolization of the feeding arteries. The prognosis is variable and depends on how advanced the symptoms are at presentation. Existing symptoms tend to be permanent. According to their size, these AVFs may be radiographically classified into three types. Type 1 AVFs are small, type 2 AVFs are medium size and are the most commonly found, and type 3 AVFs are giant and are fed by multiple arteries. The venous drainage of these malformations is usually to the veins on the surface of the spinal cord. These may be very large and at times extend the entire length of the spinal cord. A variation of these AVFs are fistulas between radiculomeningeal arteries and veins with subsequent drainage into veins on the surface of the spinal cord. These AVFs are more common in males and tend to present with a progressive radiculopathy at the level where the fistula is located. If untreated, paraplegia probably ensues in most patients. The symptoms are probably caused by venous hypertension. In these cases, the AVF is not directly seen, but MR imaging shows widening of the spinal cord, T2 hyperintensity, and enhancement after contrast administration. Most of these fistulas are found from the midthoracic to the upper lumbar levels. Embolization of the feeding pedicles is the treatment of choice.

CASE 2

Clinical History: You are shown two patients. The first one (Figs. A–C) presents with increasing lower extremity weakness. The second (Figs. D–F) presents with weakness and spasticity in all four extremities.

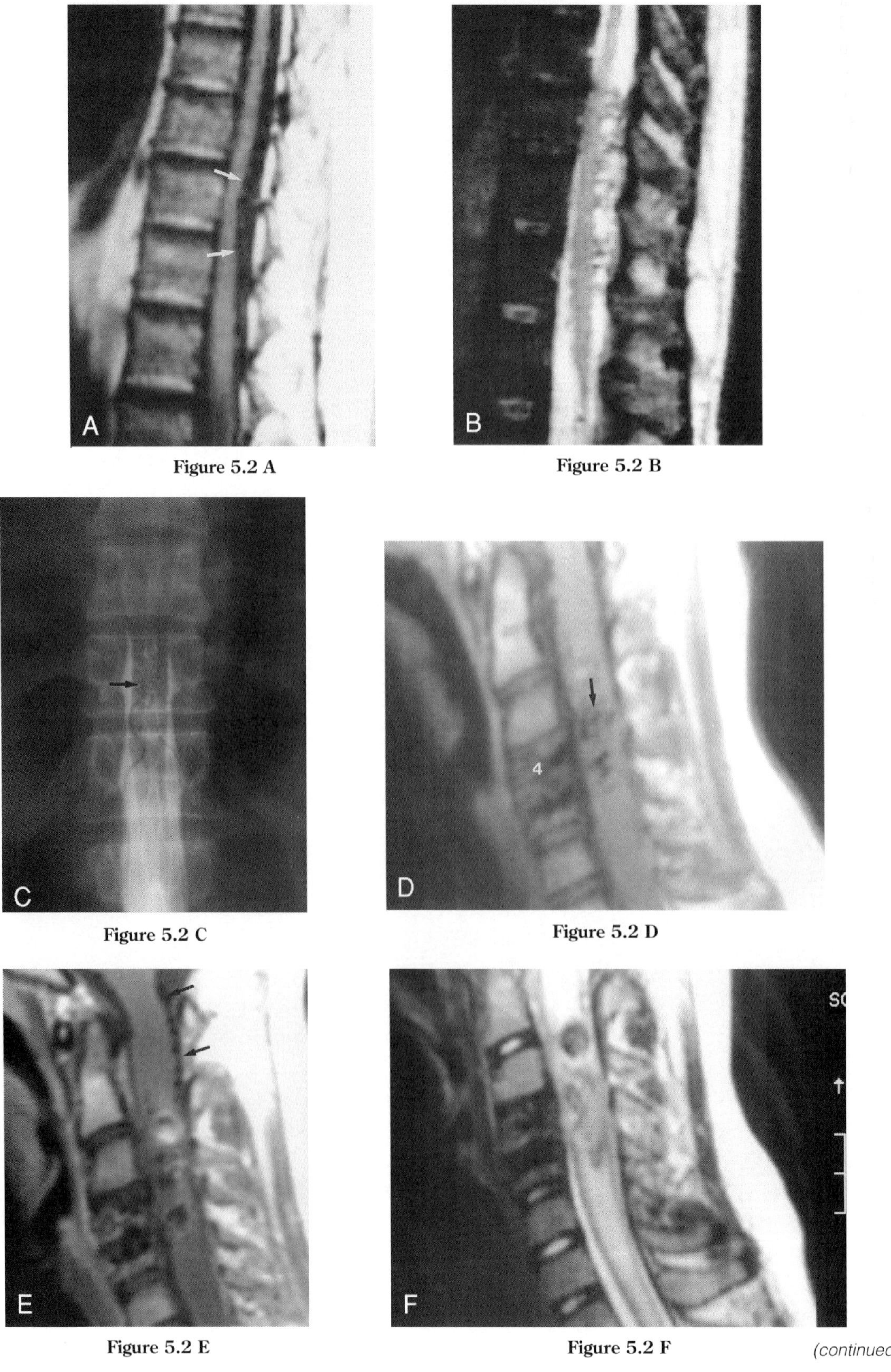

Figure 5.2 A

Figure 5.2 B

Figure 5.2 C

Figure 5.2 D

Figure 5.2 E

Figure 5.2 F

(continued)

Findings: Midsagittal noncontrast MR T1-weighted image (Fig. A) shows widening of the posterior subarachnoid space (arrows) from T9-T11. Corresponding T2-weighted image (Fig. B) shows serpiginous flow voids in the posterior subarachnoid space. Frontal radiograph (Fig. C) from a myelogram confirms tangled vessels (arrow) in the subarachnoid space. In the second patient, midsagittal MR T1-weighted image (Fig. D) shows areas of flow void (arrow) inside the spinal cord and abnormal low signal intensity in the C4 (4) vertebral body. Corresponding postcontrast T1-weighted image (Fig. E) shows some enhancement of the spinal cord lesion and of C4. Note large draining vessel (arrows) on the dorsal surface of the spinal cord. Corresponding T2-weighted image (Fig. F) shows that the intramedullary lesion is of low signal intensity as is the lesion involving C4. Note increased signal intensity of the spinal cord neighboring the lesion.

Diagnosis: Spinal cord arteriovenous malformations (AVM). The second patient has a malformation of the metameric type.

Discussion: Spinal cord AVMs are rare and comprise less than 2% of all space-occupying lesions of the spine. They are congenital in nature and generally present between 20–60 years of age. They are more common in males. The most common clinical symptoms are progressive compression of the spinal cord, radiculopathies, sphincter dysfunction, impotence, and abnormal sensation and weakness in the lower extremities. Some patients may present with the Foix–Alajouanine syndrome which is caused by a subacute necrotizing myelitis generally associated with thrombosis of spinal cord AVMs. This syndrome is characterized by progressive paresis and carries a poor prognosis. These malformations may hemorrhage and the patients present with subarachnoid hemorrhage or hematomyelia (which has a 20–30% mortality). The imaging method of choice to screen these patients is MR. It clearly shows the abnormal vessels as well as intramedullary pathology. The spinal cord may contain cysts. Angiography is the gold standard before therapy is attempted. Type 1 malformations are glomus-like and are fed by one or more arteries. Type 2 malformations (juvenile) are mass-like and are fed by innumerable arteries. Type 3 (metameric) involves not only the spinal cord but also the adjacent vertebra and paraspinal soft tissues. Some patients with metameric AVMs show cutaneous angiomatosis. Most type 2 AVMs are found in the cervical spine. Many believe that embolization should be the first line of treatment. The risk of permanent complications is small (6%), and more than one-half of patients report amelioration of their symptoms. Because many of these AVMs recur, some authors prefer surgical treatment even after successful embolization. MR angiography, predominantly using phase-contrast techniques, may demonstrate these malformations.

CASE 3

Clinical History: This lesion was incidentally found during a work-up for back pain.

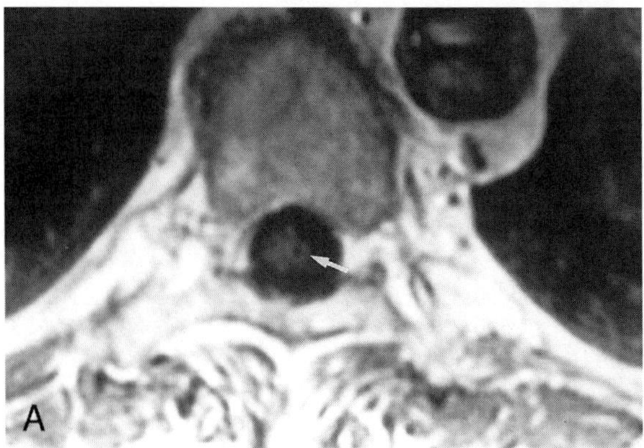

Figure 5.3 A

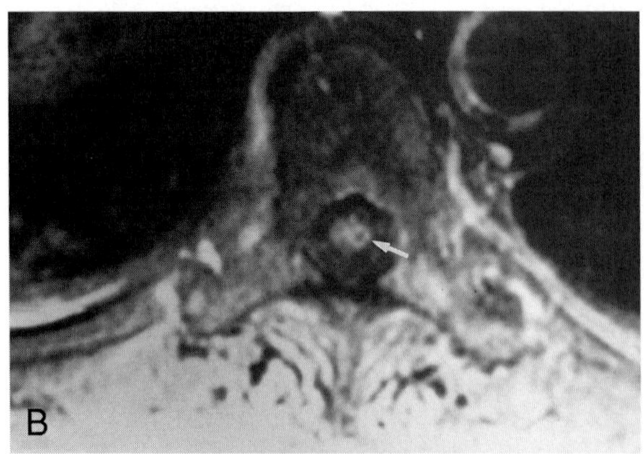

Figure 5.3 B

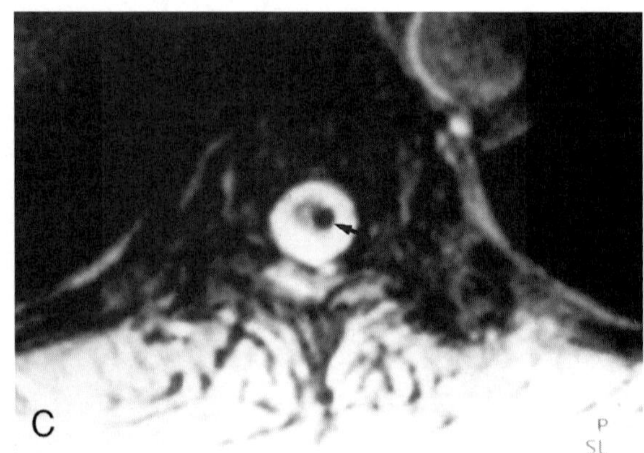

Figure 5.3 C

Findings: Axial MR noncontrast T1-weighted image (Fig. A) shows a focal lesion (arrow) of low signal intensity in the lower thoracic spinal cord. Corresponding postcontrast T1-weighted image (Fig. B) shows some mild and peripheral enhancement of the lesion (arrow). Corresponding T2*-weighted image (Fig. C) shows the lesion (arrow) to be of low signal intensity. Note "blooming" of the lesion, suggesting calcification or old blood products.

Differential Diagnosis: Spinal cord arteriovenous malformation, spinal cord cavernous angioma (presumed).

Diagnosis: Spinal cord cavernous angioma (presumed).

Discussion: Spinal cord cavernous hemangiomas are rare and their exact incidence is not known. They are said to comprise between 5–10% of all spinal cord vascular malformations. Histologically, they are composed of dilated vascular sinusoids devoid of smooth muscle and elastic fibers. There are no normal intervening neural tissues and there is abundant surrounding hemosiderin deposition. These malformations are confined to the spinal cord. Common clinical symptoms include progressive paraparesis, sensory abnormalities, pain, and occasionally hematomyelia and subarachnoid hemorrhage. However, some patients may be asymptomatic if the lesion is small. Myelography and postmyelography CT show only mild expansion of the spinal cord. At times, CT may show intramedullary calcifications. MR is the imaging method of choice. They are hypointense on both T1- and T2-weighted sequences. Their hypointensity is augmented on gradient echo imaging, reflecting the presence of magnetic susceptibility from hemosiderin. Minimal enhancement after contrast administration may be seen. Surgical resection is the method of choice.

CASE 4

Clinical History: You are shown three patients. The first (Figs. A and B) woke up unable to move the lower extremities after surgery for an abdominal aorta aneurysm. The second (Figs. C–E) presents with sudden onset of lower extremity paresis. The third (Fig. F) is a child paraplegic after being involved in a car accident.

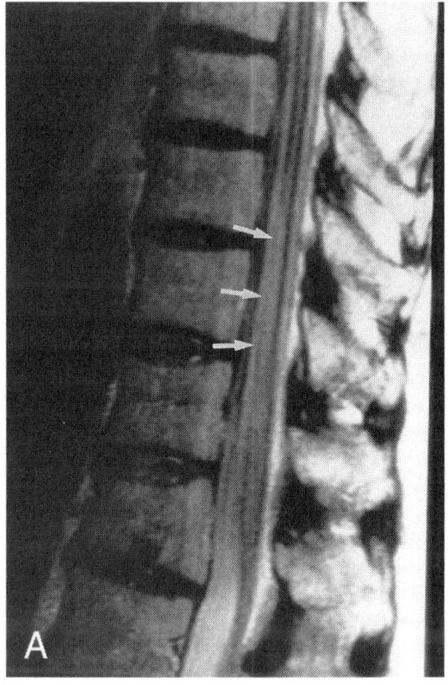

Figure 5.4 A

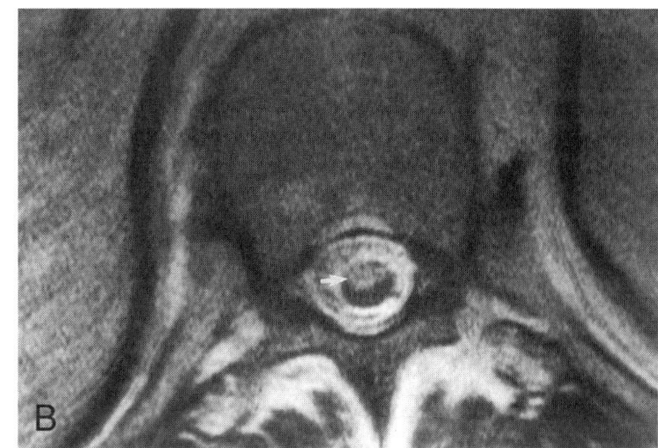

Figure 5.4 B

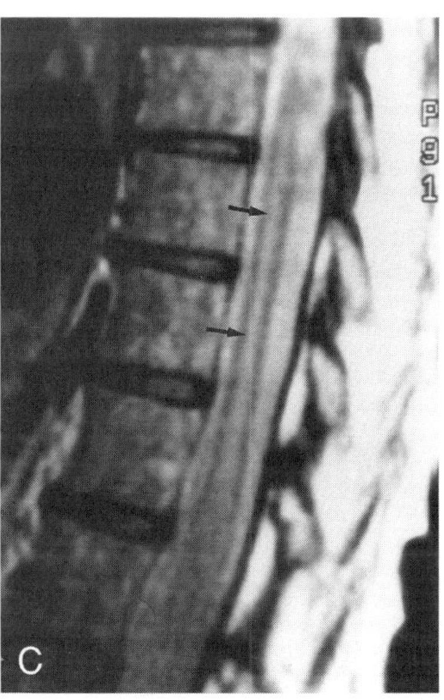

Figure 5.4 C

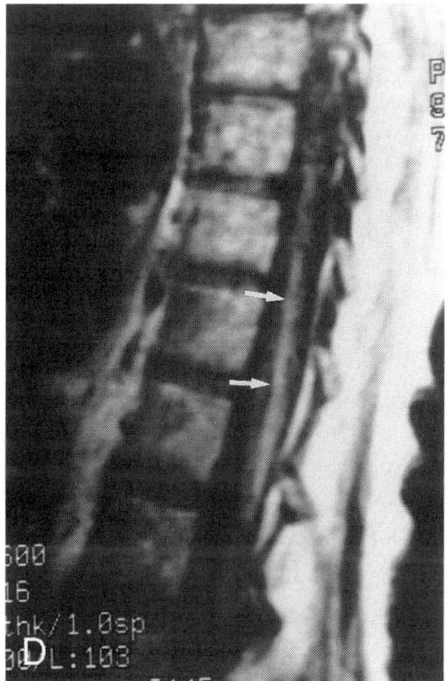

Figure 5.4 D

(continued)

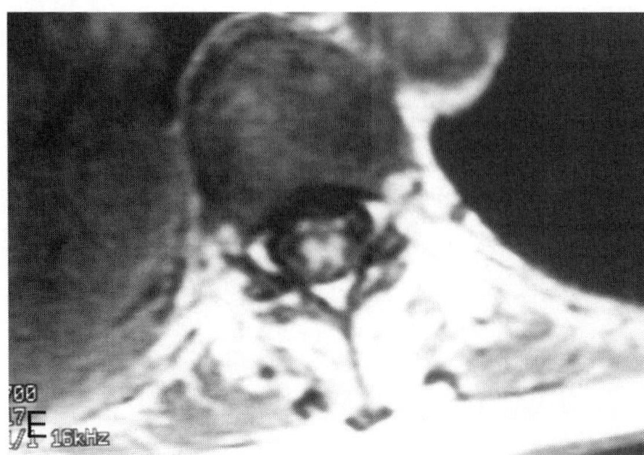

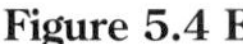

Figure 5.4 E

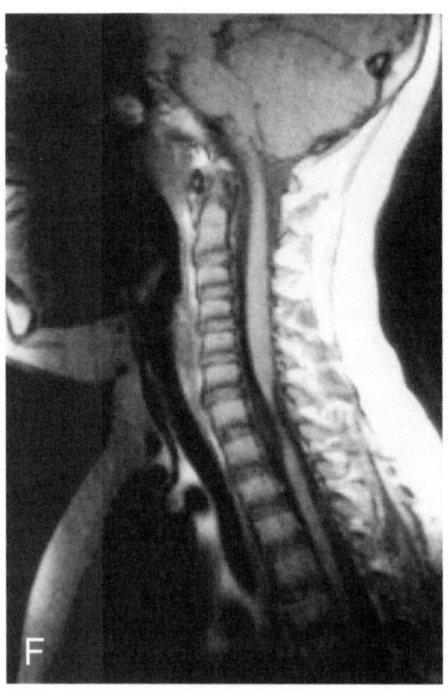

Figure 5.4 F

Findings: Midsagittal proton density MR image (Fig. A) shows increased signal intensity (arrows) in the ventral aspect of the distal spinal cord. Axial MR T2-weighted image (Fig. B) confirms that the signal abnormality (arrow) is confined to the anterior two-thirds of the spinal cord. In the second case, midsagittal MR proton density image (Fig. C) shows increased and abnormal signal intensity (arrows) in the lower spinal cord. Corresponding postcontrast T1-weighted image (Fig. D) shows enhancement (arrows) of the abnormality. Axial postcontrast T1-weighted image (Fig. E) shows enhancement of the gray matter within the spinal cord. In the third patient, midsagittal MR T1-weighted image (Fig. F) shows severe atrophy of the spinal cord at C7-T2 levels.

Diagnosis: Acute spinal cord infarctions (first and second cases) and chronic sequela of spinal cord infarction (third case).

Discussion: Spinal cord infarctions are rare and mostly occur in patients with hypertension, diabetes, trauma, sickle cell disease, Caisson disease, and atherosclerosis. They may also follow surgery for treatment of aortic aneurysm and hypotensive events. Most patients are over 60 years of age and there is no gender predilection. The patients generally present with acute onset of paraplegia and bowel and bladder dysfunction. Most spinal cord infarctions are secondary to occlusion of the largest anterior spinal artery (artery of Adamkiewicz). Dissecting aortic aneurysms with left-sided false lumen may lead to occlusion of this artery which most commonly arises on the left from T8 to L4. Venous infarctions may also occur and their onset is insidious. Venous infarctions are associated with arteriovenous fistulas, hypercoagulable states, and fibrocartilaginous emboli. These infarctions present with symptoms identical to those found in patients with subacute necrotizing myelopathy (Foix-Alajouanine syndrome). The anterior spinal artery supplies most of the cord's gray matter and the anterior two thirds of its cross section. Occlusion of this artery produces abnormalities which are more prominent at the level of the distal portions of the perforating branches. Therefore, the gray matter is first affected. In addition, the gray matter is more vulnerable to ischemia because it is relatively hypermetabolic when compared to the spinal cord white matter. MR is the imaging method of choice. On T1 weighted images the involved cord may thicken and show subtle hyperintense or hypointense regions. The anterior 2/3's of the spinal cord may be bright on T2 weighted images. These regions may enhance after contrast administration. Enhancement may be more prominent in the swollen gray matter resulting in the so-called "owl eyes" appearance on axial postcontrast T1-weighted images. The imaging features of spinal cord infarction are quite typical excluding other etiologies for the patients symptoms. In cases of chronic spinal cord infarctions, there is severe atrophy of the spinal cord. In children, the cervico-thoracic is a watershed region and is specially vulnerable to ischemia. This ischemia may follow traumatic breech deliveries or other types of injuries.

CASE 5

Clinical History: 12-year-old boy with a 6-month history of back pain, lower extremity weakness, and bowel/bladder dysfunction.

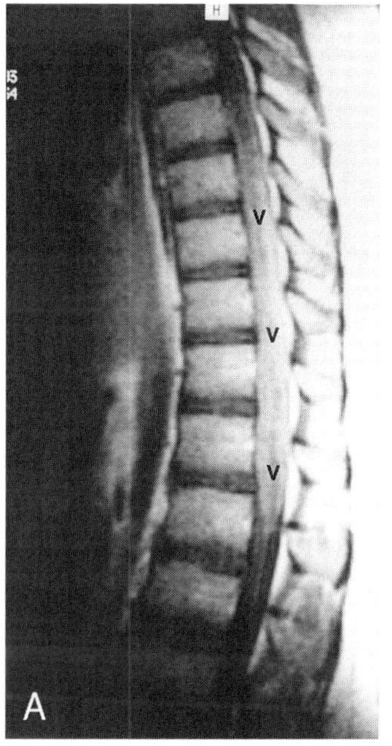

Figure 5.5 A

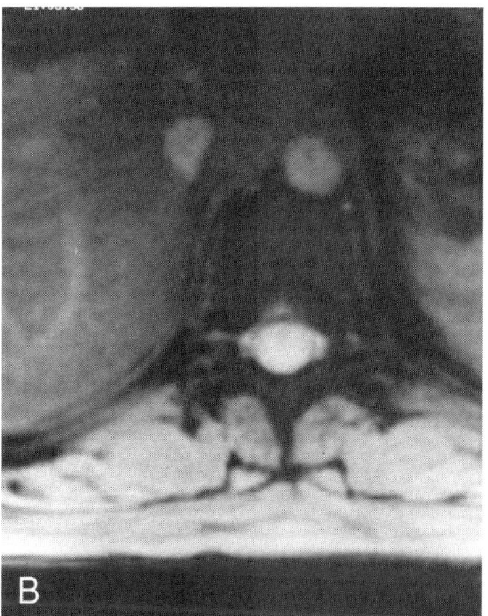

Figure 5.5 B

Findings: Midsagittal postcontrast MR T1-weighted image (Fig. A) shows diffuse and marked enhancement (V) of the thoracic spinal cord which is also expanded. Axial MR T2-weighted image (Fig. B) shows that the spinal cord is diffusely hyperintense and is swollen. (Case courtesy S.K. Mukherji, M.D., Chapel Hill, NC.)

Diagnosis: Vasculitis (granulomatous angiitis) involving the spinal cord.

Discussion: Vasculitis involving the spinal cord is relatively rare and generally occurs in the presence of involvement of the brain. Isolated vasculitis to the spinal cord is very rare. Vasculitis that can involve the spinal cord includes granulomatous angitis, antiphospholipid syndrome, scleroderma, Sjögren disease, polyarteritis nodosa, and rheumatoid arthritis. Infectious causes include the human immunodeficiency virus (HIV), tuberculosis, and cytomegalovirus. Chagas disease may also result in a vasculitis which may involve the spinal cord. Sarcoidosis may result in direct infiltration of the spinal cord or in a vasculitis. Rhabdomyolysis and paraneoplastic syndromes may affect the spinal cord in an identical fashion to a vasculitis. Granulomatous angitis is a rare disorder which may be primary or occur in association with lymphoma, sarcoidosis, herpes virus infections, and HIV. Patients with spinal cord involvement present with back pain, progressive myelopathy, elevated proteins in cerebrospinal fluid, and a normal sedimentation rate. MR is the imaging method of choice for the evaluation of these patients. The findings are nonspecific and include increased T2 signal intensity and widening of the spinal cord. Generally, there is no enhancement after contrast administration. The correct diagnosis requires biopsy. Treatment with steroids or cytotoxic drugs may lead to rapid stabilization or disappearance of the symptoms. The long-term prognosis of these patients is uncertain.

Clinical History: Elderly patient who presents with acute upper lumbar spine pain.

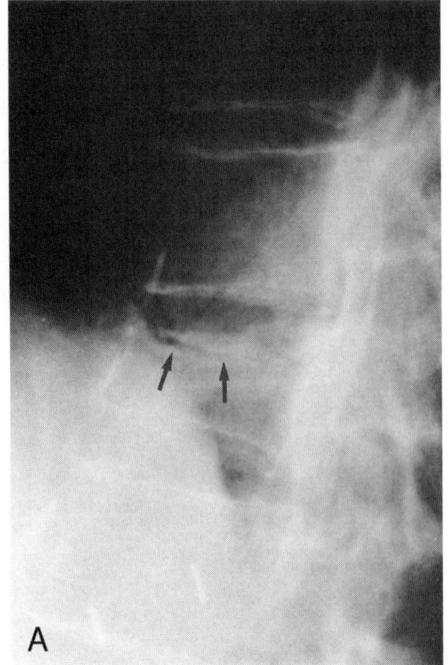

Figure 5.6 A

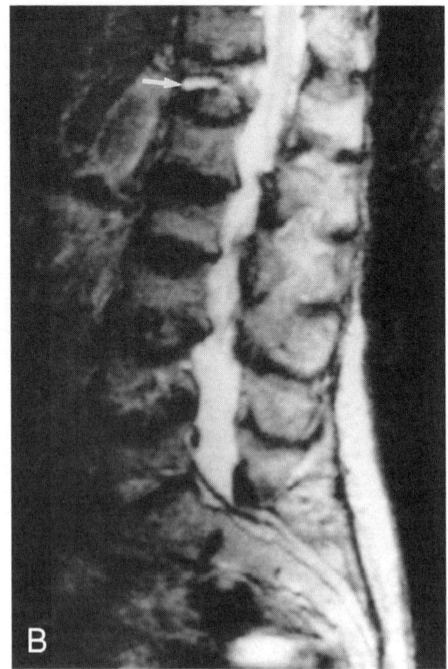

Figure 5.6 B

Findings: Lateral radiograph (Fig. A) shows a partially collapsed T12 vertebral body containing a cleft (arrows) filled with gas. Midsagittal MR T2-weighted image (Fig. B) shows that the signal intensity of the affected vertebral body is low but that the cleft (arrow) is hyperintense.

Differential Diagnosis (For Gas in a Vertebral Body): Infection and Schmorl's nodes, aseptic necrosis of a vertebral body (Kummell disease).

Diagnosis: Aseptic necrosis of a vertebral body (Kummell disease).

Discussion: In this rare disease, an insult (generally trauma) results in a vascular injury which leads to aseptic necrosis and collapse of a vertebral body. This collapse may occur after a symptom-free period of months to years after the initial injury. Other underlying etiologies are pancreatitis, Gaucher disease, and the result of spinal angiography. Most patients are middle aged or older and there is no gender predilection. The most affected region is the lower thoracic and upper lumbar spine. Although generally only one vertebra is involved, collapse of several vertebrae has been documented. Radiographs usually demonstrate gas within a collapsed vertebral body. This gas may extend into the paraspinal soft tissues. The collapsed vertebra(e) may result in compression of the spinal cord. The vacuum (gas) cleft may be visible as low signal intensity on MR T1- and T2-weighted images. On T2-weighted images, the affected vertebra is generally of low signal intensity, a feature that distinguishes Kummell disease from collapse due to metastasis. With metastasis, the affected vertebra(e) is usually of high signal intensity. After contrast administration, enhancement may occur in Kummell disease.

Clinical History: This patient presented with sudden onset of mid-back pain and lower extremity weakness.

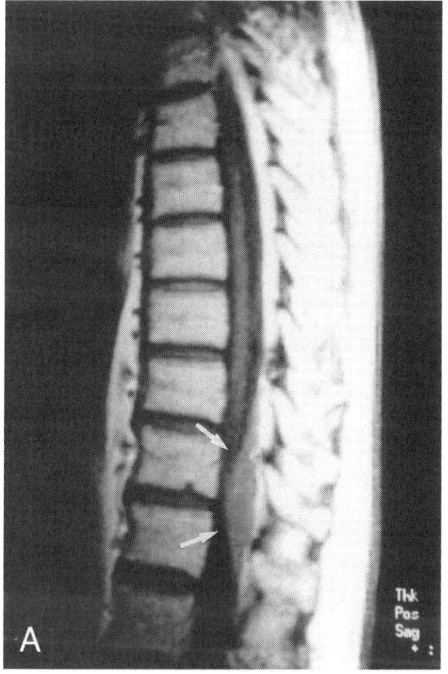

Figure 5.7 A

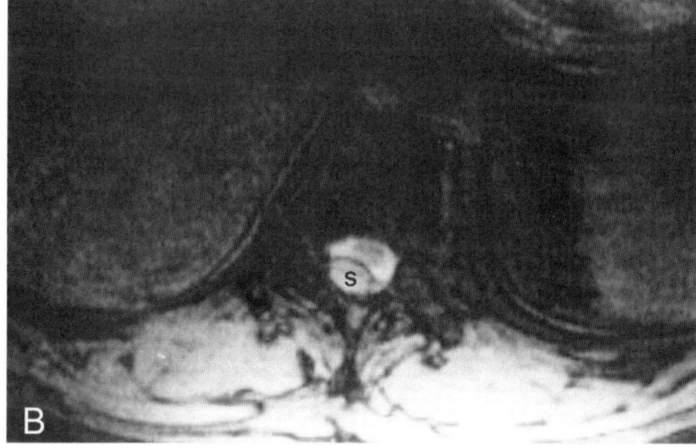

Figure 5.7 B

Findings: Midsagittal MR T1-weighted image (Fig. A) shows a dural-based abnormality (arrows) of intermediate signal intensity. The lesion did not enhance after contrast administration. Axial T2-weighted image (Fig. B) shows the extramedullary abnormality (S) to be of high signal intensity.

Differential Diagnosis: Epidural hematoma, spinal subdural hematoma (surgically proven).

Diagnosis: Spinal subdural hematoma (surgically proven).

Discussion: Acute spinal subdural hematomas are much less common than epidural ones (see Case #8). Spinal subdural hematomas may, however, expand rapidly, resulting in acute symptoms caused by compression of the spinal cord. At times, the clinical course of these hematomas may be insidious. The most common predisposing etiologies include coagulopathies and trauma. Because these hematomas occur deep to the dura, correct preoperative localization informs the surgeon of the need to open the dura to adequately drain the collection. These hematomas are more common in the dorsal and lateral aspects of the spinal canal (but may also be circumferential) and may involve the cervical or thoracic regions or the entire length of the spine. By CT, subdural hematomas are seen as areas of increased density abutting the bone. Differentiating them from epidural hematomas may not be feasible using this imaging technique. MR is the imaging method of choice for the evaluation of these patients. The hematoma has a crescentic configuration and displaces the epidural fat away from it. It is of very low signal intensity on gradient echo images. It tends to involve long segments of the spine but occasionally may involve short lengths. Subarachnoid hematomas are uncommon in the spine because of the dynamic flow of cerebrospinal fluid which prevents their formation.

Clinical History: You are shown two patients. The first (Figs. A–C) was receiving warfarin sodium for deep venous thrombosis and presented with acute lumbar back pain and weakness in the lower extremities. The second (Figs D–F) presented with acute back pain.

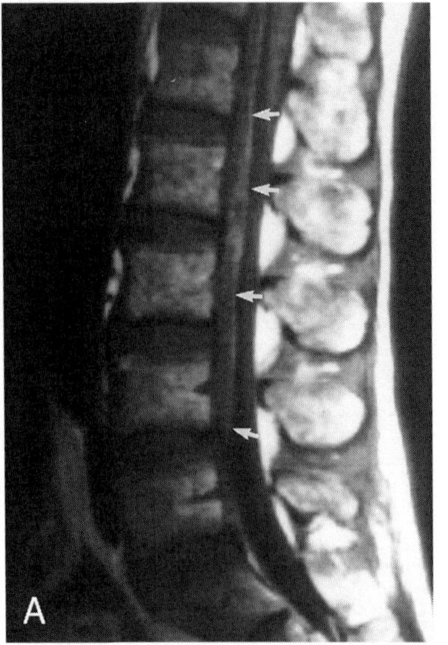

Figure 5.8 A

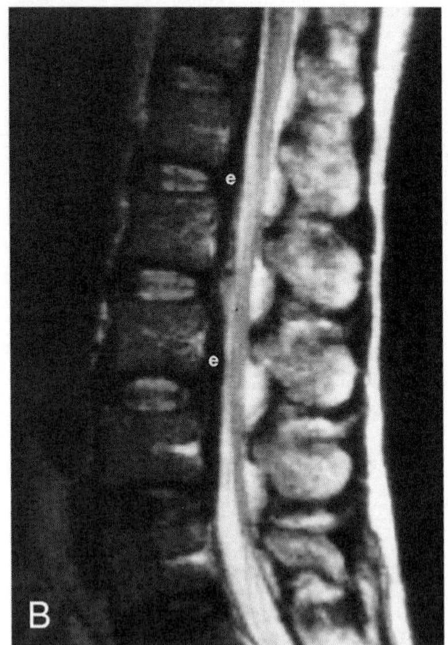

Figure 5.8 B

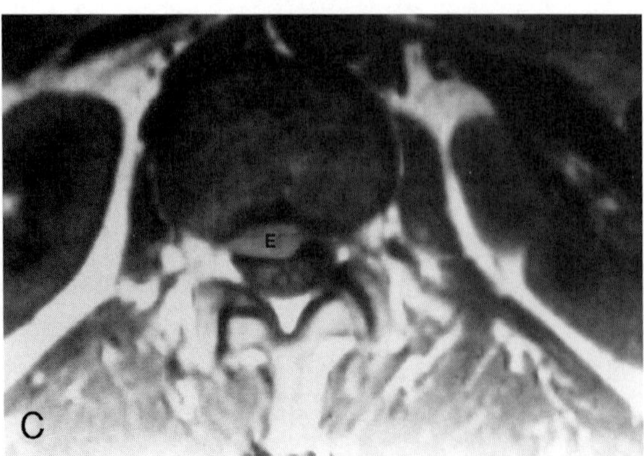

Figure 5.8 C

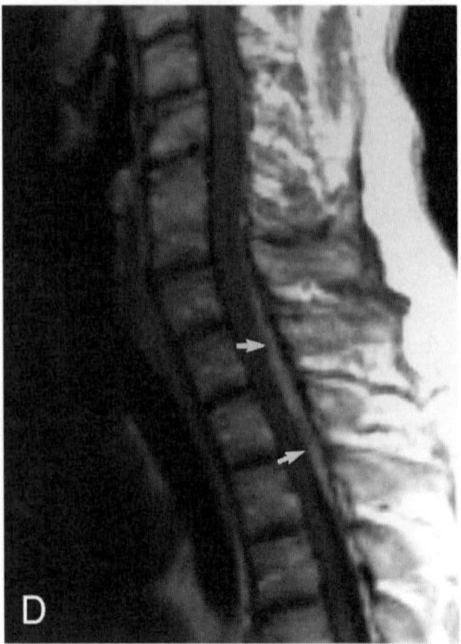

Figure 5.8 D

(continued)

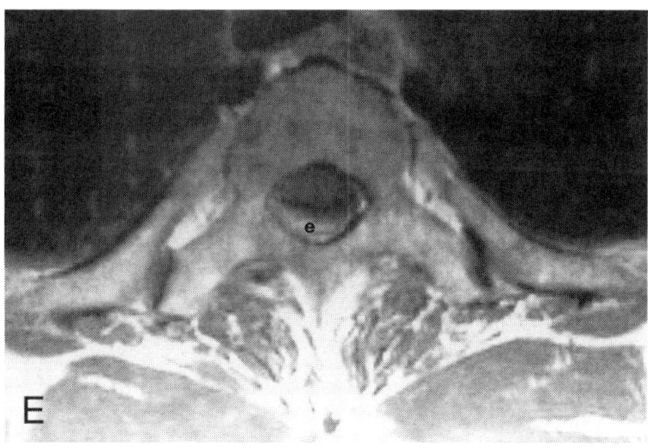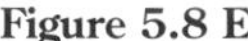

Figure 5.8 E

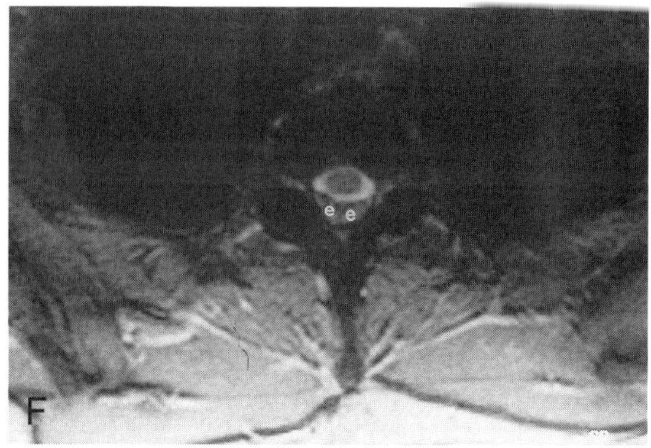

Figure 5.8 F

Findings: In the first patient, a midsagittal MR T1-weighted image (Fig. A) shows a lesion (arrows) of mixed signal intensity in the ventral epidural space extending throughout the lumbar spine. Corresponding T2-weighted image (Fig. B) shows the lesion (e) to be hypointense. Axial MR T1-weighted image (Fig. C) shows the extradural location of the lesion (e) which is of increased signal intensity. In the second patient, midsagittal MR T1-weighted image (Fig. D) shows the presence of an extradural linear (arrows) abnormality of increased signal intensity. Axial T1-weighted image (Fig. E) confirms that the bright lesion (e) is located outside of the spinal cord, which is slightly anteriorly displaced. Axial T2*-weighted image (Fig. F) shows a bilobed configuration of the hypointense lesion (e) suggesting its epidural location.

Differential Diagnosis: Subdural hematoma.

Diagnosis: Spinal epidural hematomas (surgically proven).

Discussion: Spontaneous spinal epidural hematomas are very uncommon. The estimated prevalence of this disease is 0.1 patient per 100,000 patients per year. This disease is slightly more common in males age 40–60 years. In more than one-half of patients, an etiology is never found. Predisposing factors include coagulopathies, trauma, spinal puncture, arteriovenous malformations, hemangiomas, hypertension, pregnancy, old age, infection, spinal surgery, forceful sneezing, and lupus erythematosus. The source of bleeding is generally a lacerated venous epidural plexus. Most patients with spinal epidural hematomas present with acute onset of symptoms, including pain and compressive myelopathy. Spinal epidural hematomas are more common in the thoracic region, particularly along the dorsal and lateral aspects of the spinal canal. In the lumbar spine, posterior epidural hematomas are commonly the result of lumbar punctures in patients with associated coagulopathies. However, epidural hematomas may be located ventrally and simulate herniated disks (see Case #12, Chapter 1). MR is the imaging method of choice in these patients. Acutely, on T1-weighted images, the hematoma is isointense to the spinal cord. On T2-weighted images it is bright. On gradient echo images, the acute hematoma is of low signal intensity. In the subacute period, the signal intensity becomes high on both T1- and T2-weighted images. They tend to have a convex border projecting into the spinal canal and completely obliterate the epidural fat, a finding that distinguishes them from spinal subdural hematoma (see Case #7). They tend to be short. Surgical decompression may be indicated.

CASE 9

Clinical History: African-American patient with a systemic disorder who suffers from periodic pain in the bones.

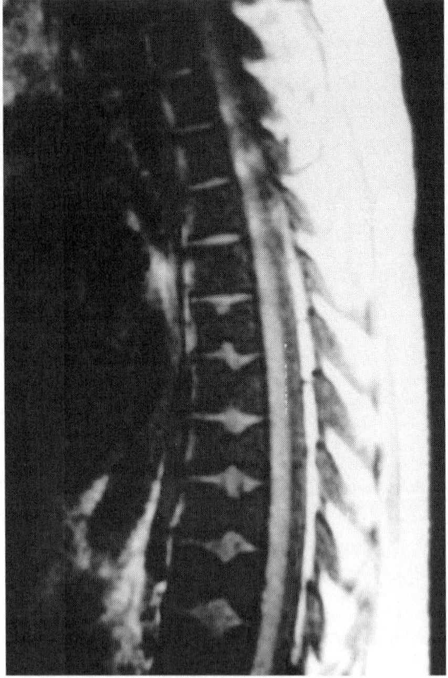

Figure 5.9

Findings: Midsagittal MR T1-weighted image shows low signal intensity in the bone marrow of all vertebrae and depression of the mid aspect of end-plates, particularly in the mid- to lower thoracic region.

Diagnosis: Sickle cell anemia.

Discussion: As a response to the long duration of the anemia, there is hypercellularity of the bone marrow in patients with this disease. The bone marrow spaces may be widened and the cortices of those bones thinned. On radiographs, there may be accentuation of the secondary trabeculae. There are infarctions involving the vertebral end-plates, which lead to their central depression. This results in so-called "H-shaped" or "fish" vertebrae on radiographs. Intraosseous herniation of the intervertebral disks (Schmorl's nodes) may also be responsible for these vertebral abnormalities. On radiographs, the vertebrae may show increased density. Osteomyelitis and diskitis may also occur in these patients.

chapter 6

TRAUMATIC INJURIES

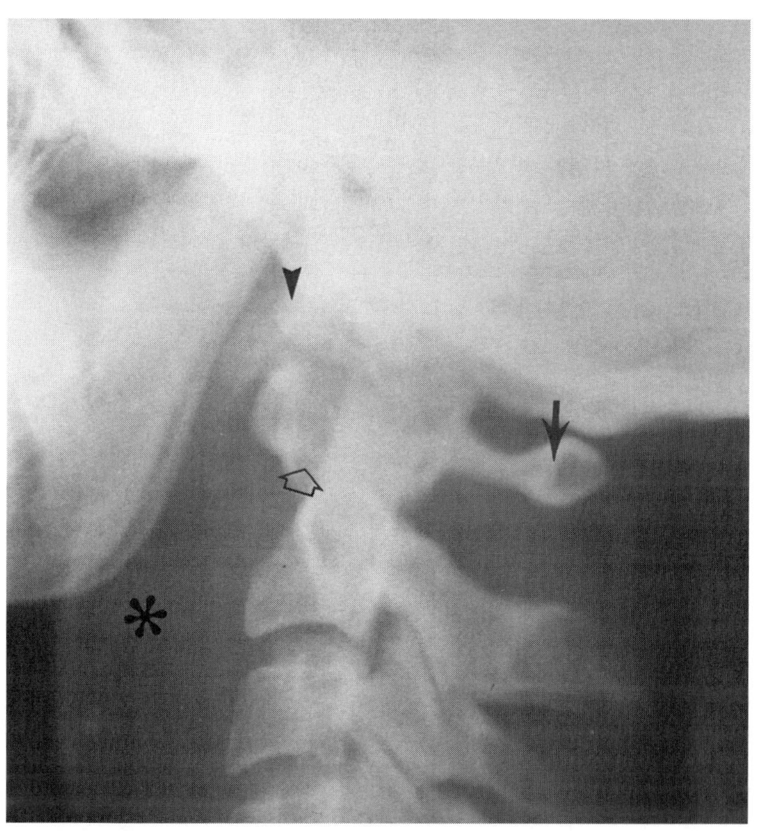

CASE 1

Case History: This patient was ejected from an automobile. She had an ISS (injury severity score) of 17 and GCS (Glasgow-coma score) of 3. You are shown lateral radiographs of her cervicocranium (Figs. A, B) and a lateral radiograph (Fig. C) of a non-trauma patient, which demonstrates a normal cervicocranial prevertebral soft tissue contour and a normal occipito-atlantal relationship.

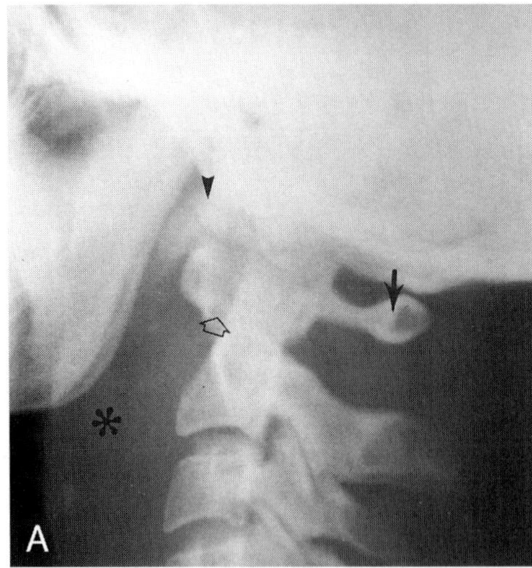

Figure 6.1 A

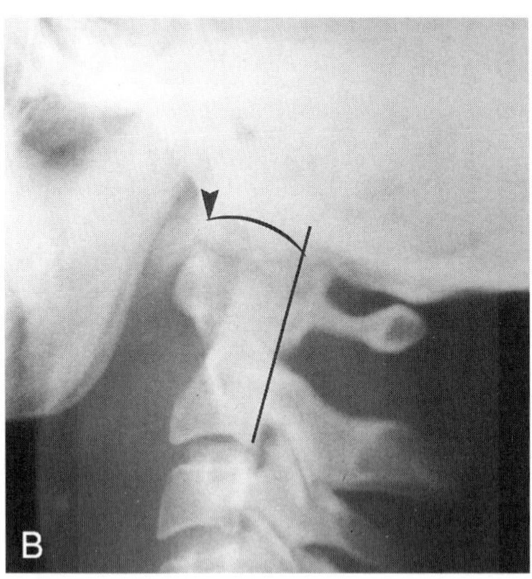

Figure 6.1 B

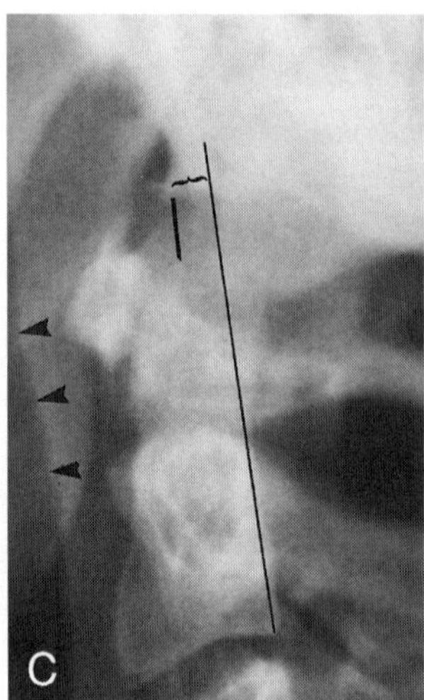

Figure 6.1 C

Findings: Lateral radiograph of the cervicocranium (Fig. A) shows marked cervicocranial prevertebral soft tissue swelling (asterisk). Although relatively underexposed, it is possible to recognize that the anterior atlantodental interval (open arrow) is wide, the spinolaminar line of C1 (arrow) is anterior to the arch of the posterior spinal line, and the basion (arrowhead) is abnormally situated with respect to C2.

Differential Diagnosis: Occipitoatlantal dislocation; occipitoatlantal subluxation.

Diagnosis: Occipitoatlantal subluxation.

Discussion: Occipitoatlantal subluxation (OAS) is a partial dislocation of the occipitoatlantal articulations. It is much less common and its radiographic signs are less obvious than the occipitoatlantal dislocation (OAD). Most patients with OAD die at, or shortly following, the injury, whereas the majority of patients with OAS survive and with either no, or relatively minor, neurologic deficits.

The traditional methods proposed to identify occipitoatlantal articulation injury include the Power ratio and the "X" line of Lee. Each is dependent upon a recognizable opisthion and a spinolaminar line of C1. The opisthion may not be identifiable in as many as 47% of patients, and failure of fusion of the posterior arch of C1 is a less frequent variant, precluding the use of these methods.

The basion-axial interval (BAI), the distance between the basion and the upward extension of the posterior axial line (long line), is an easy and reliable method of assessing the occipitoatlantal relationship in patients of all ages. The basion-dental interval (BDI), the distance between the basion and the tip of the dens, is reliable in patients 12 years of age or older. Normally, neither the BAI nor the BDI should exceed 12 mm as determined on a lateral radiograph of the cervicocranium obtained at a target film distance of 1 meter. In the case presented, the BAI exceeds 12 mm (Fig. B, arrowhead to solid line). Fig. C shows the normal BAI (—), BDI (short line), each being less than 12 mm, and a normal contour of the cervico-cranial prevertebral soft tissues (arrowheads).

Widening of the anterior atlantodental space greater than 3 mm in adults indicates disruption of the transverse atlantal ligament, which is not an integral component of occipitoatlantal dissociation. The diffuse prevertebral soft tissue swelling represents hemorrhage into the retropharyngeal soft tissues from, in this instance, both the OAS and rupture of the transverse atlantal ligament.

On a lateral radiograph, occipitoatlantal dislocation is characterized by frank dislocation of the occipital condyles with respect to the superior articulating facets of the lateral masses of C1. The dislocation, like the subluxation, may be directly anterior, distracted, anterior and distracted, and rarely posterior.

CASE 2

Case History: This adult patient was involved in a motor vehicle accident in which her head was thrown into severe hyperextension. She complained of severe pain at the base of the skull and had marked tenderness to palpation. She had no neurologic signs or symptoms. You are shown two lateral radiographs of the cervicocranium (Figs. A, B) and two axial post-myelogram CT images of C1 (Figs. C, D).

Findings: Fig. A shows a faint vertical lucent defect in the inferior cortex in each side of the posterior arch of C1 (arrowheads). Additionally, the dorsal portion of the posterior arch of C1 is angled caudally. Fig. B shows a fracture of the superior cortex of one side of the posterior arch of C1 (arrowhead). Figs. C and D demonstrate minimally displaced fractures of the right (Fig. C) and left (Fig. D) sides of the posterior arch of C1 (arrows). The anterior arch of C1 is intact (Fig. D).

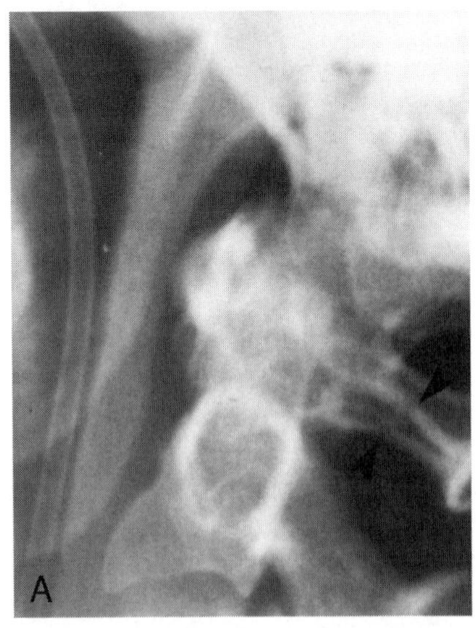

Figure 6.2 A

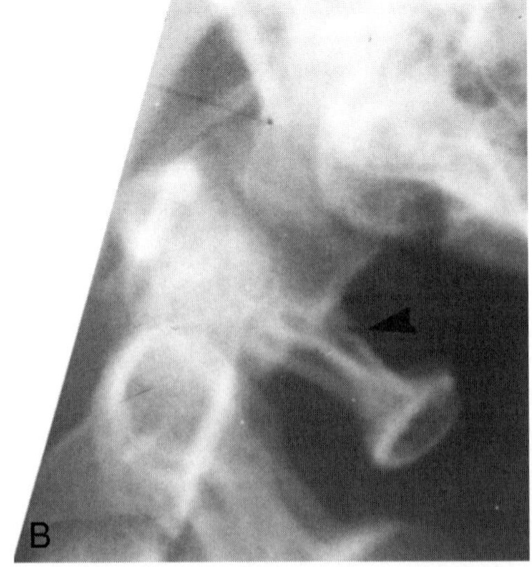

Figure 6.2 B

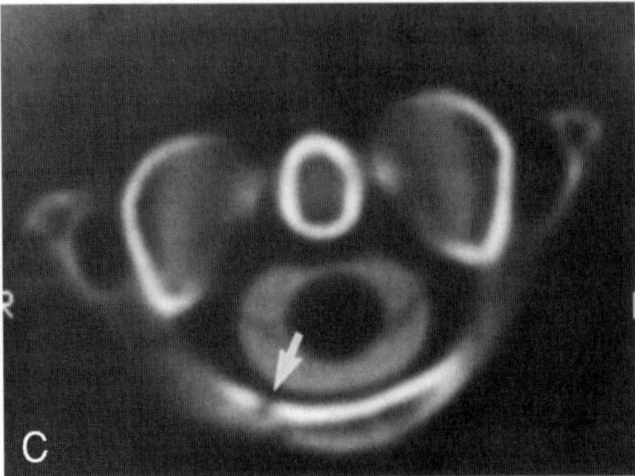

Figure 6.2 C

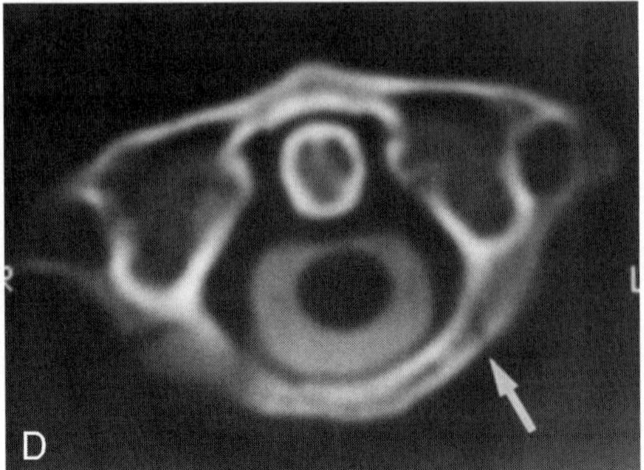

Figure 6.2 D

Differential Diagnosis: Jefferson bursting fracture; isolated fracture, posterior arch, C1.

Diagnosis: Isolated fracture, posterior arch, C1.

Discussion: Isolated fracture of the posterior arch of C1 is one of the family of cervical spine injuries caused by hyperextension during which the posterior arch of C1 is crushed between the occipital bone and the spinous process of C2. This injury usually occurs as a single fracture but has been seen in association with extension teardrop fracture of C2 and traumatic spondylolisthesis of C2, either individually or in concert.

The only differential diagnosis is the Jefferson bursting fracture (JBF). Both JBF and isolated fracture of the posterior arch of C1 have fracture(s) of the posterior arch of C1. Identification of the Jefferson bursting fracture of C1 rests upon demonstration of secondary evidence of an anterior arch of C1 fracture (lateral displacement of the lateral masses of C1 on an open-mouth projection) or by direct evidence of an anterior arch fracture of C1 by axial CT. The absence of the latter, as shown in Figs. C and D, indicates that this patient has an isolated fracture of the posterior arch of C1.

CASE 3

Case History: This adult complained of severe pain in the upper cervical area after a motor vehicle accident.

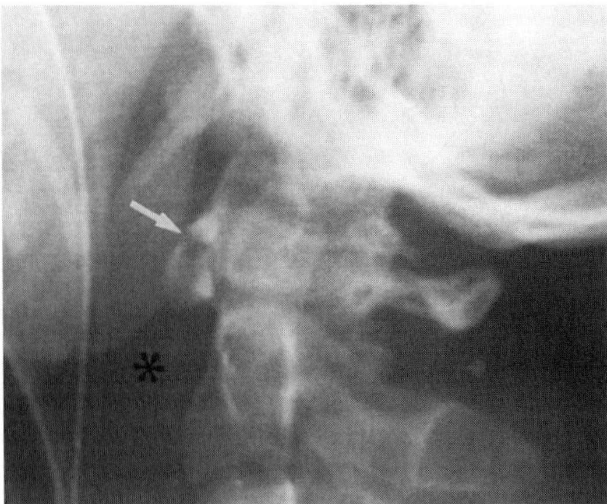

Figure 6.3

Findings: Lateral radiograph of the cervicocranium shows a transverse defect (arrow) with irregular, non-sclerotic margins in the anterior tubercle of C1. Prevertebral soft tissue swelling (asterisk) is reflected by the anterior displacement of the nasogastric tube.

Differential Diagnosis: Ununited secondary ossification center of the anterior tubercle of C1; acute avulsion fracture of the anterior tubercle of C1.

Diagnosis: Acute avulsion fracture, anterior arch of C1.

Discussion: Acute avulsion of the anterior tubercle (arch) of C1 is one of the family of predominant hyperextension injuries of the cervical spine. The fracture results from a traction force applied to anterior arch of C1 through the intact fibers of atlantoaxial ligament (rostral extension of the anterior longitudinal ligament). The fracture commonly involves not only the anterior tubercle, but also the anterior arch which, because of its posterior-lateral extension from the tubercle to the lateral masses is obscured by the superimposed lateral masses. Consequently, the only portion of this fracture that is visible on the lateral cervical radiograph is that involving the anterior tubercle. This fracture usually involves the inferior pole of the anterior tubercle, but can involve the mid portion or, as in this instance, the superior portion. The history of an acute injury, the radiograph characteristics of the margins of the defect, and the signs of cervicocranial prevertebral soft tissue swelling all indicate an acute fracture. CT or MR imaging will confirm the diagnosis, if necessary.

Smooth, faintly sclerotic margins of an anterior tubercle defect with normal cervicocranial prevertebral soft tissue contour are consistent with an ununited secondary ossification center or, less likely, an old ununited avulsion fracture.

CASE 4

Case History: You are shown the lateral radiograph of the cervicocranium (Fig. A) and the "open-mouth" radiograph (Fig. B) of one patient, the lateral radiograph (Fig. C) and axial CT images (Fig. D) of the cervicocranium of a second patient, both of whom sustained major trauma to the top of the head in different roll-over motor vehicle accidents. Both patients complained of severe upper neck pain and limitation of motion at the base of the skull. Fig. E is from a normal individual and is offered for comparison purposes.

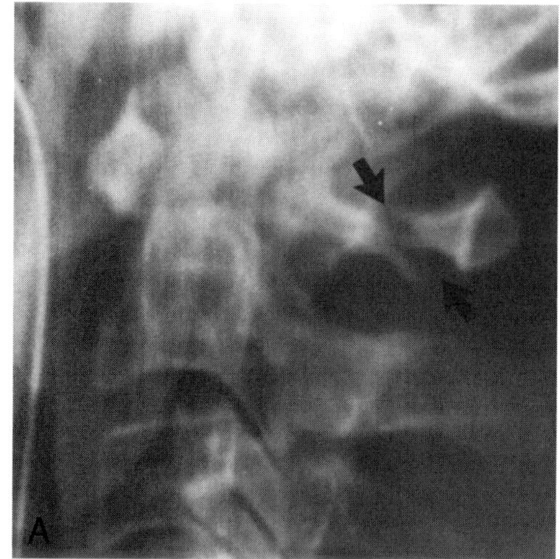

Figure 6.4 A

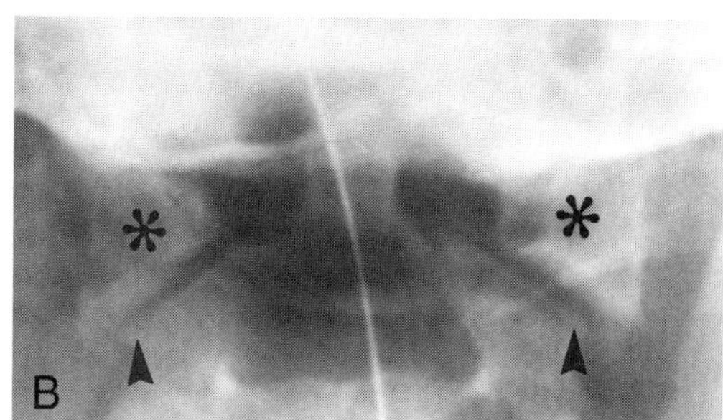

Figure 6.4 B

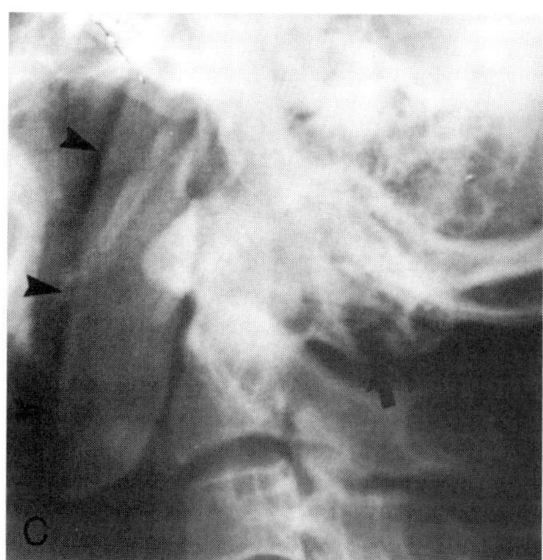

Figure 6.4 C

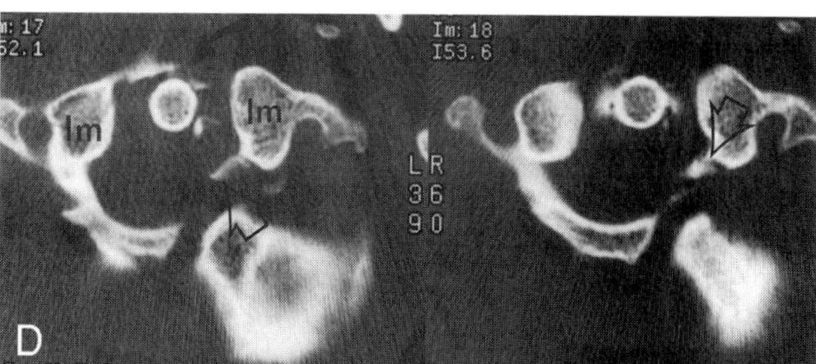

Figure 6.4 D

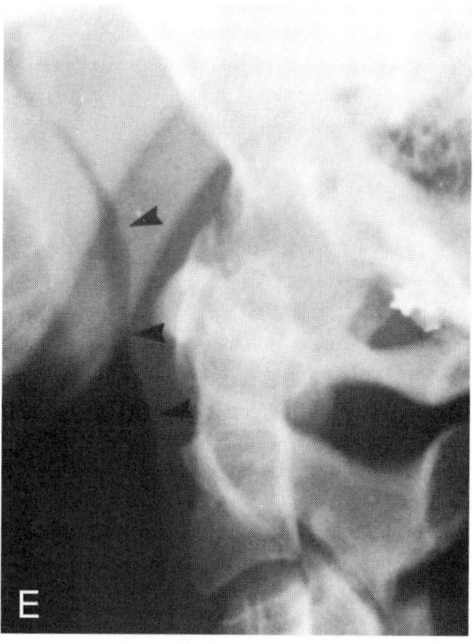

Figure 6.4 E

Findings: Fig. A shows a fracture of the posterior arch of C1 (arrows). The presence of the nasogastric tube precludes evaluation of the cervicocranial prevertebral soft tissue (CCPVST) contour. The "open mouth" radiograph (Fig. B) shows bilateral displacement of the lateral masses of C1 (asterisks) with respect to the dens and to the superior facets of C2 (arrowheads).

Lateral radiograph of the cervicocranium of the second patient (Fig. C) shows fractures of the posterior arch of C1 (arrow) and a grossly abnormal CCPVST shadow in that, not only is it much wider than normal but, and more importantly, its air-soft tissue interface is anteriorly convex (arrowheads). (An example of the normal CCPVST contour is seen in Fig. E, arrowheads.) The axial CT images (Fig. D) show a fracture of the left anterior (curved arrow) and the posterior (open arrows) arches of C1 as well as bilateral lateral displacement of the lateral masses (lm) of C1 with respect to the dens.

Diagnosis: Jefferson bursting fracture (JBF).

Discussion: The JBF is one of the two injuries of the cervical spine caused by "axial-loading" or vertical compression MECHANISM OF INJURY. By definition, the JBF is limited to the axis vertebra. The injuring force, usually applied to the vertex of the skull, is transmitted to the convex occipital condyles which are seated in the bi-concave superior articulating surface of the lateral masses of C1. Consequently, the force to the occipital condyles drives the lateral masses of C1 laterally, resulting in fractures of the anterior and posterior arches of C1. Jefferson's original description of this injury postulated a fracture of each side of both the anterior and posterior arches of C1. However, CT has demonstrated, as in Fig. D, that only unilateral fracture of both the anterior and posterior arches is sufficient to produce a JBF. As in Fig. B, the lateral displacement of the lateral masses may be symmetrical or, if the impacting force is excentrically oriented, lateral mass displacement may asymmetrical with the side of greatest displacement of the lateral mass reflecting the direction of excentric force. JBF is frequently associated with concomitant fractures of an occipital condyle, particularly on the side of greatest impact between the occipital condyle and the lateral mass of C1. When lateral mass displacement is sufficiently great, the transverse atlantal ligament is torn, resulting in antero-posterior instability at the atlanto-axial level.

When the axial loading force to the cervical spine spares the atlas, the force is transmitted to the lower cervical spine and may result in a burst, bursting, or dispersion fracture.

CASE 5

Case History: This fireman fell from the second floor on to soft ground in such a way that his head and upper cervical spine were forced into hyperextension. He complained of severe pain, tenderness, and loss of motion in the upper cervical area, but had no neurologic signs or symptoms. You are shown a lateral radiograph of the cervicocranium (Fig. A) and axial CT images of C2 (Fig. B).

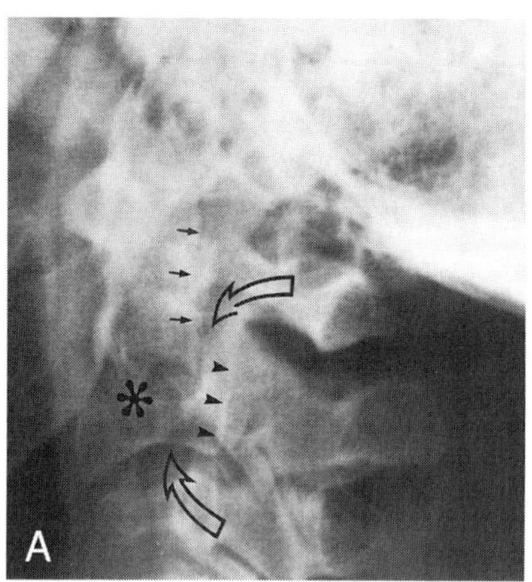

Figure 6.5 A

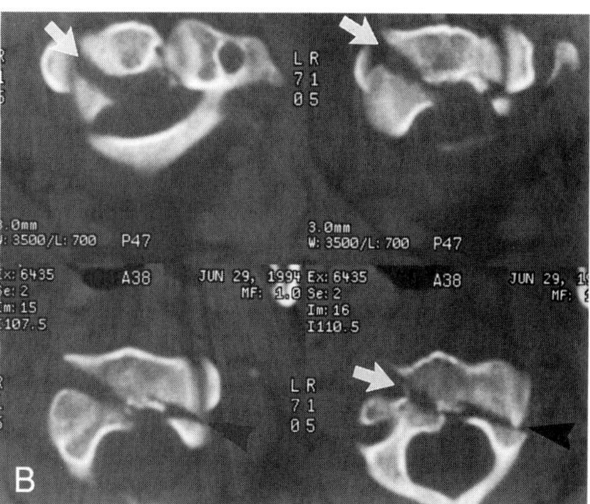

Figure 6.5 B

Findings: Fig. A shows a fracture in the coronal plane of the posterior aspect of the axis body which extends into its inferior end-plate (open arrows). At the site of the upper arrow, the posterior axial cortex is disrupted and discontinuous with the posterior cortex of the dens (small arrows). The axial body fragment (asterisk) is rotated anteriorly. The posterior axial body cortex (arrowheads) remains in its normal position with respect to the posterior elements of C2 and to the posterior cortex of C3. Fig. B shows an obliquely oriented fracture in the coronal plane of the right side of the axis body (arrow) and a coronally oriented fracture on the left (arrowheads). The concept of bilateral atypical traumatic spondylolisthesis is ideally demonstrated in Fig. B, image 16.

Differential Diagnosis: Type I, II, III traumatic spondylolisthesis; bilateral atypical traumatic spondylolisthesis.

Diagnosis: Bilateral atypical traumatic spondylolisthesis of C2.

Discussion: Issues regarding traumatic spondylolisthesis are found in the discussion of Case #22.

The term "atypical" traumatic spondylolisthesis is ascribed to coronal fractures of the posterior portion of the axis body. The atypical location of the fracture may be unilateral or, as in this instance, bilateral. When unilateral, the contralateral fracture is typically located in the pars. Because of the orientation and location of the atypical fractures, the weight of the head may result in a shearing force to the anterior fragment, mediated through the oblique fracture line(s), resulting in potentially greater instability and more difficult immobilization of the atypical, rather than the typical, traumatic spondylolisthesis.

Rotation of the anterior axial fragment indicating disruption of the second intervertebral disk makes this a Type II atypical traumatic spondylolisthesis discussed in Case #6.

CASE 6

Case History: This restrained passenger in a high speed, abrupt deceleration motor vehicle accident experienced severe pain in the upper cervical spine when her head was thrown into hyperextension. You are shown a lateral radiograph of the cervicocranium (Fig. A) and an axial CT image of C2 (Fig. B).

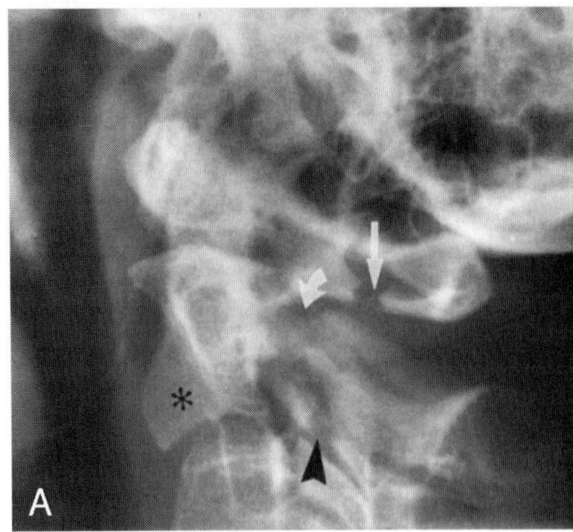

Figure 6.6 A

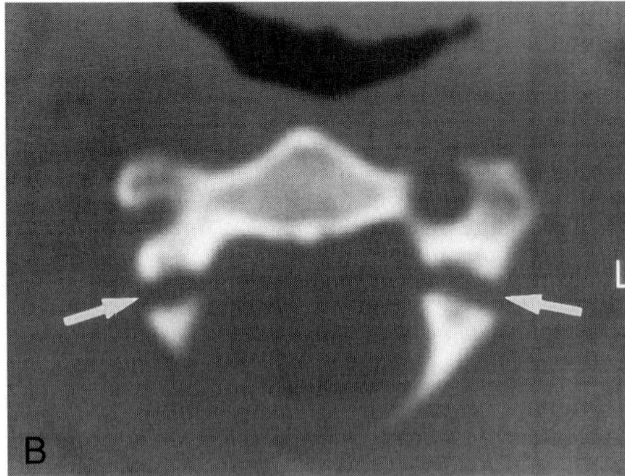

Figure 6.6 B

Findings: Fig. A shows a fracture of the posterior arch of C1 (arrow). Of greater significance is the fracture of the pars interarticularis on one side of C2 (curved arrow) and a fracture of the pars and the inferior facet of C2 on the other (arrowhead). Additionally, the axis body (asterisk) is anteriorly displaced with respect to C3, indicating disruption of the second intervertebral disk. Axial CT image (Fig. B) shows the fractures (arrows) in the pars interarticularis.

Differential Diagnosis: Type I, II, III traumatic spondylolisthesis; atypical traumatic spondylolisthesis.

Diagnosis: Type II traumatic spondylolisthesis of C2; isolated fracture of the posterior arch of C1.

Discussion: Traumatic spondylolisthesis is one of the family of cervical spine injuries caused by predominant hyperextension. It is generally accepted that traumatic spondylolisthesis results when the hyperextension force is received by the pars interarticularis of C2. The pars is the segment of the posterior arch of C2 between its superior and inferior articulating facets. The hyperextension mechanism of injury is confirmed by the fracture of the posterior arch of C1. Traumatic spondylolisthesis is not a bilateral "pillar" fracture of C2 as is occasionally, inaccurately stated.

Traumatic spondylolisthesis is defined as Type I, in which there is no evidence of disruption of the C2 intervertebral disk. Type II is when there is a change in height and/or configuration of the C2 disk space or displacement of the axis body indicating disruption of the second disk. Type III has the characteristics of Type II plus a C2-3 bilateral interfacetal dislocation which results from rebound severe hyperflexion. Type III is rare and is both mechanically and neurologically unstable. Type I is mechanically and neurologically stable, whereas Type II is considered mechanically unstable but neurologically stable. The absence of brainstem/cord injury is attributed to the favorable spinal canal–cord ratio at the level of C2 and the fact that the bilateral pars fractures result in "auto-decompression" of the spinal canal.

Atypical traumatic spondylolisthesis is the term given to traumatic spondylolisthesis when one, or both fracture sites involve the posterior aspect of the axis body rather than the pars. Atypical traumatic spondylolisthesis is discussed in Case #5.

CASE 7

Case History: This 67-year-old woman was involved in a relatively minor motor vehicle accident in which she sustained blunt trauma to the face. She complained of severe pain in the upper cervical region without neurologic signs or symptoms. You are shown a lateral radiograph of her cervicocranium (Fig. A). You are also shown a lateral radiograph of a different patient (Fig. B) who was involved in a major accident in which he experienced severe neck pain and signs and symptoms of a cervical myelopathy.

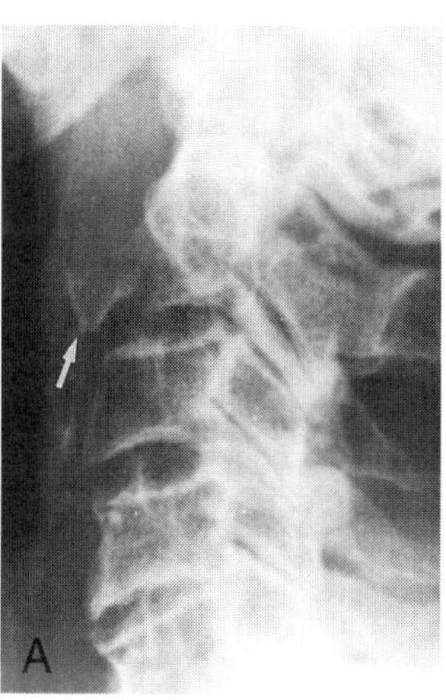

Figure 6.7 A

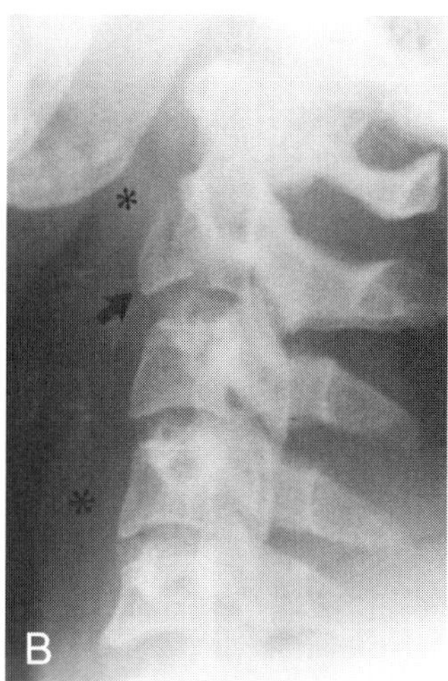

Figure 6.7 B

Findings: Generalized osteopenia shown in Fig. A is consistent with the patient's age and gender. A triangular separate fragment (arrow), whose vertical height is equal to its transverse dimension and which comprises the antero-inferior corner of C2 is distracted and rotated. There is minimal prevertebral soft tissue swelling.

The avulsed fracture fragment of C2 (arrow) in Fig. B has the same characteristics as that seen in Fig. A. A difference in this patient is the marked, diffuse prevertebral soft tissue swelling (asterisks).

Differential Diagnosis: Hyperextension dislocation (HD); extension teardrop fracture.

Diagnosis: Extension teardrop fracture of C2.

Discussion: Extension teardrop fracture is one of the family of injuries caused by predominant hyperextension. The fragment is avulsed by fibers of the anterior longitudinal ligament that inserts on the antero-inferior aspect of each vertebral body, particularly at C2. The physical characteristics of the avulsion fragment and its site of origin are pathognomonic of an extension teardrop fracture. The clinical and radiologic findings in the first patient (Fig. A) are those classically ascribed to this injury. It has been shown that extension teardrop fracture may also involve any cervical vertebra and that approximately 11% of patients with extension teardrop fractures present with cervical myelopathy. These patients are typically young adults and 80% of them have marked diffuse prevertebral soft tissue swelling (Fig. B). Extension teardrop fractures typically occur as isolated injuries, but may involve more than one cervical vertebra. Extension teardrop fractures have been associated with Type II or Type III dens fracture, traumatic spondylolisthesis, isolated fractures of the posterior arch of C1, or any combination of these.

Extension teardrop fractures, when associated with marked diffuse prevertebral soft tissue swelling, are distinguished radiographically from HD by the site of origin and the physical dimensions of the avulsed fracture fragment (Case #11).

CASE 8

Case History: This elderly woman sustained blunt trauma to the neck after a fall down a flight of stairs. She complained of severe pain in the upper neck with limitation of movement of her head. She had no neurologic deficits. You are shown a lateral radiograph of her cervicocranium (Fig. A) and the "open-mouth" projection (Fig. B).

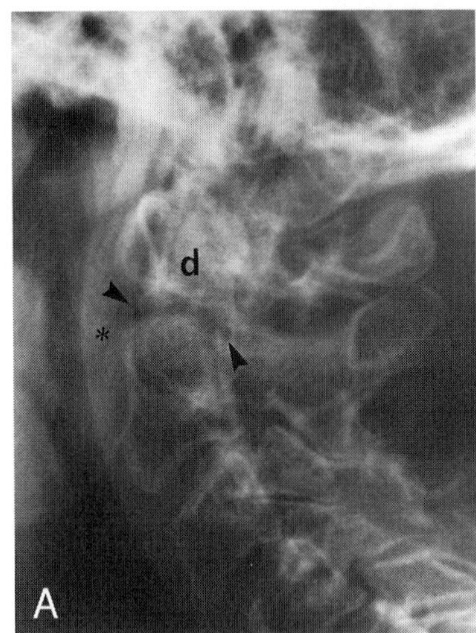
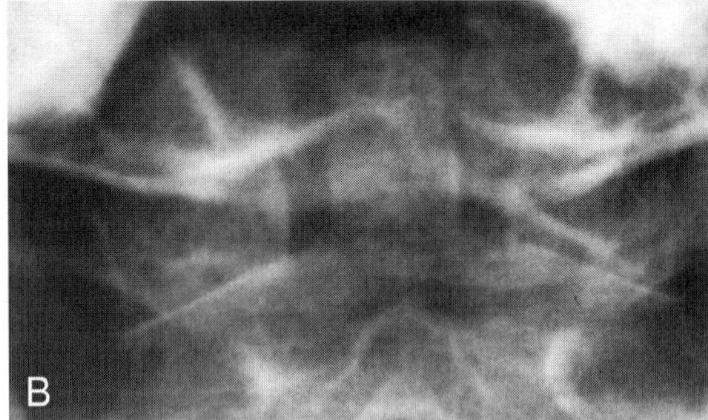

Figure 6.8 A   **Figure 6.8 B**

Findings: Lateral radiograph of the cervicocranium (Fig. A) shows posterior displacement of the dens (d) with respect to the axis body. The anterior and posterior cortices of the base of the dens are disrupted (arrowheads). The fracture line, which is rostral to the superior arch of the axis ring, is wider anteriorly than posteriorly. The cervicocranial prevertebral soft tissue shadow (asterisk) is abnormal, being convex inferior to the anterior tubercle of the axis. The "open-mouth" projection (Fig. B) fails to show the fracture because of the posterior rotation of the rostral fragment with respect to the axis body and because of the absence of lateral displacement of the dens.

Differential Diagnosis: Type III dens fracture; Type II dens fracture.

Diagnosis: Type II (high) dens fracture.

Discussion: A discussion of dens fractures appears in Case #9. With respect to the patient presented in this case, the location of the fracture at the base of the dens and rostral to the superior arch of the axis ring defines it as a Type II injury. Posterior rotational displacement of the dens and the configuration of the fracture line reflect a hyperextension mechanism of injury. Because of their location, the Type II dens fractures are considered mechanically unstable. Contrary to the Type III dens fracture, the Type II is associated with an approximate 30% incidence of nonunion. The ununited rostral fracture fragment is referred to as "os odontoideum." Failure of the dens to unite with the axis body provides the opportunity for abnormal range of motion of the head and atlas and a potential for brainstem injury following even relatively minor trauma.

As mentioned in Case #9, the Type III dens fracture, by definition, must disrupt the axis ring on the lateral cervical spine radiograph indicating that the fracture involves the axis body rather than the odontoid process.

CASE 9

Case History: This man fell from a tree, landing on his head and shoulders. He complained of severe pain at the base of the skull and limitation of movement of the head. He had no neurologic signs or symptoms. You are shown a lateral radiograph of his cervicocranium (Fig. A) and axial (Fig. B), sagittal (Fig. C), and coronal (Fig. D) CT images as well as a surface-rendered 3-D CT image (Fig. E) of the axis.

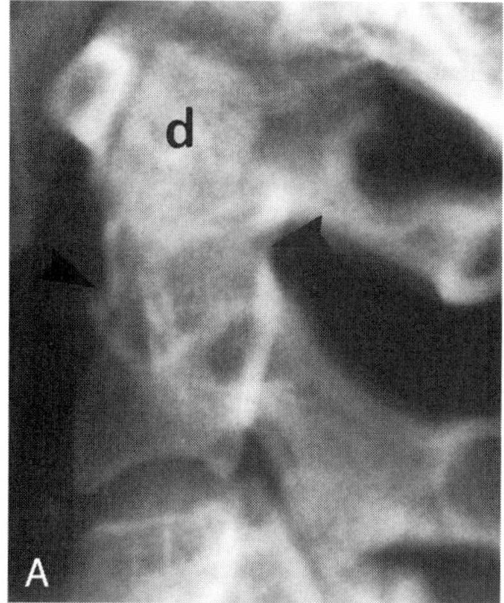

Figure 6.9 A

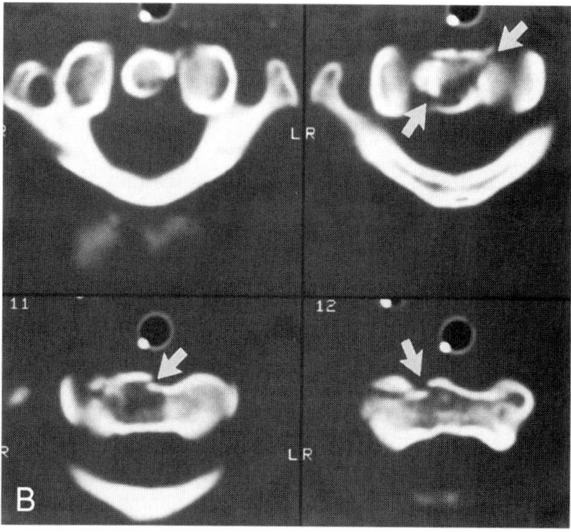

Figure 6.9 B

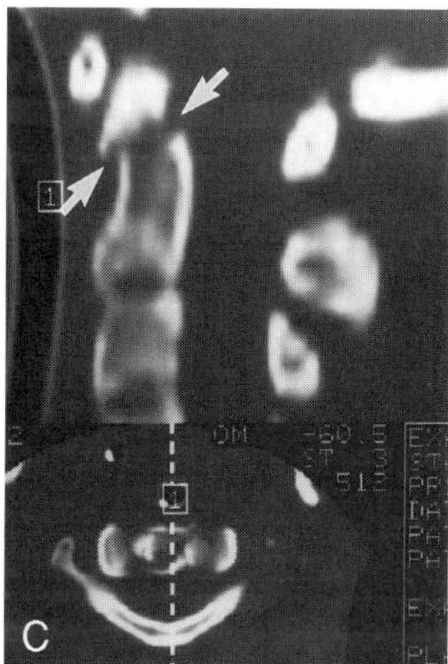

Figure 6.9 C

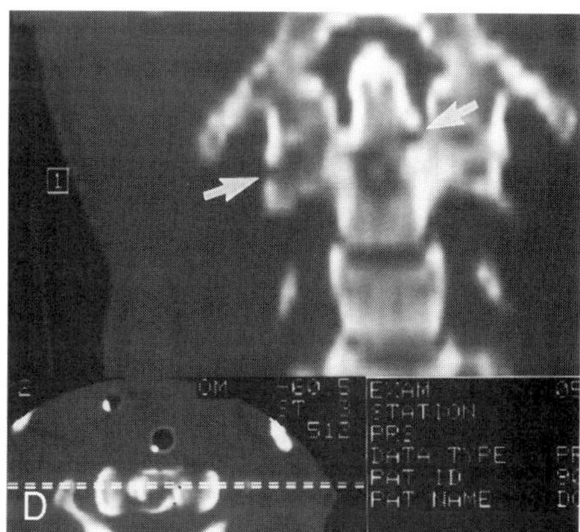

Figure 6.9 D

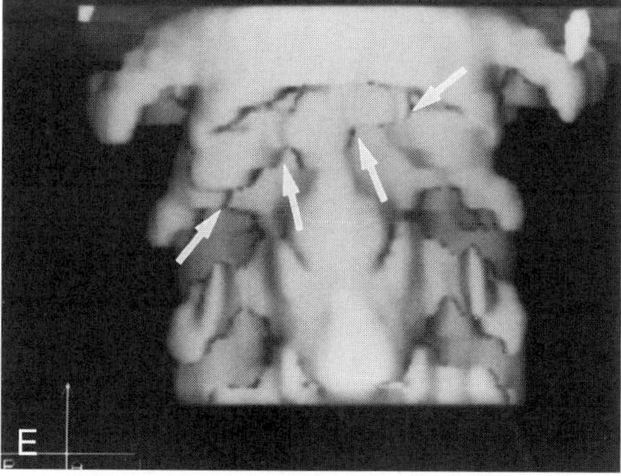

Figure 6.9 E

(continued)

Findings: Lateral radiograph (Fig. A) of the cervicocranium shows disruption of the anterior and posterior arches (arrowheads) of the axis ring and anterior displacement of the dens (d) with respect to the body. Axial CT images (Fig. B) show comminution of the axis body (arrows) inferior to the base of the dens. The distribution of the fracture line (arrows) within the axis body is shown in sagittal (Fig. C) and coronal (Fig. D) CT reformations and in the surface-rendered 3-D CT image (Fig. E) (arrows).

Differential Diagnosis: High (Type II) dens fracture; low (Type III) dens fracture.

Diagnosis: Low (Type III) dens fracture.

Discussion: Dens fractures were classified as Type I (superolateral aspect of the tip of the dens avulsed by the alar "check" ligaments), Type II (base of dens), and Type III (superior portion of the axis body inferior to the odontoid process). Because many authors believe that the Type I dens fracture occurs only very rarely, Type II and Type III fractures are now designated "high" and "low," respectively. Recently, the Type I dens fracture has been documented as a very rare injury whose mechanism of injury is either lateral tilt or rotation of the head in a direction opposite the side of the avulsion fracture. The mechanism of injury of the Type II and Type III fractures may be hyperflexion, hyperextension, or lateral tilt. The mechanism of injury may be inferred by the position of the dens with respect to the axis body (as in the patient illustrated with anterior displacement of the dens), suggesting a hyperflexion injury.

The low dens fracture breaks the axis ring, an inverted water-drop shaped density the anterior arc of which represents the anterior cortex of the axis pedicles; the superior arc, the cortex of the groove between the base of the dens and the medial aspect of the superior articulating facets of C2; and the posterior arc, the posterior cortex of the axis body. The postero-inferior aspect of the "ring" is incomplete in approximately 50% of normal patients due to superimposition of the foramen transversarium. "Fat-axis body" is a term sometimes applied to a low dens fracture when the rostral fragment is anteriorly displaced, as in the case shown. Because the low dens fracture involves principally cancellus bone, proper management results in fracture healing, and nonunion does not occur with the frequency typical of the Type II (high) dens fracture.

The distinction between the high (II) and low (III) dens fractures rests solely on the location of the fracture site. The Type II fracture is confined to the odontoid process, whereas the Type III involves the axis body inferior to the base of the dens. Rarely, a fracture line may begin at the base of the dens anteriorly and exit through the posterior arc of the axis ring, for example, a Type II–III fracture, which has no unique clinical consequences.

Because of the frequency of nonunion, the Type II dens fracture is considered mechanically unstable. The Type III dens fracture is considered mechanically stable. The spinal cord–canal ratio tends to spare the spinal cord in all but the most severely displayed dens fractures and, consequently, most dens fractures are neurologically stable.

CASE 10

Case History: Each of these patients sustained blunt trauma to the neck in motor vehicle accidents. Each patient complained of severe neck pain, limited motion of the neck, and tenderness. None had a neurologic deficit. You are shown multiple images of patient 1 (Fig. A–E), patient 2 (Fig. F–J), and patient 3 (Fig. K–P).

Patient 1

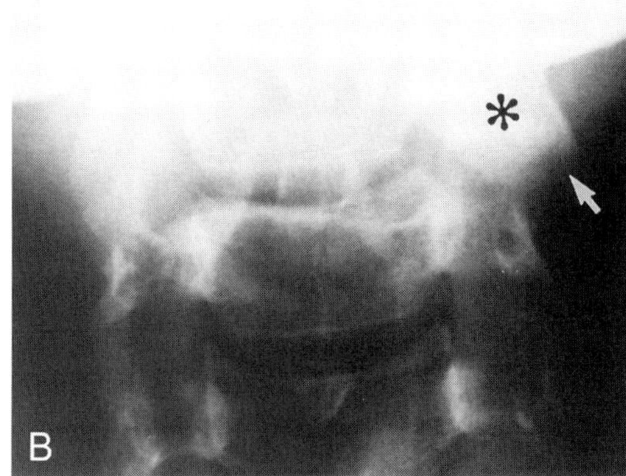

Figure 6.10 A

Figure 6.10 B

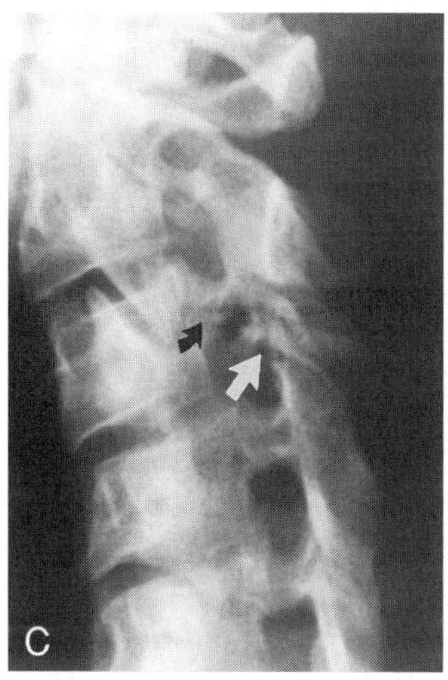

Figure 6.10 C

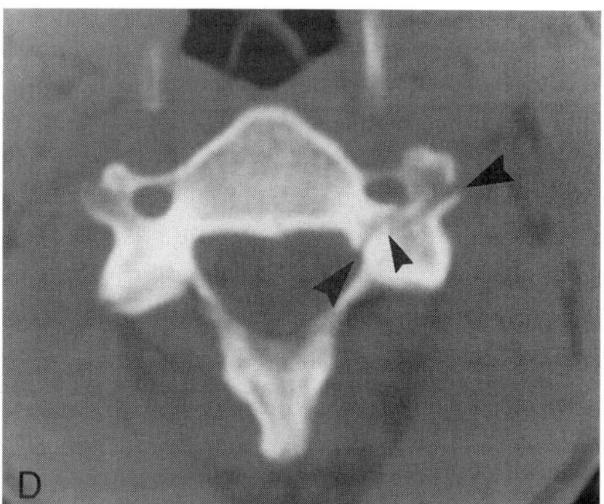

Figure 6.10 D

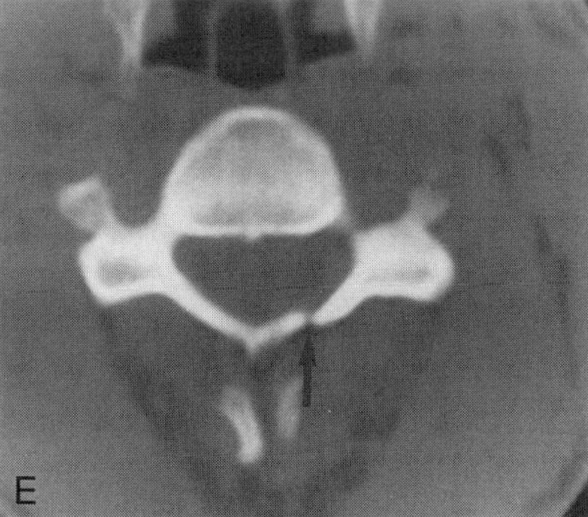

Figure 6.10 E

(continued)

Patient 2

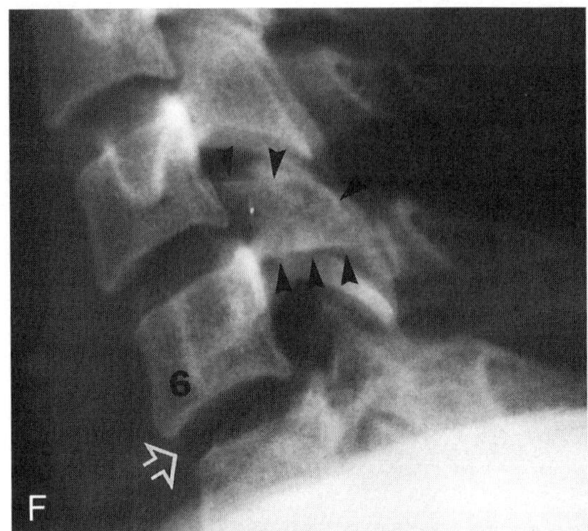

Figure 6.10 F

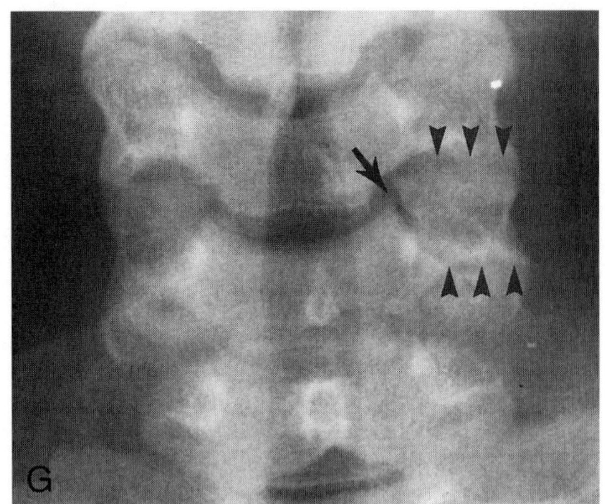

Figure 6.10 G

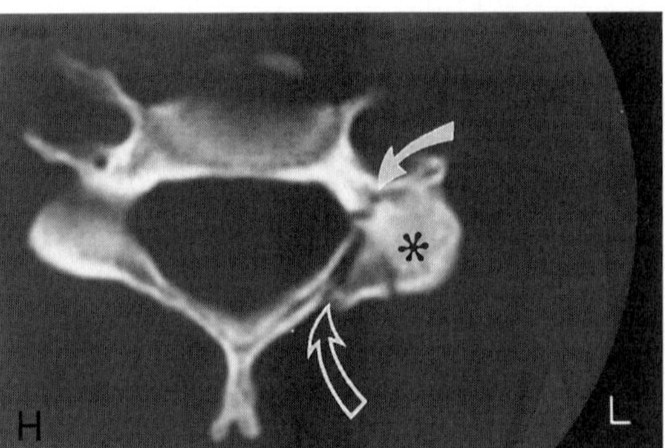

Figure 6.10 H

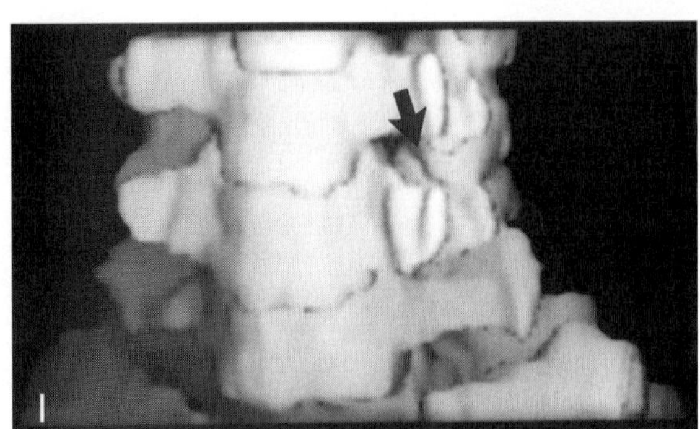

Figure 6.10 I

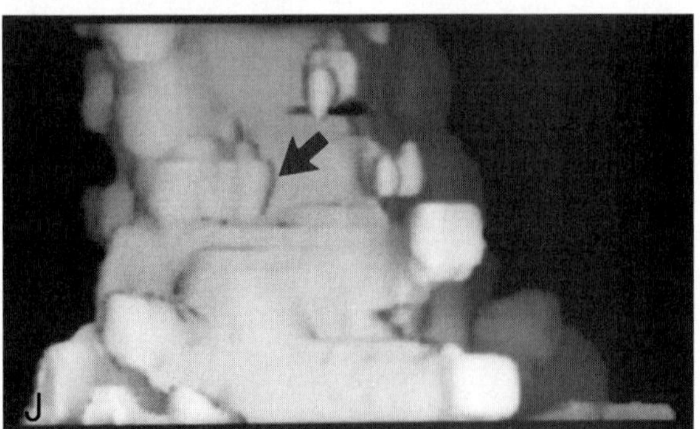

Figure 6.10 J

Patient 3

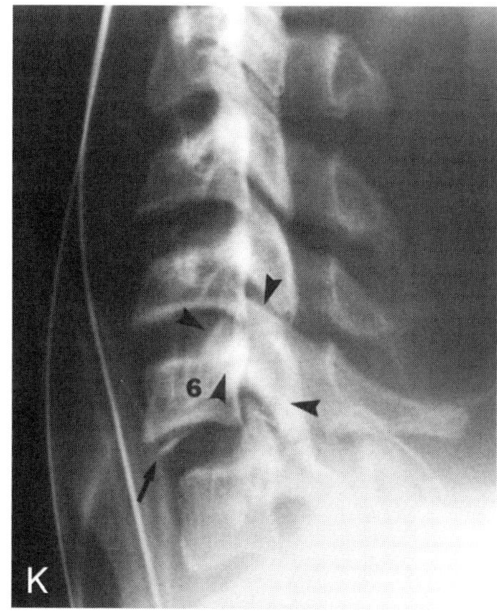

Figure 6.10 K

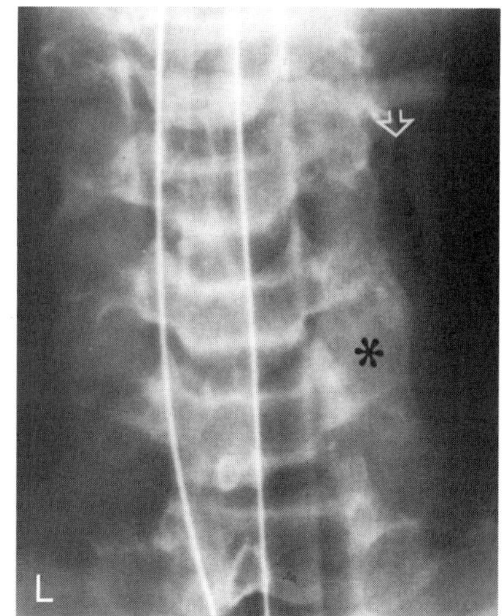

Figure 6.10 L

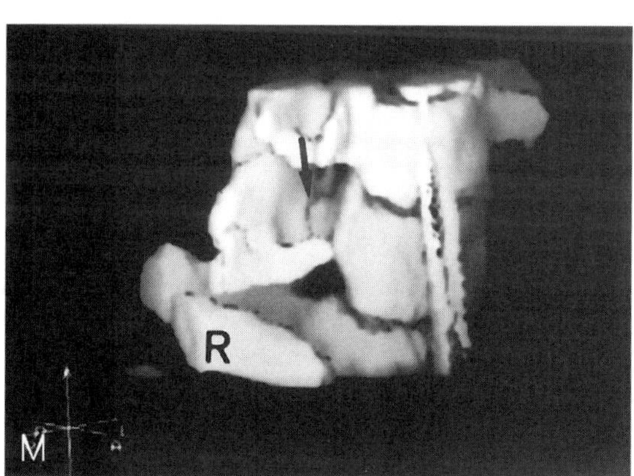

Figure 6.10 M

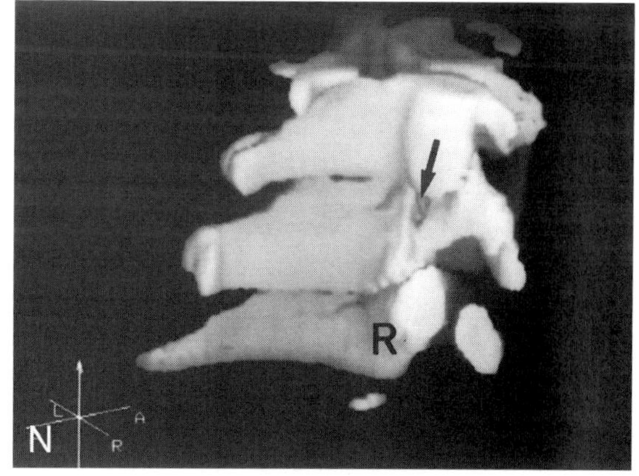

Figure 6.10 N

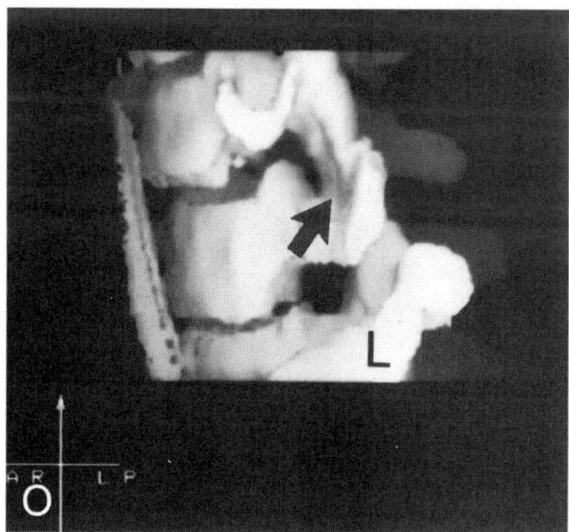

Figure 6.10 O

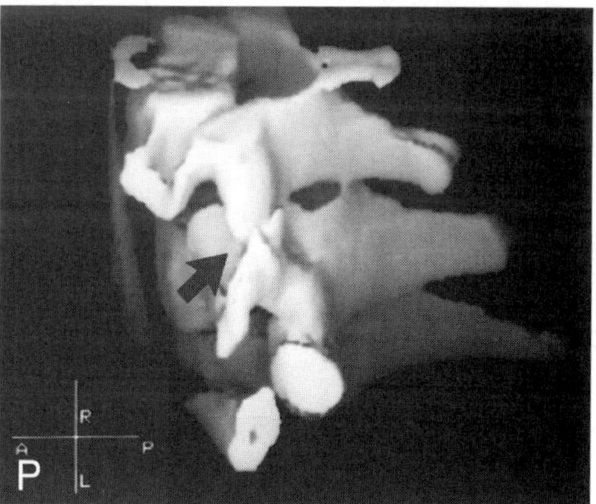

Figure 6.10 P

(continued)

Findings: Patient 1 (Fig. A–E): Lateral radiograph of the cervical spine from C1-5 (Fig. A) shows reversal of cervical lordosis, intact vertebral bodies, and normally maintained disk spaces. Of importance is the observation that one of the articular masses of C3 (arrowheads) is changed in its orientation with respect to the contralateral mass. On the AP view of the C3-4 level (Fig. B), the left articular mass of C3 (asterisk) is laterally displaced, resulting in disruption of the outer margin of the lateral column (white arrow). The left oblique view (Fig. C) of the same patient shows a minimally displaced fracture of the pedicle (curved arrow) and a comminuted fracture of the left lamina (white arrow) of C3. Axial CT images of C3 show a fracture of the left pedicle which extends into the adjacent transverse process (Fig. D, arrowheads) and into the left lamina (Fig. E, arrow).

Patient 2: On the lateral radiograph (Fig. F), the C6-7 disk space is slightly narrowed (open arrow) and the body of C6 is slightly anteriorly translated. Of importance is the finding that one of the articular masses (arrowheads) is displaced posteriorly and rotated anteriorly. In the AP radiograph (Fig. G), an oblique fracture defect (arrow) involves the region of the left pedicle. The facets (arrowheads) of the laterally displaced and the anteriorly rotated left articular mass give the appearance of one-half of a bow-tie (the "bow-tie" sign). Axial CT (Fig. H) of the same patient shows the pedicle (curved arrow) and comminuted laminar (curved open arrow) fractures which result in the lateral mass (asterisk) becoming a free-floating fragment capable of rotation and displacement as seen in the lateral (Fig. F) and AP (Fig. G) radiographs. The surface-rendered 3-D images show the left pedicle (Fig. I, arrow) and laminar (Fig. J, arrow) fractures.

Patient 3: Lateral radiograph (Fig. K) shows a slight anterior translation of the body of C6 with an avulsion fracture (arrow) of the anterior aspect of its inferior end-plate, indicating a hyperextension mechanism of injury, narrowing of the C6-7 disk space, and abnormal orientation of one of the articular masses of C6 (arrowheads). The frontal radiograph (Fig. L) shows disruption of the left lateral column at the C6 level (asterisk) but without a "bow-tie" sign. Subcutaneous emphysema of the left side of the neck (open arrow) is secondary to a laceration. Surface-rendered 3-D images show the right pedical (Fig. M, arrow) and laminar fractures (Fig. N, arrow) and the left unilateral interfacetal dislocation (Figs. O and P, arrows).

Differential Diagnosis: Anterior subluxation, unilateral interfacetal dislocation, bilateral interfacetal dislocation, pedicolaminar fracture separation (PLFS).

Diagnosis: Pedicolaminar fracture-separation (PLFS).

Discussion: Fracture of the ipsilateral pedicle and lamina of the same vertebra (Types I, II, III) and pedicolaminar fractures associated with contralateral interfacetal joint dislocation (Type IV) have been principally described in French language literature as "fracture-separation du masse articulare." The Type IV injury was originally described by Forsythe (1963) and subsequently by others as "hyperextension fracture–dislocation." English language articles propose a continuous circular mechanism of injury in hyperextension. The French language authors propose a simultaneous hyperextension and rotation mechanism of injury with one lateral mass on the side of the direction of rotation impacting the subjacent articular mass, resulting in an ipsilateral pedical and laminar fracture and, in the most severe form, an interfacetal dislocation on the contralateral, distracted side.

The clinical significance of PLFS, particularly in those types of injuries with vertebral body anterior translation, is recognition of PLFS as a predominantly hyperextension injury rather than hyperflexion as implied by the anterior translation of the vertebral body. The appropriate mechanism of injury is established by displacement and rotation of the involved articular mass in both the AP and lateral cervical spine radiographs and the absence of any other sign of hyperflexion. The clinical importance of an accurate diagnosis (and mechanism of injury) assures appropriate surgical management.

Anterior subluxation, which may be associated with a minor anterior translation, is characterized by signs of hyperflexion, namely a hyperkyphotic angulation at the level of posterior ligament complex tear, "fanning," and signs of bilateral interfacetal joint subluxation. Unilateral interfacetal dislocation is also associated with anterior translation usually greater than that found in anterior subluxation, and is characterized by the signs of hyperflexion previously described coupled with signs of rotation from the level of the interfacetal dislocation rostrally. Bilateral interfacetal dislocation is distinguished from PLFS by anterior translation of the involved vertebral body equal to or greater than the AP diameter of that vertebral body, frank interfacetal dislocation, and signs of posterior ligament complex disruption.

CASE 11

Case History: This unbelted car passenger was thrown forward, striking his face on the dashboard at the time of impact of a high velocity abrupt deceleration accident. The patient had facial lacerations and complained of upper extremity paresthesia. You are shown a lateral cervical spine radiograph (Fig. A) and an MR image (Fig. B) obtained shortly after admission. Fig. C is from an MR study of a different patient with the same type of injury and is shown to illustrate the pathology of hyperextension dislocation. Fig. D shows hyperextension dislocation in an adolescent.

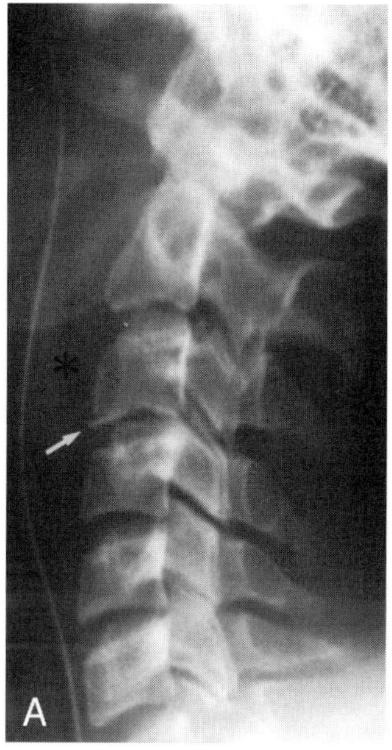

Figure 6.11 A

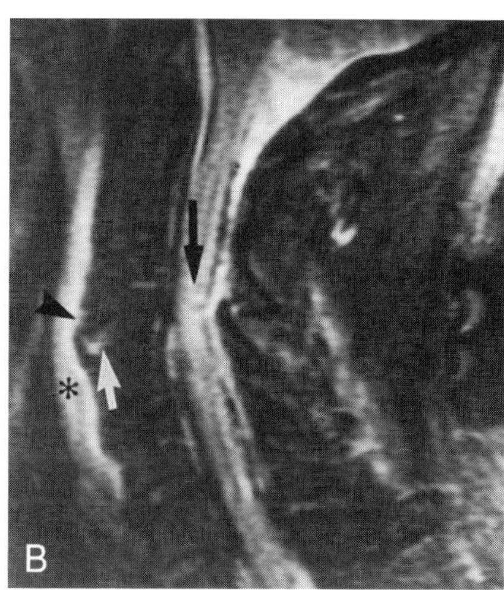

Figure 6.11 B

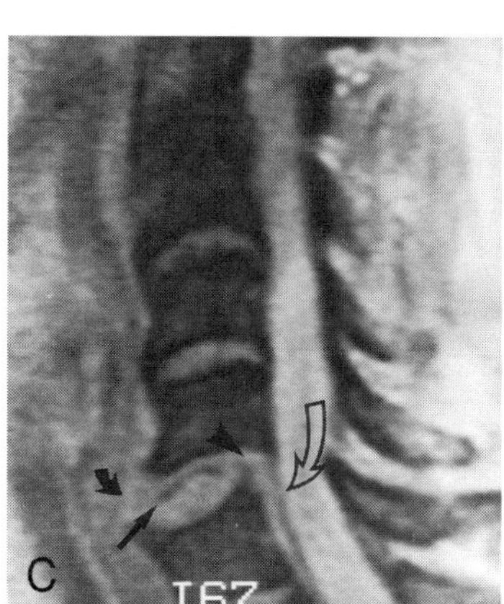

Figure 6.11 C

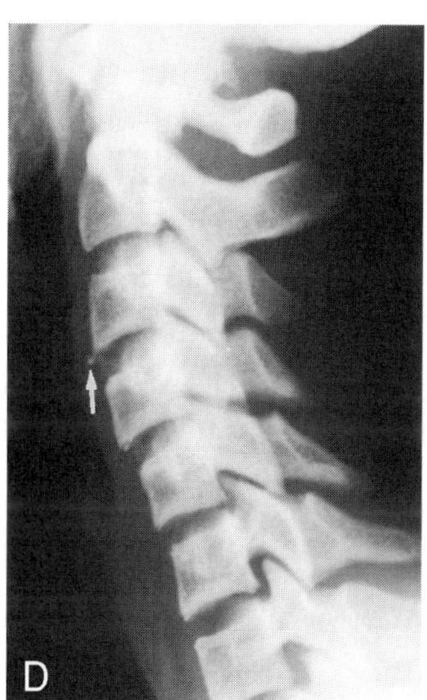

Figure 6.11 D

(continued)

Findings: Lateral cervical spine radiograph (Fig. A) shows marked diffuse prevertebral soft tissue swelling (asterisk) evidenced by the anterior location of the nasogastric tube rostral to its entry into the esophagus. The visualized cervical vertebrae are normally aligned. An avulsion fracture fragment (arrow), whose long axis exceeds it vertical height, arises from the anterior aspect of the inferior end-plate of C3. The MR study (Fig. B) shows blood and edema in the retropharyngeal space (asterisk). The blood, which comes from the longus capitis and colli muscles being torn during hyperextension, is the basis of the prevertebral soft tissue swelling seen on the lateral cervical spine radiograph. In this patient, the anterior annulus, including the Sharpey fibers, is intact, resulting in an avulsion fracture (arrowhead). The high intensity signal in the disk (white arrow) represents blood and edema within the torn intervertebral disk. Spinal cord compression has resulted in edema (black arrow) in the center of the cord, which is the genesis of the acute central cord syndrome.

Diagnosis: Hyperextension dislocation (HD) of C3.

Discussion: Hyperextension dislocation of the cervical spine is the name given to the soft tissue member of the family of injuries caused by predominant hyperextension. HD is not "a" or "the" hyperextension injury of the cervical spine. HD is a radiologic paradox because there is no sign of dislocation of any of the cervical vertebrae on the lateral cervical spine radiograph. This injury was designated hyperextension dislocation by orthopedic surgeons in the 1940s after observation of the cine-radiographic monitoring of anesthetized animal experiments designed so that the face of a subject struck a wall following a high speed sled travel. At the time of impact, the head and upper cervical vertebra went into severe hyperextension. Upon dissipation of the impacting force, the head and cervical vertebrae returned, by "rebound" or "recoil," to normal alignment.

Clinically, patients with HD characteristically present with signs of facial trauma and some degree of acute central cervical cord syndrome. Radiographically, the cervical vertebrae are normally aligned. All mature adult patients with HD have marked, diffuse cervical prevertebral soft tissue swelling that is at least 1 cm in width anterior to the mid-point of the anterior cortex of the body of C3 and that extends to the level of the basion. In approximately two-thirds of adult patients with HD, the intact Sharpey fibers of the annulus cause the avulsion fracture described previously, which is characteristic of HD in both location and configuration. Fig. C illustrates the pathophysiology of HD when the anterior annulus is torn (curved arrow). Blood (arrow) is present in the torn and widened intervertebral disk. The posterior annulus is torn (arrowhead) and the posterior longitudinal ligament (open curved arrow) is avulsed from the subjacent vertebra. Fig. D illustrates the appearance of HD in adolescent patients in whom the ununited ring apophysis is avulsed (arrow) and displaced by the intact Sharpey fibers of the annulus. As in this instance, soft tissue swelling may be minimal, and adolescent patients with HD may not experience cord injury.

Case History: This patient, who was a restrained passenger in a motor vehicle accident, complained of severe left sided neck pain aggravated by motion and tenderness on the left side of the neck, but had no other neurologic symptoms.

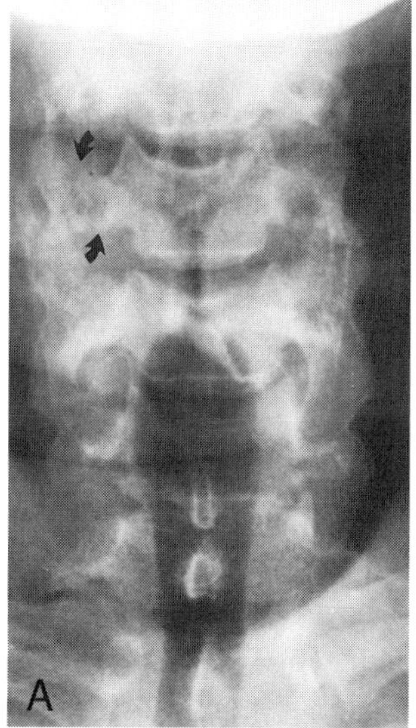

Figure 6.12 A

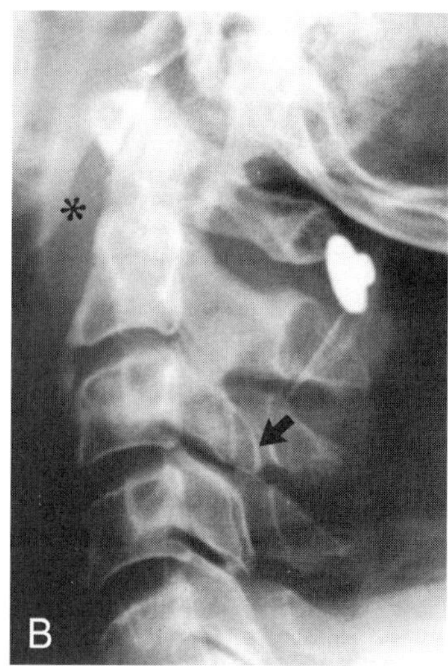

Figure 6.12 B

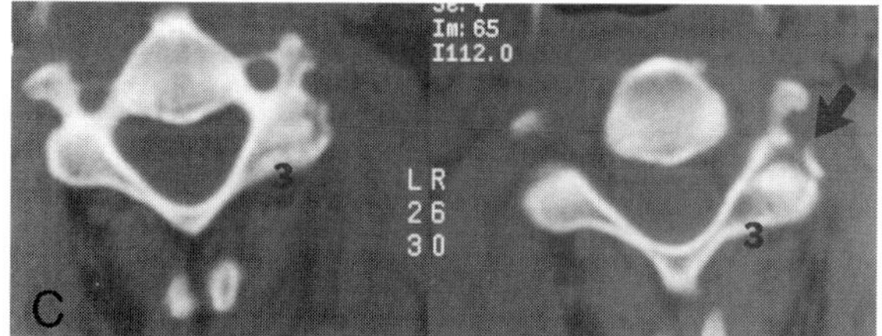

Figure 6.12 C

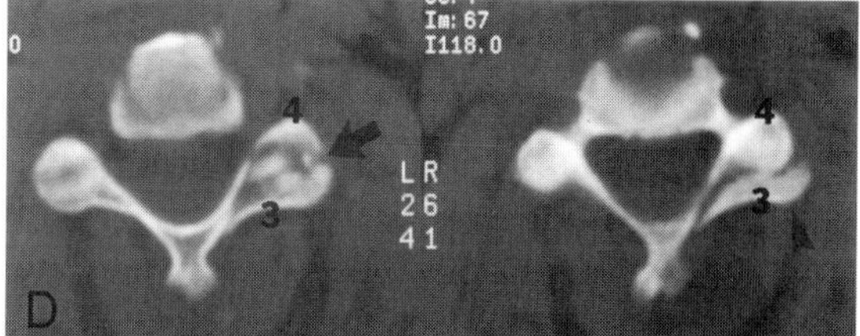

Figure 6.12 D

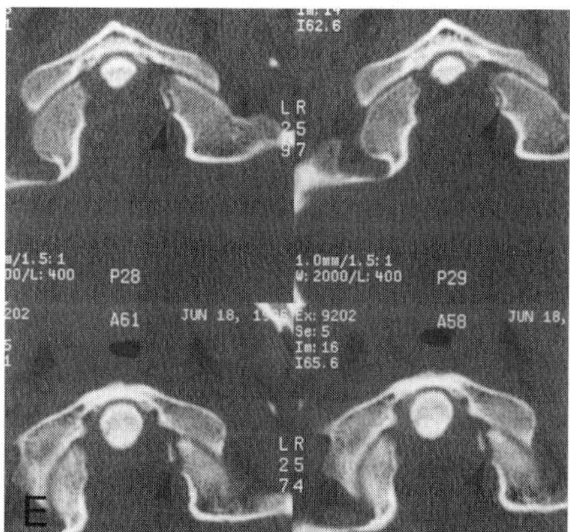

Figure 6.12 E

(continued)

Findings: Frontal radiograph of the cervical spine (Fig. A) shows a minimally displaced fracture of the lateral aspect of the left articular mass of C3 (curved arrows). Lateral projection (Fig. B) reveals the posterior cortical margin of one of the articular masses of C3 to be posteriorly displaced (arrow) with respect to its contralateral member. The lack of superimposition of the posterior cortical margins of the lateral masses at the same level is called the "double outline" sign. A second finding on this projection is an abnormal cervicocranial prevertebral soft tissue contour (asterisk) inferior to the anterior tubercle of C1. Old calcification in the anterior annulus of the second intervertebral disk is an incidental finding of no significance pertaining to the acute injury. Axial CT scans of the C3-4 level (Figs. C, D) demonstrate a comminuted fracture of the left articular mass of C3 (arrow) with lateral displacement of the separate major fragment (arrowhead, 8.D, image 67) (C3=3, C4=4). Axial CT images at the occipito-atlantal level (Fig. E) show a comminuted fracture of the left occipital condyle (arrowhead).

Differential Diagnosis: (1) Lower cervical spine: pillar fracture; pedicolaminar fracture-separation (PLFS). (2) Cervicocranium: occipital condylar fracture(s); lateral mass of C1 fracture(s); false positive cervicocranial prevertebral soft tissue contour.

Diagnosis: (1) Pillar fracture, left, C3. (2) Left occipital condylar fracture.

Discussion: This case was chosen primarily for the pillar fracture because it demonstrates the classic signs of this injury. The occipital condylar fracture is, for this educational exercise, an extra added benefit. The abnormal contour of the cervicocranial prevertebral soft tissue shadow does, however, emphasize the need to be constantly alert for the possibility of a coexistent second injury in the cervical spine. Most authorities agree that the pillar fracture is caused by simultaneous hyperextension and rotation with the suprajacent lateral mass impacting on the superior facet of the subjacent mass on the side of the direction of rotation, resulting in a vertically oriented fracture through the subjacent mass. The impacting force drives the separate fragment(s) posteriorly and laterally. Others suggest the pillar fracture is caused by lateral tilt. Because the articular masses are anatomically located posterolaterally with respect to the vertebral bodies, and because of the typical orientation of the articular mass fracture line and the characteristic posterolateral displacement of the separate fragment(s), the pillar fracture is the result of simultaneous hyperextension and rotation with the fracture occurring in an articular mass on the side of the direction of rotation.

On a frontal projection of the cervical spine, one may expect to find changes in the lateral column (that portion of the cervical spine lateral to the vertebral bodies in the frontal projection). The lateral column represents the articular masses and appears as a solid bone with an apparently continuous, smoothly undulating lateral cortical margin resembling bamboo. The outer margin of the lateral column represents the cortex of the superimposed lateral masses. Normally, the superior and inferior margins of the lateral masses, that is, the superior and inferior margins of the interfacetal joints, are obscured by the density of the superimposed articular masses. Thus, the lateral column should be devoid of lucent defects, either interfacetal joint margins or fractures. In Fig. A, disruption of the normally intact outer margin of the lateral column and the curved, lucent fracture in the column itself, is abnormal and, given the case history, must be considered a minimally laterally displaced fracture fragment. Posterior displacement of the separate fragment results in its posterior cortical margin being posterior and parallel to that of the contralateral mass on the lateral radiograph (Fig. B), e.g., the "double outline" sign. Occasionally, it is possible to recognize a fracture defect in the inferior facet of the fractured mass. The pillar fracture is usually obvious on the appropriate oblique projection. CT is indicated to define the fracture limited to the articular mass (pillar) and to distinguish it from the pedicolaminar fracture–separation. MR imaging is not indicated because the pillar fracture is typically not associated with neurologic deficits. Because of the mechanism of injury, acute traumatic disk herniation is rare. The integrity of the articular mass anatomy being maintained, even though fractured, indicates the pillar fracture is mechanically stable.

Convexity of the cervicocranial prevertebral soft tissue shadow inferior to the anterior tubercle of C1 in the presence of blunt trauma to the cervical spine must be considered as representing a retropharyngeal hemorrhage. Because there is no sign of occipito-atlantal dissociation, Jefferson bursting fracture, dens fractures, or traumatic spondylolisthesis, and because the anterior atlantodental interval is normal, the only remaining diagnostic options for the abnormal soft tissue contour are fractures of an occipital condyle or a lateral mass of C1. Identification of and distinction between these options is most efficiently obtained by CT. In the absence of a neurologic deficit, MR imaging is not indicated.

The fact that, in this patient, the occipital condylar fracture and the pillar fracture are on the same side confirms a simultaneous hyperextension and rotation mechanism of injury.

CASE 13

Case History: This driver of a tractor trailer was involved in a rollover accident. He climbed out of the cab but complained of severe neck pain. He had no neurologic signs or symptoms. You are shown frontal (Fig. A), lateral (Fig. B), and left anterior oblique (Fig. C) radiographs of the cervical spine. You are also shown a lateral radiograph (Fig. D) and axial CT images (Fig. E) of a different construction worker who experienced severe cervical spine pain and tenderness after a fall. The construction worker, similar to the truck driver, had no neurologic deficit.

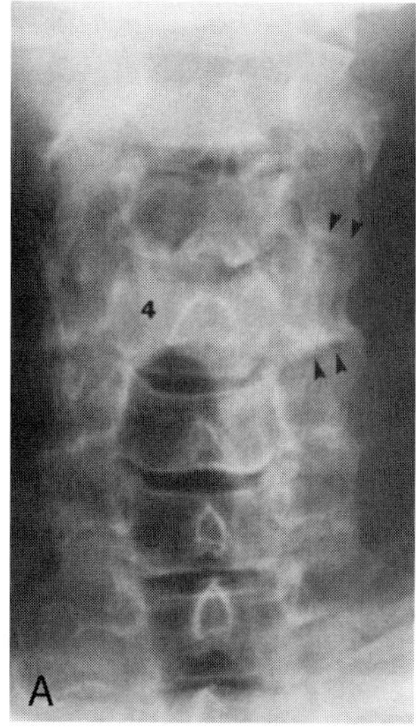

Figure 6.13 A

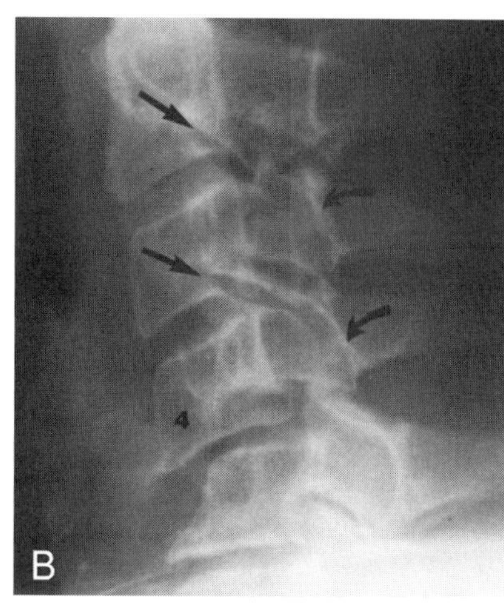

Figure 6.13 B

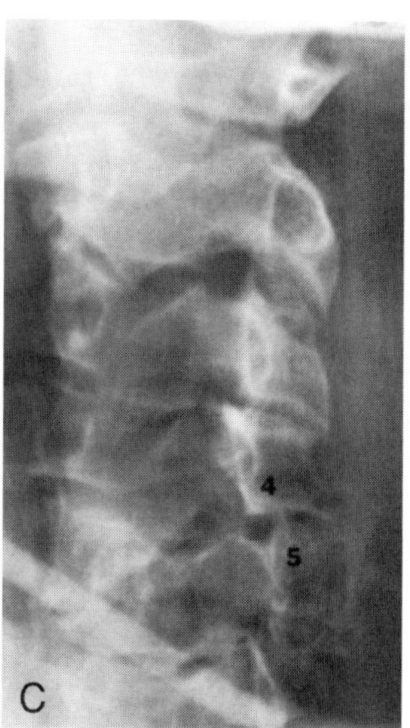

Figure 6.13 C

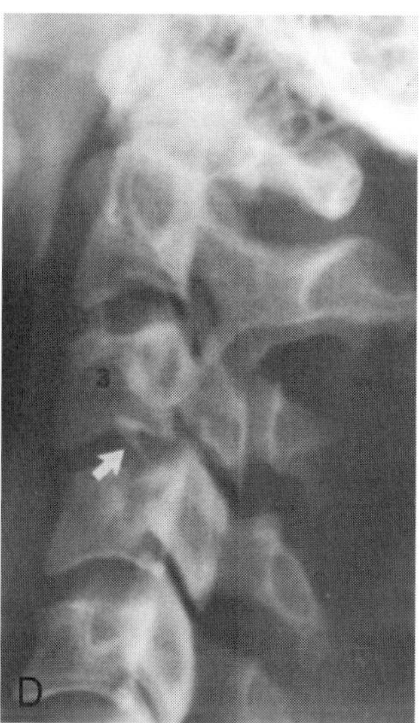

Figure 6.13 D

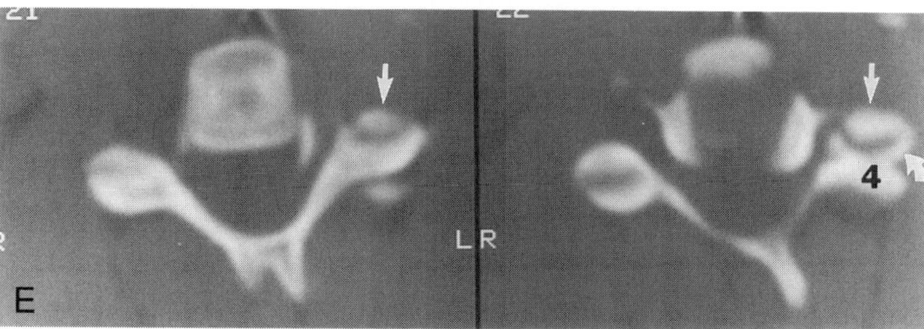

Figure 6.13 E

(continued)

Findings: Frontal radiograph of the cervical spine (Fig. A) in the first patient demonstrates displacement of the spinous processes from C4 upward to the left of midline. The left lateral column, at the same level, shows transverse lucent defects with smoothly sclerotic margins (arrowheads) which represent the C3-4 and C4-5 interfacetal joint spaces. Lateral radiograph (Fig. B) shows anterior translation of C4 (4) approximately 4 mm with respect to C5. The more rostral cervical vertebrae have accompanied C4. Additionally, C4 and all of the vertebrae above it show that their articular masses and interfacetal joints (arrows) in one side superimpose upon the vertebral bodies while, on the opposite side, the posterior cortical margins of the articular masses (curved arrows) are superimposed upon the spinolaminar line obliterating the laminar space. There is no visible fracture and soft tissue swelling is minimal. Oblique projection (Fig. C) shows the left articular mass of C4 (4) is dislocated anteriorly with respect to that of C5 (5).

Lateral radiograph (Fig. D) in the second patient shows similar findings from C3 (3) upwards. However, in addition, the superior articular process of the articular mass of C4 on the side of dislocation constitutes a separate fragment (white arrow). Axial CT (Fig. E) shows the left articular mass of C3 (curved arrow) dislocated anterior to that of C4 (4) and, anterior to it, a left C4 superior articular process fragment (straight arrows).

Differential Diagnosis: Anterior subluxation (AS), bilateral interfacetal dislocation (BID), pedicolaminar fracture separation (PLFS), and unilateral interfacetal dislocation (UID).

Diagnosis: Unilateral interfacetal dislocation (UID).

Discussion: UID, also sometimes referred to as the "locked" or "jumped" vertebra, is the result of simultaneous hyperflexion and rotation resulting in distraction on the side opposite to the direction of rotation. The rotation, combined with hyperflexion, causes dislocation of one (rarely two) interfacetal joint(s) on the distracted side. On the opposite side, at the level of the interfacetal dislocation, the interfacetal joint is usually subluxated secondary to hyperflexion. Dislocation of the articular mass itself is usually not visible on the oblique radiograph. However, the laminae, which extend posteromedially from the articular masses to meet at the midline forming the spinolaminar line, are clearly visualized *en face* in the normal "shingles-on-the-roof" configuration. On the appropriate oblique projection, the lamina at the level of the dislocated articular mass is anteriorly displaced with respect to the subjacent lamina, resulting in disruption of the "shingles-on-the-roof" alignment.

UID is considered mechanically and neurologically stable because of the presence of the dislocated articular mass within the inferior portion of the adjacent intervertebral foramen. UID rarely results in spinal cord injury. CT is appropriate to exclude an associated articular mass fracture which, if major, changes the stable UID to an unstable unilateral interfacetal fracture-dislocation. The differential diagnoses cited are based solely upon the anterior translation of the involved vertebra and is discussed in Case #15.

CASE 14

Case History: This gymnast was quadriplegic after a fall in which he landed on the back of his head. You are shown AP and lateral cervical spine radiographs (Fig. A and B), two axial CT images of the midcervical spine (Fig. C), and AP and lateral cervical spine radiographs of a different patient with a similar injury (Figs. D, E).

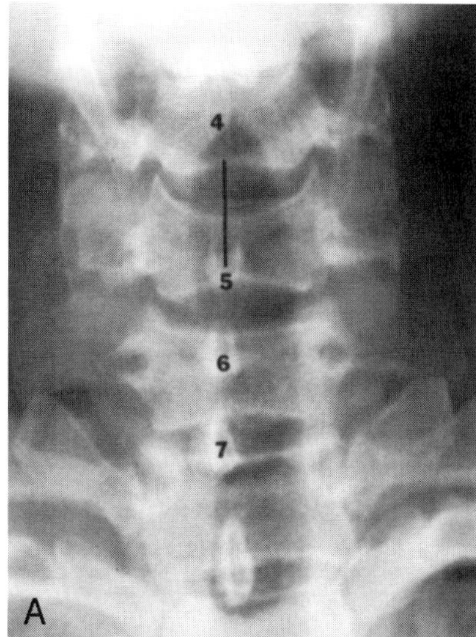

Figure 6.14 A

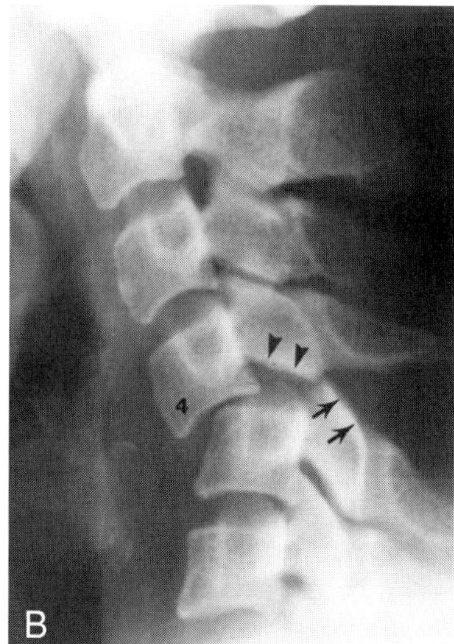

Figure 6.14 B

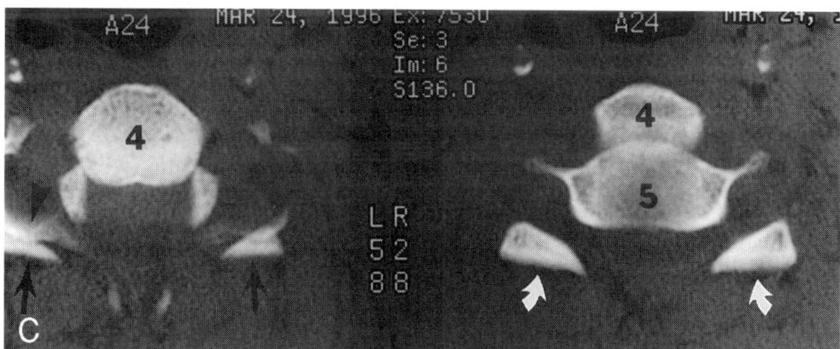

Figure 6.14 C

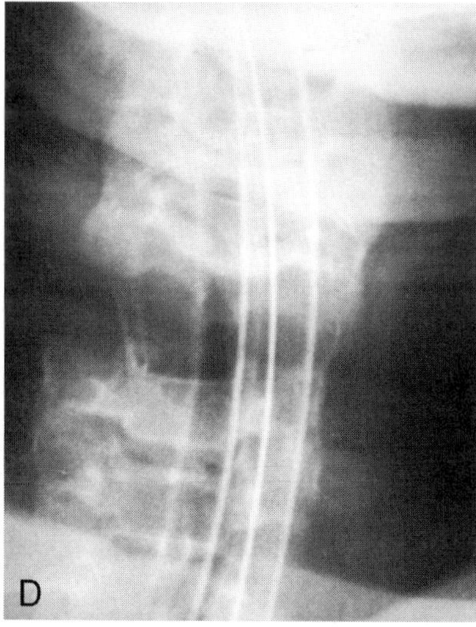
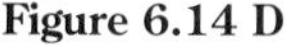

Figure 6.14 D

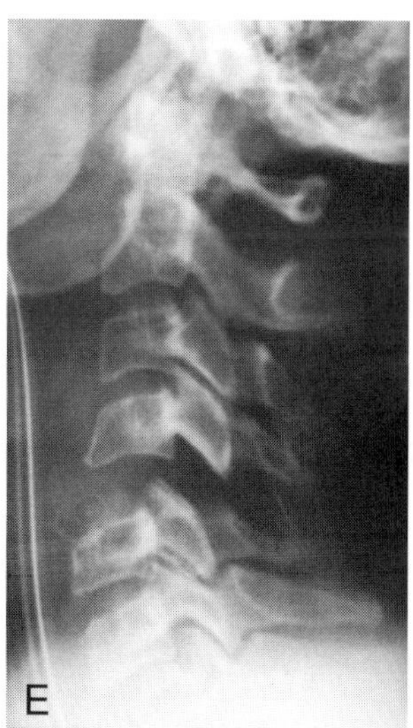

Figure 6.14 E

(continued)

Findings: On the AP cervical spine radiograph (Fig. A), the C4-5 interspinous distance is abnormally wide (vertical line). On the lateral radiograph (Fig. B), a severe hyperkyphotic angulation is present at C4-5 and C4 (4) is anteriorly rotated and displaced with respect to C5 by a distance equal to half the AP diameter of the vertebral body. The articular masses of C4 (including their inferior facets [arrowheads] are completely dislocated with respect to the articular masses of C5 (arrows). The interlaminar and interspinous spaces are abnormally wide ("fanning"). Left side image in Fig. C shows the articular masses of C4 (arrowheads) to lie anterior to those of C5 (arrows) and the body of C4 (4) to be anteriorly displaced with respect to the uncinate processes of C5 (5). Right side image in Fig. C shows the body of C4 anteriorly displaced with respect to that of C5 and the uncovered ("naked") superior facets of C5 (curved arrows).

Diagnosis: Bilateral interfacetal dislocation (BID).

Discussion: The severe hyperkyphotic angulation at the level of injury is due to distraction of the posterior and middle columns and reciprocal compression of the anterior column of the spine, all indicating a hyperflexion mechanism of injury. BID is one of the two injuries caused by hyperflexion, the other being anterior subluxation (hyperflexion sprain). In this patient, the relationship of C4 to C5 on the lateral radiograph shows that stability of the cervical spine at the level of the BID is disrupted as a result of dislocation of the articular masses of C4 with respect to those of C5. Additionally, "fanning" indicates that the interspinous and interlaminar ligaments and the ligamentum flavum are torn. Articular mass dislocation also causes disruption of the articular joint capsules. Anterior translation of the C4 vertebral body indicates the posterior longitudinal ligament, the intervertebral disc, and the anterior longitudinal ligament are all torn. Therefore, at the level of a BID, there is neither skeletal nor ligamentous stability. Because the AP diameter of the spinal canal at the level of dislocation is reduced by approximately 50%, the spinal cord is compressed between the spinolaminar line of the dislocated vertebra and the posterosuperior cortex of the subjacent vertebral body. Therefore, BID is mechanically (structurally) and neurologically unstable. For this reason, the term "doubly locked vertebra" sometimes used in reference to BID is not only pathologically inaccurate, but also clinically misleading.

Tiny impaction fracture fragments that arise from the free margins of the dislocated interfacetal joints, commonly found at surgery, are of no clinical significance. Major interarticular mass fractures, contrarily, are rare in BID. Therefore, CT contributes no additional information to that available from radiographs of the cervical spine. Conversely, MR imaging is essential to assess the type and extent of spinal cord and ligamentous injuries, and integrity of the vertebral arteries.

More commonly in children than adults, BID may result from a distractive force, in which event the signs of hyperflexion are replaced by those of distraction (Figs. D, E).

Case History: The patient is a 30-year-old passenger who was in a stopped car when it was struck from behind by another vehicle.

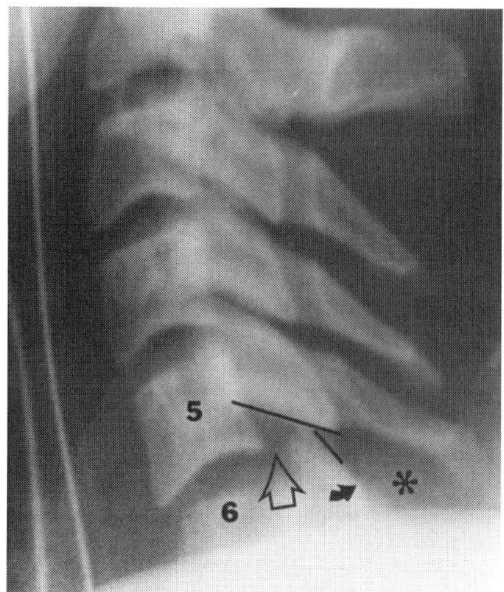

Figure 6.15

Findings: Lateral cervical spine radiograph shows hyperkyphotic angulation at C5-6 with anterior translation of C5, widening of the space between the body of C5 (5) and the superior articular process of C6 (6) (open arrow), incongruity of the C5-6 interfacetal joints (lines) with partial uncovering of the superior facets of C6 (curved arrow), and widening of the interlaminar and inter-spinous spaces ("fanning," asterisk).

Differential Diagnosis: Anterior subluxation (AS), unilateral interfacetal dislocation (UID), bilateral interfacetal dislocation (BID), pedicolaminar fracture–separation (PLFS).

Diagnosis: Anterior subluxation of C5.

Discussion: Anterior subluxation (hyperflexion sprain), one of the family of cervical spine injuries caused by predominant hyperflexion, is the flexion component of the whiplash injury. The mechanism of injury (MOI) described in the clinical presentation is the most common etiology of AS. The pathology of AS consists of tearing of the posterior ligament complex (interspinous and interlaminar ligaments, the ligamentum flavum, and the capsule of the apophyseal joints) and, sometimes, partial tearing of the posterior longitudinal ligament and the posterior aspect of the annulus fibrosus—all of which result from distraction of the posterior and middle columns of the spine during hyperflexion. Anterior translation of the subluxated vertebra is an inconsistent finding and, when present, is typically less than 3 mm. Prevertebral soft tissue swelling, when present, is minimal and is not important to the diagnosis. Widening of the interspinous space on the anteroposterior (AP) radiograph is simply the reflection of distraction of the posterior column during hyperflexion. In the AP view, this is not specific for AS, occurring in BID as well. When equivocal, AS may be confirmed by controlled lateral flexion and extension radiographs. CT plays no role in the diagnosis, but MR imaging is the definitive examination. AS is initially mechanically and neurologically stable but is complicated by failure of the posterior ligament complex to heal ("delayed instability") in approximately 50% of patients.

Anterior translation of the subluxated vertebra, when present, is the only feature of AS that is common to UID, BID, and PLFS. UID is characterized by anterior translation, usually 3 mm or greater but less than half the AP diameter of a cervical vertebral body, and is coupled with signs of rotation at, and above, the level of dislocation. BID is characterized by anterior translation equal to at least 50% of the AP diameter of a cervical vertebral body. PLFS refers to ipsilateral pedicle and laminar fractures resulting in the articular mass, becoming a free-floating fragment. Anterior translation is not present in all stages of PLFS. When present, it is associated with rotation and displacement of the free-floating articular mass in both the AP and the lateral cervical spine radiograph. Displacement of the articular mass distinguishes PLFS, a predominantly hyperextension injury, from AS, UID, BID, all of which are due to predominant hyperflexion.

Case History: This Australian clay miner was shoveling wet clay out of a ditch. In attempting to throw the next shovel full of clay, the shovel stuck in the clay and instead of hyperextending his cervical spine during the shoveling process, his head and upper cervical spine were abruptly pulled into severe hyperflexion by the shovel being stuck in the clay. The miner felt a sharp pain in the cervicothoracic region and, on physical examination, complained bitterly of tenderness to palpation over the lower cervical spinous processes. He was neurologically asymptomatic. You are shown a neutral lateral radiograph of the cervicothoracic junction (Fig. A) and a lateral radiograph of the same area obtained in flexion (Fig. B).

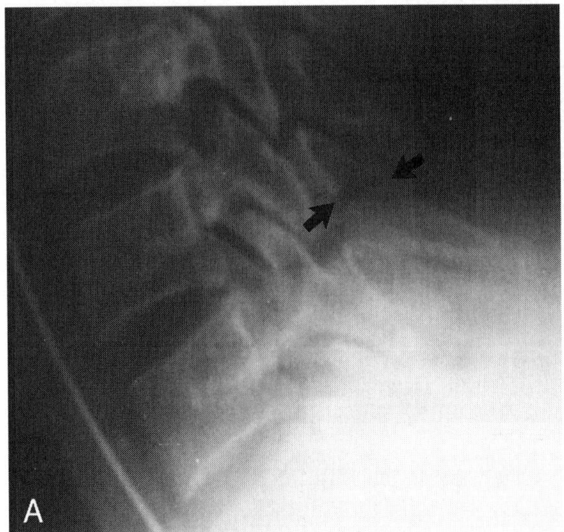

Figure 6.16 A   Figure 6.16 B

Findings: Fig. A shows an oblique fracture (arrows) traversing the base of the spinous process of C6. In all other respects, the visualized cervical segments are normal. The cervicocranial prevertebral soft tissue shadow is normal as reflected by the position of the nasogastric tube relative to the lower cervical vertebral bodies. In Fig. B, flexion to the limit of the patient's pain tolerance resulted in anterior translation of the anterior and middle columns of C6 while the spinous process fragment maintained its normal relationship to that of C7, resulting in distraction of the fragments and widening of the fracture line (open arrow).

Diagnosis: Clay shoveler's fracture of C6.

Discussion: The clay shoveler's ("coal shoveler's") fracture is one of the family of cervical spine injuries caused by predominantly hyperflexion mechanism of injury. The pathophysiology of the clay shoveler's fracture is that the intact interspinous ligament causes an avulsion fracture of the suprajacent spinous process. Had the intraspinous ligament torn, the patient would have sustained anterior subluxation (see Case #15). Characteristic of avulsion fractures, the fracture line is roughly perpendicular to the direction of the avulsive force and commonly extends into the posterior portion of the lamina. The clay shoveler's fracture is mechanically and neurologically stable.

In the flexion lateral radiograph (Fig. B), the anterior fragment demonstrates all of the signs of anterior subluxation as described in Case #15.

Case History: This young man dove into a shallow body of water, striking his head on the bottom. He was instantly quadriplegic. You are shown the initial lateral cervical spine radiograph (Fig. A), axial CT images of C5-6 (Figs. B, C), and an MR image (Fig. D) obtained shortly after admission.

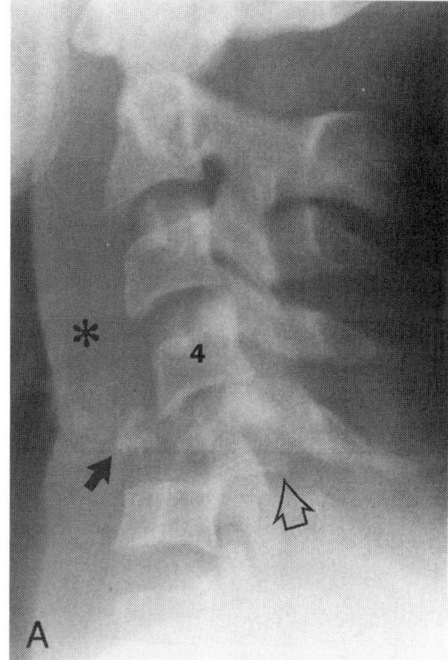

Figure 6.17 A

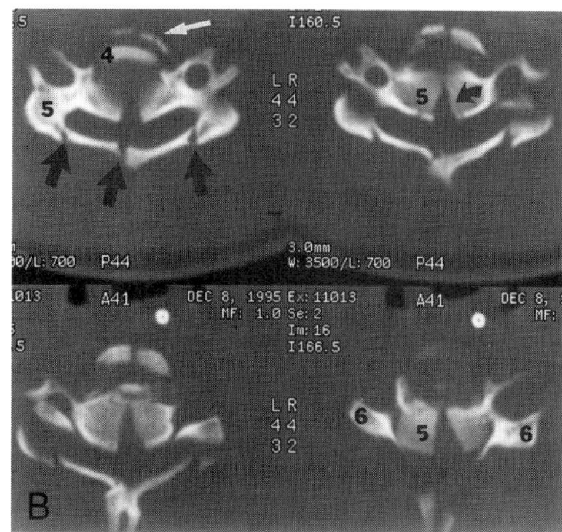

Figure 6.17 B

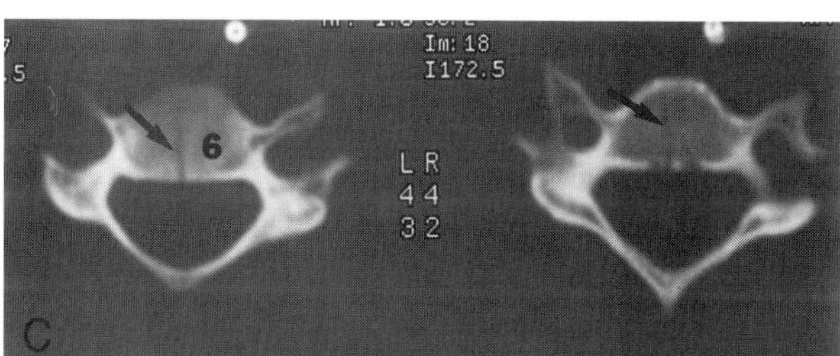

Figure 6.17 C

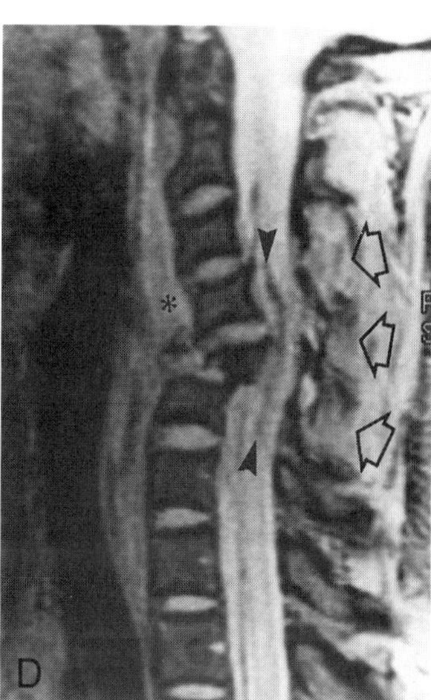

Figure 6.17 D

Findings: The most obvious finding is a severe, marked hyperkyphotic angulation of the cervical spine at the C5-6 level with the posterior portion of the C5 body (open arrow) displaced into the spinal canal by a distance greater than 50% of the AP diameter of the canal. The anterior portion of the C5 body is severely crushed by the body of C4 (4) and a large triangular fragment (arrow) has separated from the body of C5. Marked, diffuse prevertebral soft tissue swelling (asterisk) extends to the level of the anterior arch of C1. The hyperkyphotic angulation is associated with distraction of the posterior elements of C5 with respect to those of C6.

(continued)

Axial CT images (Fig. B) shows the antero-inferior corner of the body of C4 (4) interposed between the triangular fragment of C5 (white arrow) and the body of C5 (5), the latter containing a sagittal plane fracture (curved arrow) and marked posterior displacement of its fragments resulting in severe narrowing of the spinal canal. The laminae of C5 are fractured (straight arrows). Axial CT images (Fig. C) show a minimally displaced sagittal fracture (arrow) of the C6 (6) body. Sagittal MR image (Fig. D) shows, in addition to the skeletal findings described earlier, the marked antero-posterior compression of the spinal cord posterior to C5 and low intensity signal of a hemorrhagic cord injury extending from C4-C6 (arrowheads). Reflecting the hyperflexion mechanism of injury, the posterior ligament complex between C3-4, C4-5, and C5-6 is disrupted (open arrows). The prevertebral soft tissue mass of mixed signal intensity (asterisk) represents blood and edema, causing the severe prevertebral soft tissue swelling seen on the lateral cervical radiograph.

Differential Diagnosis: Bursting fracture of the lower cervical spine; flexion teardrop fracture.

Diagnosis: Flexion teardrop fracture.

Discussion: The flexion teardrop fracture is the most severe of the family of cervical spine injuries caused by predominant hyperflexion and, indeed, it is the most severe of all cervical spine injuries because, by definition, it is always associated with the acute cervical spinal cord syndrome, including instantaneous and permanent quadriplegia. The injury derives its name from the large triangular fragment arising from the anterior aspect of the involved vertebral body, which has been likened to the tear that falls on the cheek of the patient, or the patient's family, when informed of the permanent quadriplegia.

The hyperkyphotic angulation, distraction of the posterior column, including "fanning" of the interspinous and interlaminar spaces, severe subluxation or frank dislocation of the interfacetal joints, and compression of the anterior column of the involved vertebra are all characteristic of a predominant hyperflexion mechanism of injury.

The axial loading (burst, bursting, and dispersion) fracture of the lower cervical spine may resemble the flexion teardrop fracture by virtue of an anterior triangular separate fragment and retropulsion of posterior body fragments into the spinal canal. However, the bursting fracture of the lower cervical spine can be distinguished from the flexion teardrop fracture by the absence of the characteristic signs of hyperflexion described above.

CASE 18

Case History: This young adult fell from a height in such a way that she struck the ground with the top of her head. She experienced sudden, abrupt, severe pain in her midcervical region, marked limitation of motion, tenderness to palpation over the midcervical spinous processes and a myelopathy. You are shown AP (Fig. A) and lateral (Fig. B) radiographs of the cervical spine and an MR study of the cervical spine (Fig. C) obtained approximately 3 hours postadmission.

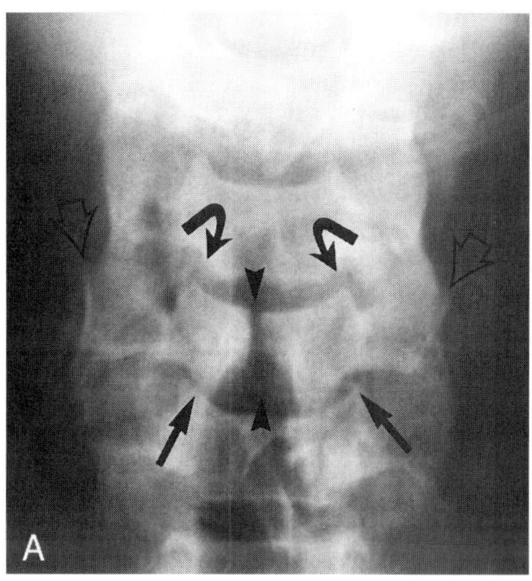

Figure 6.18 A

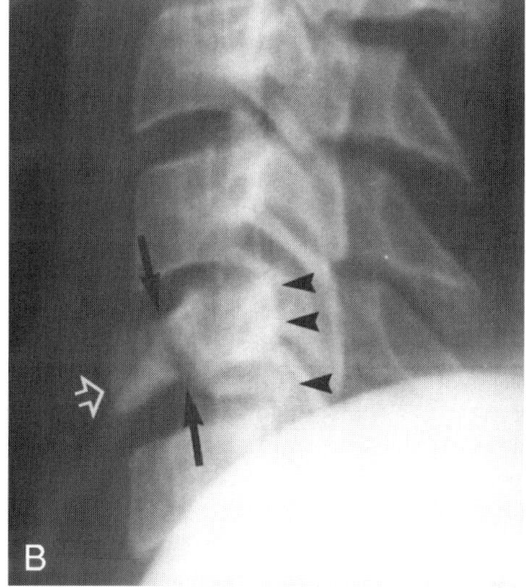

Figure 6.18 B

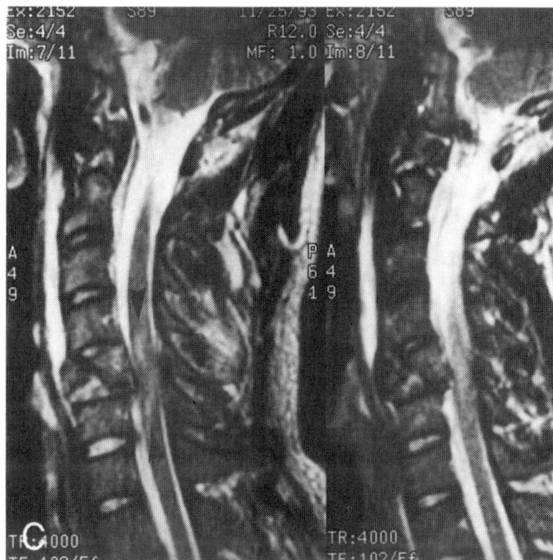

Figure 6.18 C

(continued)

Findings: AP cervical spine radiograph (Fig. A) shows a vertical fracture (arrowheads) of the body of C5. Each hemivertebral body fragment is laterally displaced with widening of the superjacent (curved arrows) and narrowing of the subjacent (straight arrows) Luschka joints. The lateral columns are disrupted bilaterally at the C6 level (open arrows). Lateral (Fig. B) radiograph shows a comminuted fracture of the body of C5 involving each end-plate (arrows) with dispersion of fragments anteriorly (open arrow) and posteriorly (arrowheads). The alignment of the cervical vertebrae is straightened and there is no distraction of the posterior elements. Midsagittal T2-weighted MR image (Fig. C) shows straightening of the cervical vertebrae with changes in the body of C5 as described on the lateral radiograph, and compression of the spinal cord by retropulsed fragments. There is high intensity (Type II, edema) injury in the spinal cord (arrowheads).

Differential Diagnosis: Simple wedge compression fracture; flexion teardrop fracture; burst fracture of the lower cervical spine.

Diagnosis: Burst fracture of the lower cervical spine.

Discussion: The burst (bursting, axial-loading, vertical compression, and dispersion) fracture of the lower cervical spine is caused by an axial-loading (vertical compression) force delivered to the vertex of the skull at the precise instant that the cervical spine is straight. This injury, as the bursting fracture of the lower lumbar spine (Case #23), is limited to those segments of the spine which may be voluntarily straightened. The pathophysiology of this injury, as recorded by cineradiography, is that of abrupt forced compression of an intervertebral disk against the intact annulus, which forces the nucleus pulposus through the inferior end-plate of the involved vertebral body. The resultant abrupt increase in pressure within the vertebral body causes it to explode, with fragments being dispersed in all directions. Axial CT shows a fracture of at least one lamina of the involved vertebra. Although the burst fracture is mechanically stable, it may be associated with the acute central cervical cord syndrome and, therefore, is considered to be neurologically unstable.

The simple wedge compression fracture of the cervical spine is distinguished from the burst fracture by a hyperkyphotic angulation at the level of injury, distraction of the posterior and middle columns, fracture of only the superior end-plate, and absence of a sagittal fracture through the vertebral body on the frontal radiograph (see Case #19). The flexion teardrop fracture is typically distinguished from the burst fracture by signs of severe hyperflexion, and by the acute cervical cord syndrome, including instant and permanent quadriplegia.

CASE 19

Case History: This wrestler experienced sudden onset of severe neck pain after being thrown in such a way that he landed striking his occiput on the mat. He had no neurologic deficit. You are shown a lateral radiograph of the lower cervical spine.

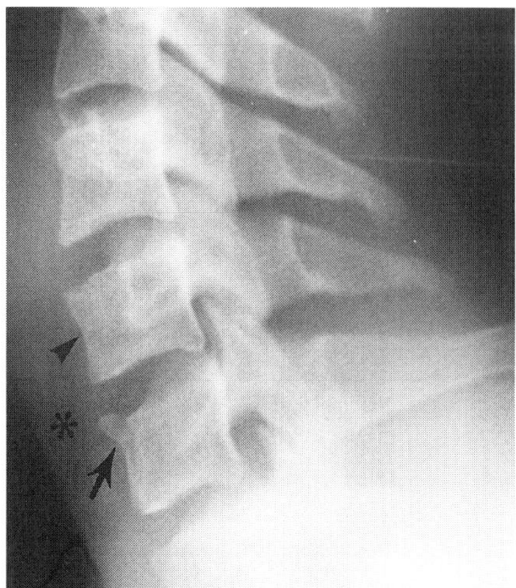

Figure 6.19

Findings: There is loss of vertical height of the anterior aspect of the bodies of C5 and C6 compared to their posterior vertical height. The superior end-plate of each is disrupted anteriorly and, concomitant with the loss of anterior vertical height, slopes antero-inferiorly. These contour changes result in an anteriorly wedged configuration of the bodies of C5 and C6. Additionally, and inherent to the loss of stature, are changes in the anterior cortex of each of these vertebral bodies. The superior portion of C5 is convex anteriorly and consequently angulated in its mid-third (arrowhead) while an incomplete fracture involves the antero-superior corner of C6 (arrow). Minimal soft tissue swelling (asterisk) is present from C4 through C6.

Differential Diagnosis: Simple wedge (compression) fracture; burst fracture of the cervical spine.

Diagnosis: Simple wedge (compression) fracture of C5 and C6.

Discussion: The simple wedge (compression) fracture is a member of the family of cervical spine injuries caused by predominant hyperflexion. During hyperflexion, the anterior column of the spine is compressed reciprocal to distraction of its posterior and middle columns. Consequently, the antero-inferior aspect of the vertebra above impacts upon the anterior aspect of the superior end-plate of the subjacent vertebra causing the simple wedge fracture. This fracture usually involves only a single vertebra but may, as illustrated, involve two or more segments. The fracture gets its name from the fact that the injury is as illustrated, that is, "simple" rather than complex, and "wedge" because of the resultant configuration of the vertebral body.

    The effect of the simple wedge fracture on the anterior cortex of the involved vertebral body is variable, as illustrated in this patient. Other findings include buckling of the superior aspect of the anterior cortex, frank impaction of the mid-portion of the cortex into the depressed superior fragment, and "step off" or "off-set." Usually there is no sign of a simple wedge fracture on the AP radiograph. Infrequently, with a simple wedge fracture, the lateral cortex of the involved vertebral body may be disrupted, buckled, or impacted. The posterior aspect of the vertebral body in a simple wedge fracture of the cervical spine is characteristically intact without retropulsion of fragment(s) into the spinal canal. Consequently, the simple wedge fracture is associated with neither spinal cord nor nerve root injury. The posterior ligament complex may be disrupted, in which event the ligamentous injury (anterior subluxation) is of greater clinical significance than the simple wedge fracture.

    On the lateral radiograph of the cervical spine, the burst (bursting, dispersion, and axial loading) fracture of the cervical spine is characterized by straightening (loss of cervical lordosis) of the cervical spine, compression of both end-plates, and displacement of fracture fragments anteriorly and posteriorly. The AP radiograph shows lateral displacement of the hemivertebral body fragments, a vertical body fracture line, and widening of the supra-adjacent and narrowing of the subjacent Luschka joints. (See Case #18). None of these signs are present in this patient and, therefore, a burst fracture is excluded.

CASE 20

Case History: This shipyard worker fell into the hold of a ship. He complained of midscapular pain and tenderness to percussion over the midthoracic spinous processes. He was neurologically intact. You are shown an AP supine chest radiograph (Fig. A), AP (Fig. B), and lateral (Fig. C) thoracic spine radiographs, axial CT (Fig. D) of the involved vertebra, and a coronal reformatted CT image (Fig. E).

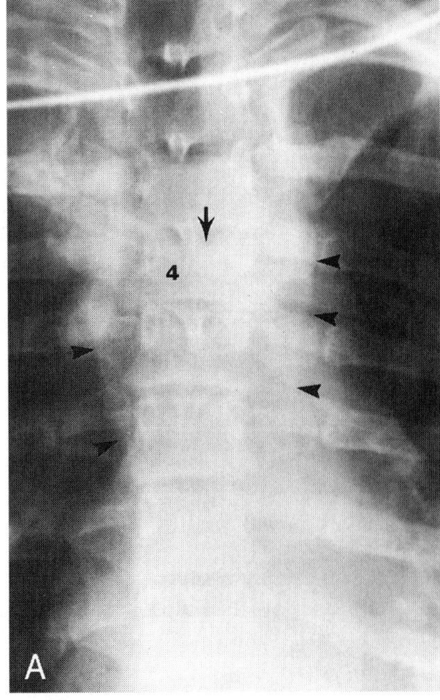

Figure 6.20 A

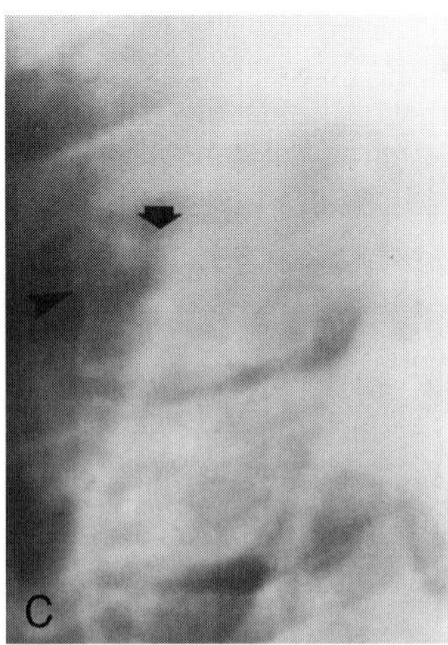

Figure 6.20 B

Figure 6.20 C

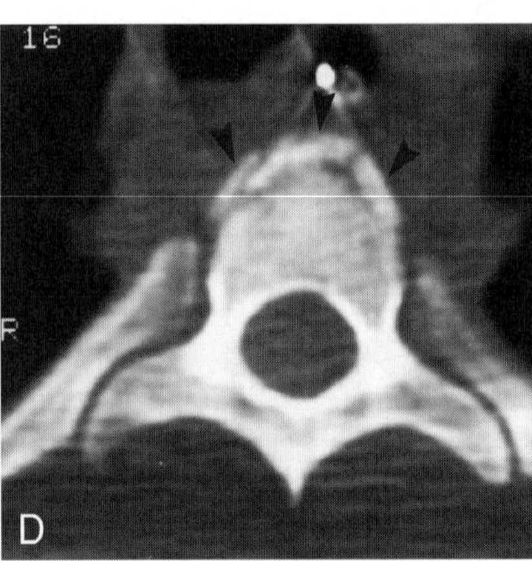

Figure 6.20 D

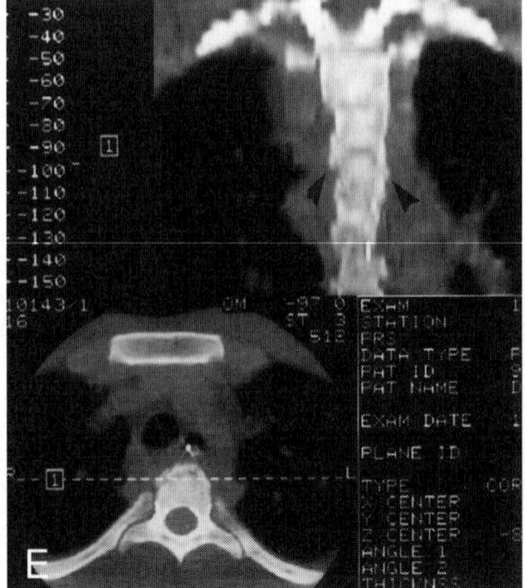

Figure 6.20 E

IMAGING OF THE SPINE: A TEACHING FILE

Findings: Supine chest radiograph (Fig. A) shows bilateral paraspinous hematoma (arrowheads) and absence of the superior end-plate of T4 (4) (arrow). The spinous processes and pedicles of the upper and midthoracic segments are normally aligned. The AP radiograph of the thoracic spine (Fig. B) shows bilateral paraspinous hematoma (arrowheads) and absence of the superior end-plate of T4 (arrow) to a better advantage. Loss of vertical height of T4 is also evident. Lateral thoracic spine radiograph (Fig. C) purposefully obtained during patient respiration ("auto-tomogram") shows depression of the superior end-plate (arrow) and buckling of the anterior cortex (arrowhead) of T4. Axial CT at the T4 level (Fig. D) shows the comminuted, anteriorly displaced fracture fragment (arrowheads) of the supero-anterior aspect of T4. The remainder of the T4 vertebral body is intact, and the spinal canal is normal. Coronal reformatted CT image (Fig. E) through the fracture shows a deformity of the superior end-plate and fractures of the superolateral cortex (arrowheads) of T4.

Diagnosis: Simple wedge compression fracture, T4.

Discussion: A simple wedge compression fracture is the most common fracture of the thoracic spine. Because of the normal thoracic kyphosis, axial loading forces accentuate the normal kyphosis resulting in a hyperflexion mechanism of injury and a compression fracture. A compression fracture of the thoracic spine is mechanically and neurologically stable. However, it is possible with a major, or severe, degree of compression to have retropulsion of posterior body fragments into the spinal canal. In the upper- and mid-thoracic segments, it is difficult to assess retropulsion on lateral radiographs and CT is indicated to assess the spinal canal. MR imaging is indicated in the presence of inappropriate pain and/or neurologic symptoms suggestive of acute traumatic herniation of an intervertebral disk.

CASE 21

Case History: This construction worker fell three stories to the ground. He was paralyzed from the T4 level. You are shown an AP supine chest radiograph (Fig. A), AP thoracic spine (Fig. B), axial CT images (Fig. C–H), and a midsagittal reformatted CT image (Fig. I).

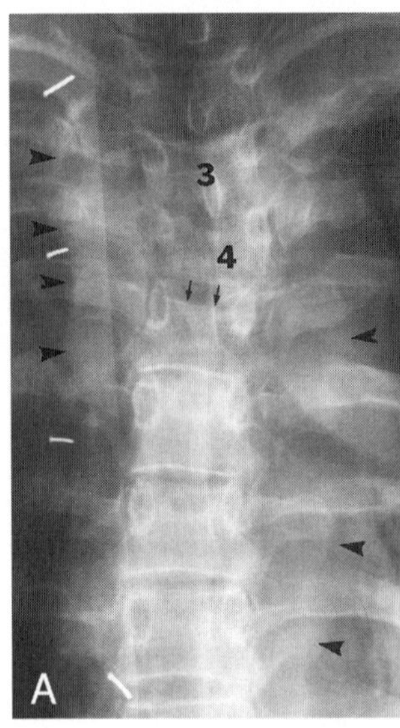

Figure 6.21 A

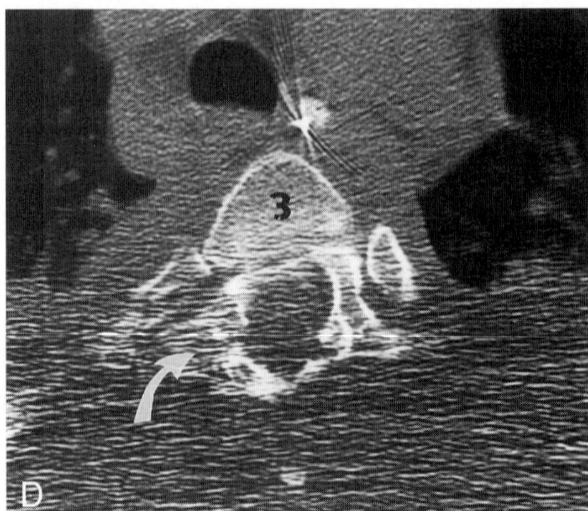

Figure 6.21 B

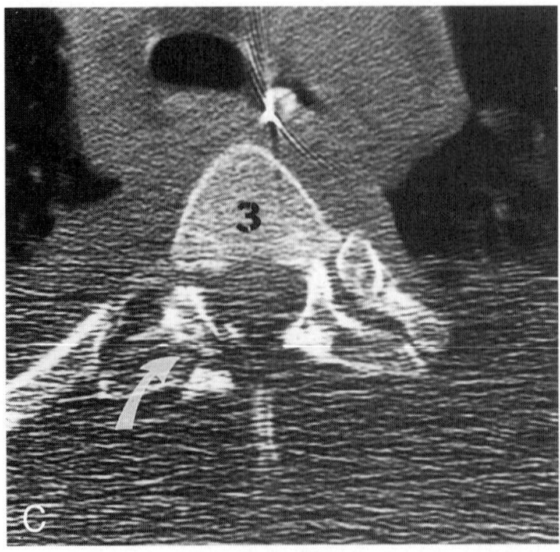

Figure 6.21 C

Figure 6.21 D

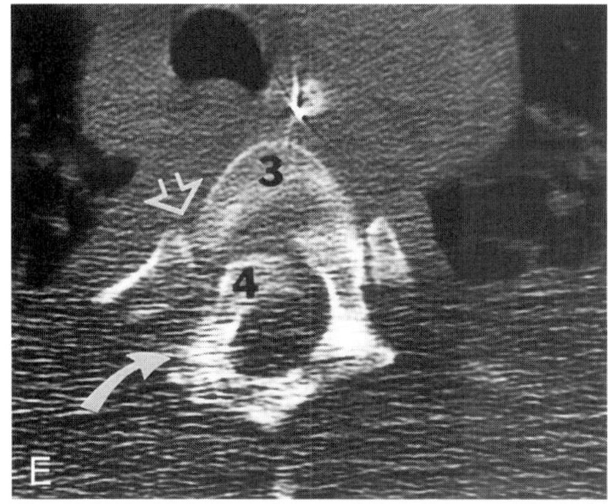

Figure 6.21 E

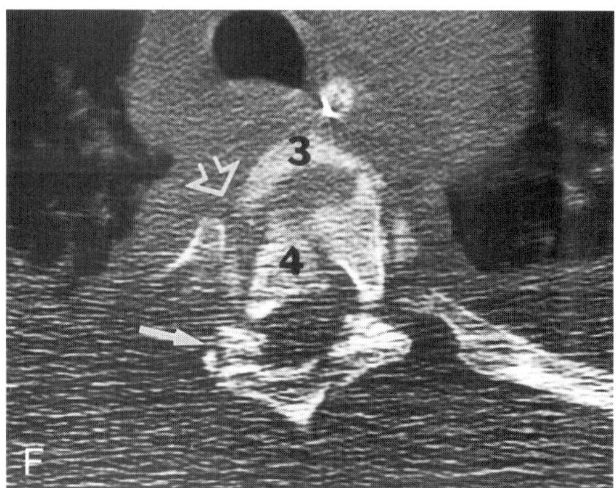

Figure 6.21 F

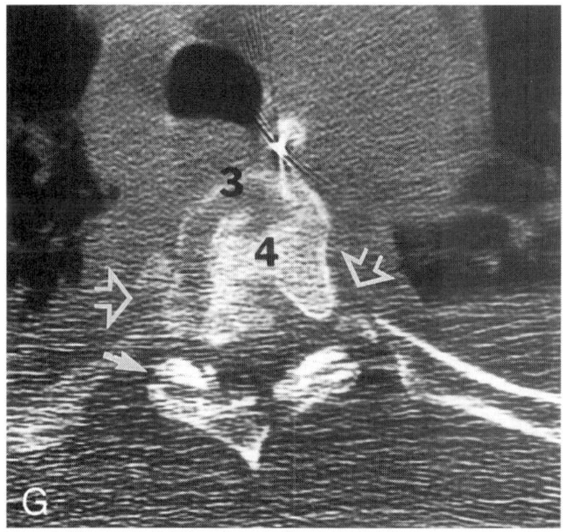

Figure 6.21 G

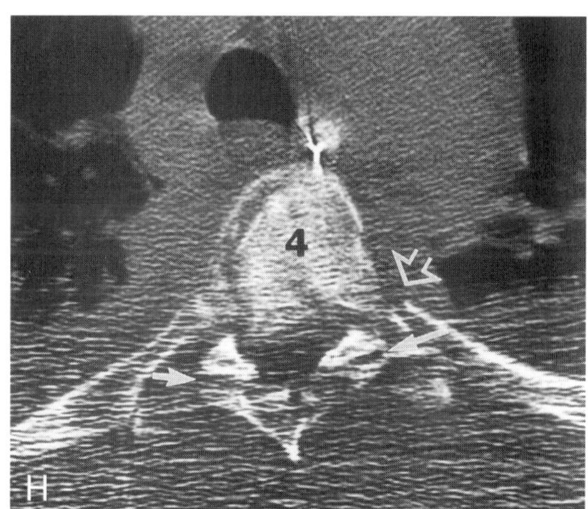

Figure 6.21 H

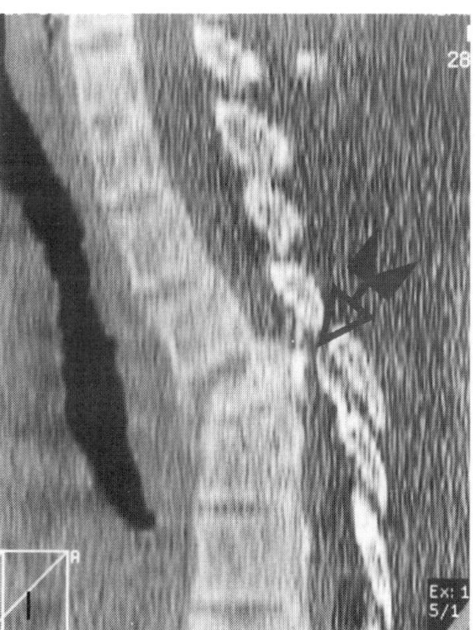

Figure 6.21 I

(continued)

Findings: The cropped AP supine chest radiograph (Fig. A) shows a bilateral paraspinal hematoma (arrowheads) and levo-scoliosis from T3–T5. The inferior end-plate of T3 (3) is not visible nor is the superior end-plate of T4 (4). T4 is also diminished in vertical height. The superior end-plate of T5 (arrows) is depressed. AP radiograph of the thoracic spine (Fig. B) shows the findings to a better advantage. The involved vertebrae were not visible on the lateral thoracic spine radiograph. Axial CT images from T3 through T4 (Figs. C–H) show severe disruption of the costovertebral (white open arrows) and apophyseal (white arrows) joints bilaterally, severe comminution of the right laminae of C3 and 4, severe comminution of the body of T4 with marked retropulsion of fragments into the spinal canal, and a left rotation of T4 with respect to T3. Mid-sagittal CT reformation (Fig. I) shows spinal canal encroachment by the retropulsed T4 posterior fracture fragments (open flagged arrow).

Diagnosis: Fracture–dislocation, T3-4.

Discussion: Fracture–dislocation of the mid and lower thoracic spine is usually evident on AP and lateral radiographs. CT and MR imaging are indicated; CT for delineation of skeletal injuries and assessment of spinal canal encroachment, and MR imaging to define the extent of spinal cord injury.

Thoracic and thoracolumbar dislocations and fracture–dislocations are, by definition, mechanically and neurologically unstable. The mechanism of injury of these injuries is predominantly simultaneous hyperflexion and rotation or shear.

CASE 22

Case History: This steeplechase horseback rider was thrown from her mount when the horse balked at a jump. The rider landed on her buttocks and experienced excruciating pain in the thoracolumbar area. You are shown AP (Fig. A) and lateral radiographs (Fig. B), and an axial CT image.

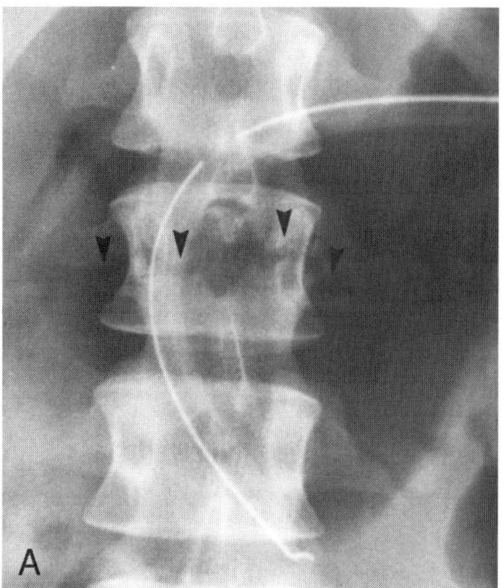

Figure 6.22 A

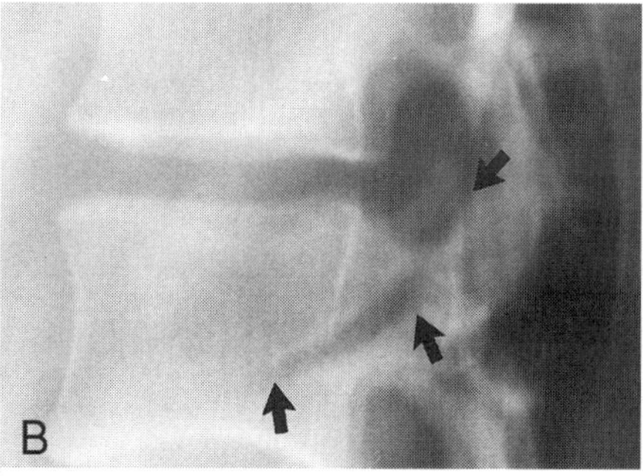

Figure 6.22 B

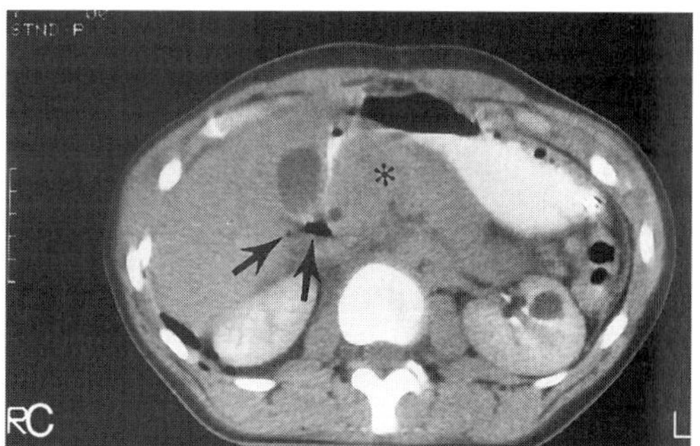

Figure 6.22 C

Findings: Frontal projection (Fig. A) of the thoracolumbar spine shows a transverse fracture to the laminae, pedicles, and transverse processes (arrowheads) of L2. Lateral radiograph (Fig. B) shows a distracted fracture of the pars interarticularis and pedicles which extends into the posterior aspect of the body of L2 (arrows). Axial CT image at a slightly higher level (Fig. C) shows enlargement of the head of the pancreas (asterisk) and periduodenal air, indicating duodenal rupture (arrows). The left renal cyst is an incidental finding.

Differential Diagnosis: Simple wedge compression fracture, L2; burst fracture, L2; Chance fracture.

Diagnosis: Chance fracture of L2.

Discussion: The Chance fracture was described by British physician G. Q. Chance in 1948 as occurring in patients involved in motor vehicle accidents while wearing only a lap seat belt. The mechanism of injury was described as severe hyperflexion with the fulcrum of flexion being the point of contact of the lap seat belt and the anterior abdominal wall. With the advent of contemporary lap-chest seat belts and air bags, the most common mechanism of injury of the Chance fracture is a fall from a height resulting in severe hyperflexion of the thoracolumbar spine.

(continued)

In the Chance fracture, signs of hyperflexion involve all three columns of the injured vertebrae, for example, distraction of the posterior and middle columns and compression of the anterior columns. The Chance fracture is found only in the thoracolumbar region (T11 through L2) because that segment of the spine, being the transition from lumbar lordosis to thoracic kyphosis, is subject to hyperflexion injuries with a primarily axial-loading force.

The Chance fracture is unique among all other thoracolumbar and lumbar spine fractures in that it is associated with an approximate 20% incidence of concomitant injury to the duodenum, pancreas, small bowel, and/or mesentery.

The similarity between simple wedge and Chance fracture lies only in those instances of the Chance fracture in which the fracture line extends to the anterior cortex with loss of vertical height. Distracted fractures of the posterior and middle columns characteristic of the Chance fracture are not present in the simple wedge compression fracture.

Distraction fractures of the posterior and middle columns of the involved vertebrae distinguish the Chance fracture from the bursting fracture on the lateral radiograph. Additionally, the Chance fracture does not involve both end-plates, which is a characteristic of the burst fracture. In the AP radiograph, the burst fracture is characterized by a vertical fracture of the vertebral body with lateral displacement of each hemi-body fragment resulting in widening of the superior, and narrowing of the inferior, Luschka joints. None of these signs are present in the Chance fracture.

CASE 23

Case History: This construction worker fell approximately 25 feet striking the ground in a sitting position. He complained of severe low back pain and paresthesias of the low back extending down the lateral aspect of each thigh. You are shown AP and lateral radiographs (Figs. A, B) of the lumbo-sacral area and axial (Fig. C) and sagittal (Fig. D) CT images of L5.

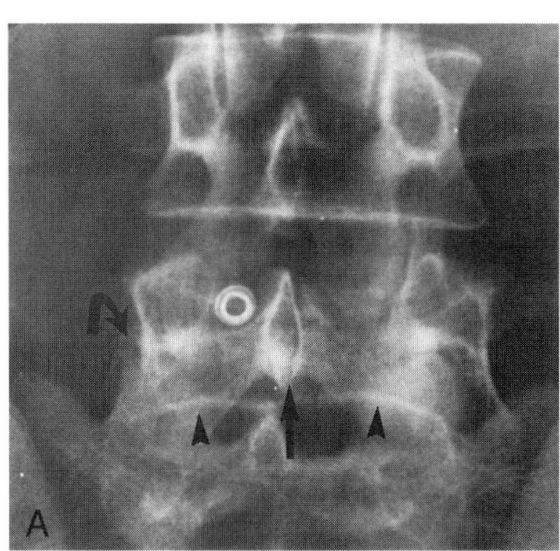

Figure 6.23 A

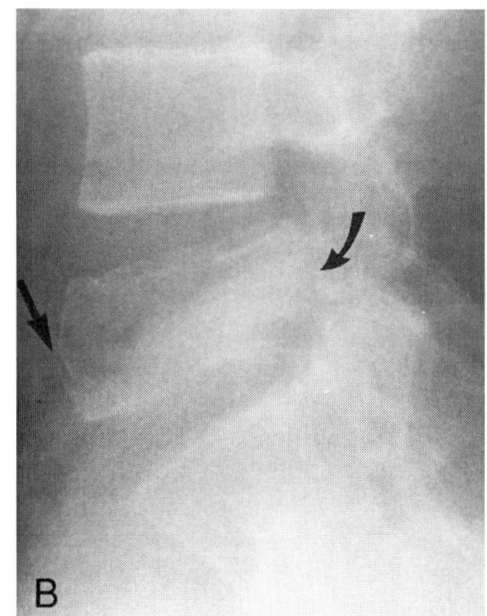

Figure 6.23 B

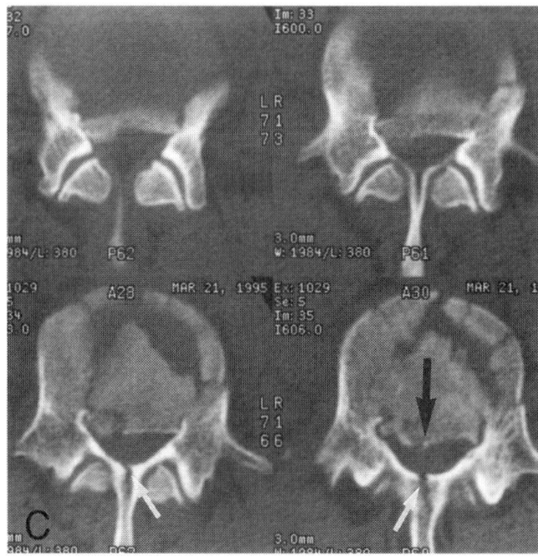

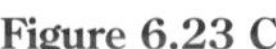

Figure 6.23 C

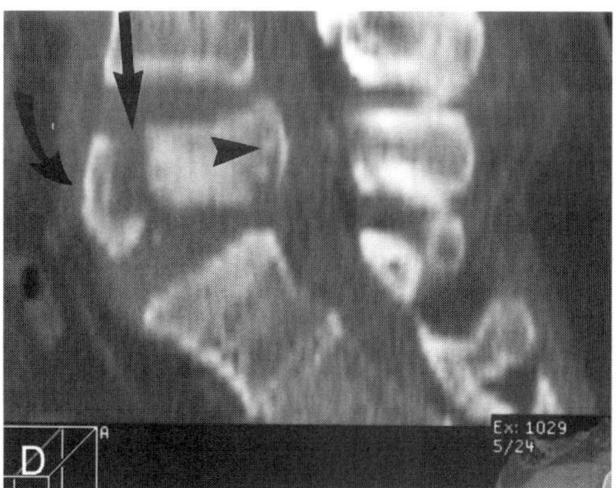

Figure 6.23 D

Findings: Fig. A shows an increased transverse diameter of L5 compared to that of L4, disruption of the right lateral cortex of the body of L5 (curved arrow), absence of its superior end-plate and concavity of its inferior (arrowheads) end-plate, and a subtle, minimally displaced fracture of its spinous process (arrow). Lateral radiograph (Fig. B) shows loss of height and disruption of both end-plates, convexity and disruption of the anterior body cortex (straight arrow), and retropulsion of the posterior aspect of the vertebral body into the spinal canal (curved arrow). Axial CT image of L5 (Fig. C) demonstrates severe comminution of the vertebral body with marked retropulsion of the posterior fragments (black arrow) and severe narrowing of the diameter of the spinal canal. A sagittally oriented fracture of the spinous process (white arrow) is also evident. The midsagittal reformatted CT image (Fig. D) confirms superior and inferior end-plate compression, demonstrates a vertical fracture through the anterior column of the vertebral body (straight arrow), anterior displacement of the anterior column fragment and its anteriorly convex cortex (curved arrow), and retropulsion of the posterior body fragment (arrowhead) into the spinal canal with resultant decrease in its diameter.

(continued)

Diagnosis: Burst fracture, L5.

Discussion: The burst (bursting, axial-loading, vertical compression, dispersion) fracture of the lumbar spine is caused by an axial-loading or vertical compression mechanism of injury. Of the various names applied to this injury, "dispersion" fracture is preferred because this name describes displacement of fragments in all directions, characteristic of this type of fracture. Bursting fractures can only occur in those segments of the spine that can be voluntarily straightened, that is, the cervical and lumbar regions. The vertical compression force must be applied to the spine at the precise instant that it is vertically straight. The pathophysiology of the burst fracture, as recorded by cineradiography in anesthetized animal experiments, is that the impacting force compresses the disk inferior to the involved vertebra. The resultant abrupt increase in intra-diskal pressure forces the nucleus pulposus to implode through the inferior end-plate into the vertebral body, resulting, in turn, in an abrupt increase in pressure within the centrum. The latter explodes the vertebral body from within outward, causing displacement of fragments in all directions. The dispersive force to the centrum is transmitted through the pedicle to the posterior arch of the involved vertebra causing a posterior arch fracture of the laminae or, as in this patient, the spinous process. The fragments retropulsed into the spinal canal may injure the spinal cord or the cauda equina as in this patient. A burst fracture usually is neurologically unstable.

chapter 7

POSTSURGICAL CHANGES (CERVICAL AND THORACIC)

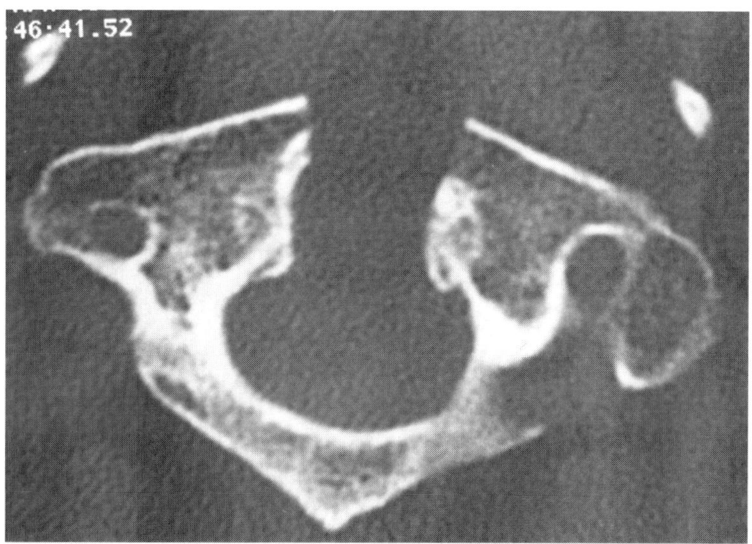

CASE 1

Clinical History: You are shown two patients who underwent diskectomies. Both are asymptomatic, and these are routine postsurgery follow-up studies.

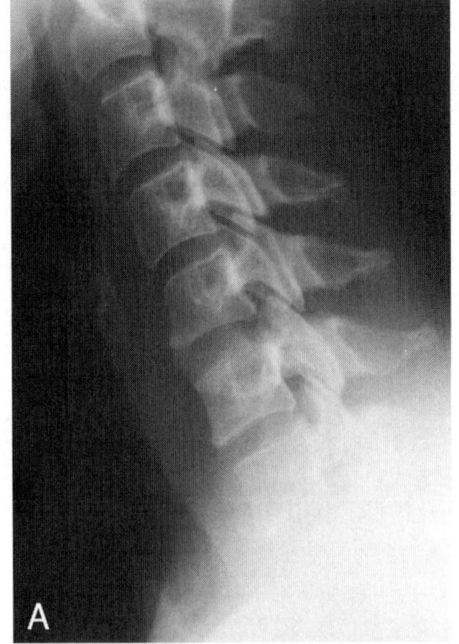

Figure 7.1 A

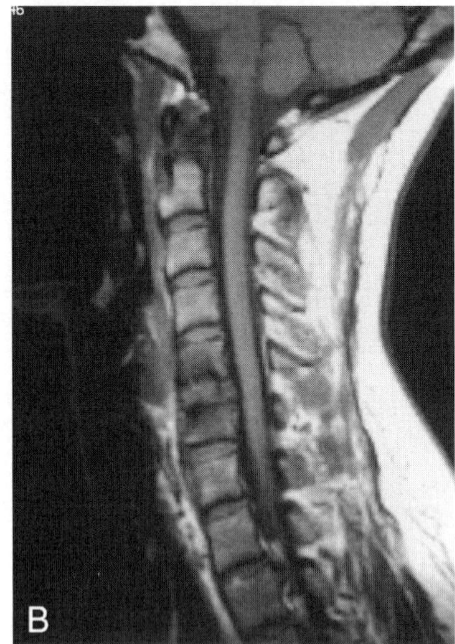

Figure 7.1 B

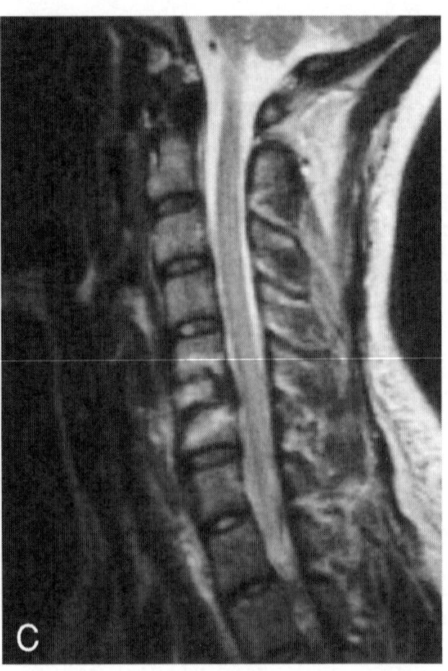

Figure 7.1 C

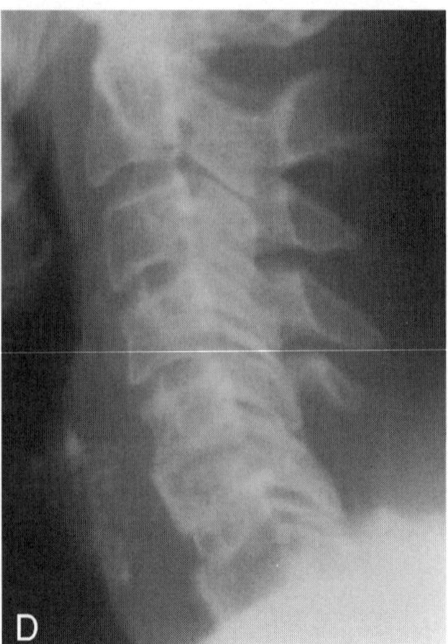

Figure 7.1 D

(continued)

   IMAGING OF THE SPINE: A TEACHING FILE

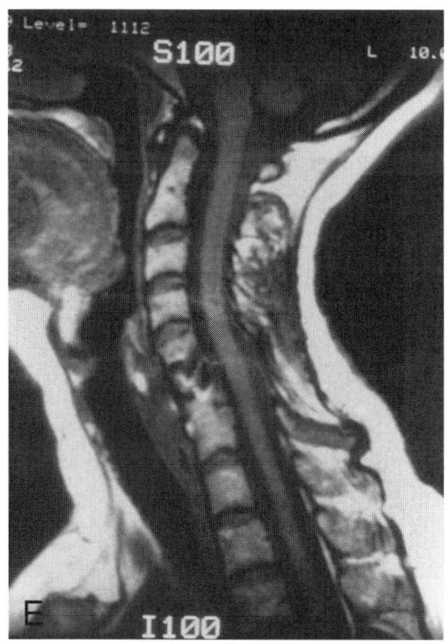

Figure 7.1 E

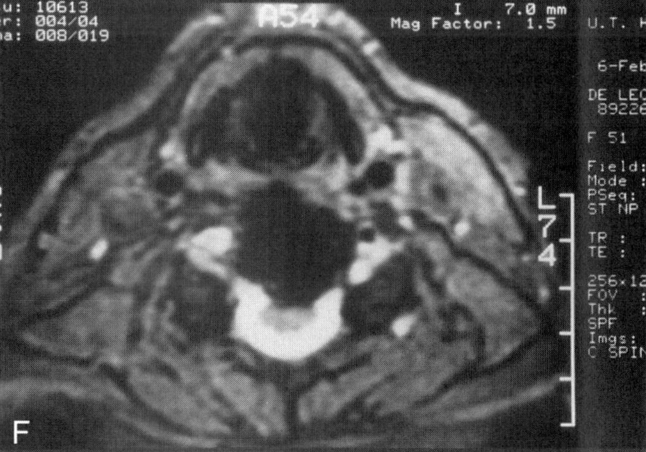

Figure 7.1 F

Findings: In the first patient, a lateral radiograph (Fig. A) shows a bone plug at C5-C6. The plug is in adequate position. Midsagittal MR T1-weighted image (Fig. B) shows the bone plug at C5-C6 with adequate diameter of the spinal canal at this level. The changes in the bone could represent edema. On a corresponding T2-weighted image (Fig. C), the bone marrow of the C5 and C6 vertebral bodies and the plug are bright. On the second patient, a lateral radiograph (Fig. D) shows surgical fusion of C5-C7. Note the absence of metal. Midsagittal MR T1-weighted image (Fig. E) shows metal-appearing artifact at the fusion levels but no significant stenosis of the spinal canal. Axial T2*-weighted MR image (Fig. F) shows considerable blooming of artifact, presumably caused by metallic particles from the drill bit. The artifact gives the appearance of compression of the ventral aspect of the spinal cord.

Diagnosis: Anterior cervical diskectomies and interbody bone fusions.

Discussion: Anterior cervical approaches offer the most direct method for decompression of the cervical spinal canal. More than 60% of patients treated this way report excellent results. The presence of myelopathy is an important indication favoring an anterior approach. Surgically, a lateral neck incision is done and all disk material and osteophytes are removed. Small anterior and posterior bone lips are left in the vertebral end-plates to prevent slippage of the bone plug. Bone grafts may come from the patient (autologous) or from a bank (allo- or homografts). There are several variations of the procedure depending on the type of graft and on the amount and shape of the bone removed from adjacent vertebrae. After surgery, patients are required to wear a brace for 6 months. Radiographically, incorporation of the plug into the neighboring vertebrae should be evident by 6 weeks. Small (not visible on radiographs) metal filings from the drill bit used to remove part of the end-plates may create metallic artifacts on MR imaging, which may obscure visualization of the spinal canal or simulate extradural abnormalities with compromise of the spinal canal diameter. The use of axial fast spin echo T2-weighted image or postcontrast axial T1-weighted image diminishes these artifacts. These artifacts are accentuated on all gradient echo images.

CASE 2

Clinical History: A 30-year-old man had an anterior diskectomy for a herniated disk. After falling down, he presents with acute cervical pain.

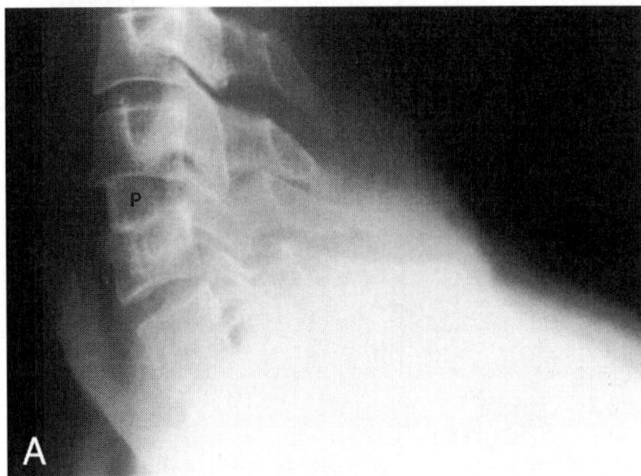

Figure 7.2 A

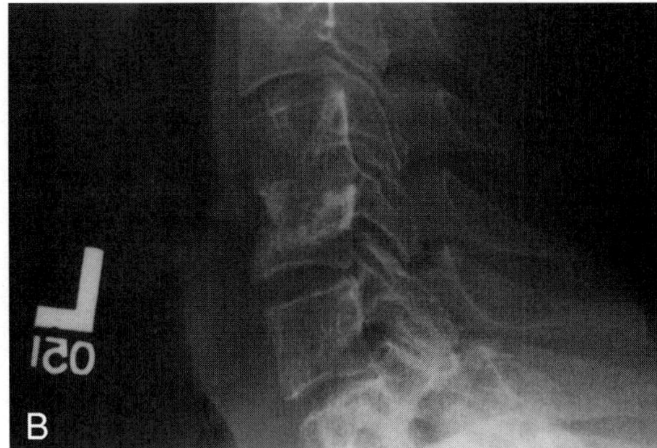

Figure 7.2 B

Findings: Lateral radiograph (Fig. A) obtained 6 months after initial surgery shows a bone plug (P) at C5-C6. The bones and plug are osteopenic. The plug has not been incorporated and there is no obvious bone fusion at this site. Corresponding radiograph (Fig. B) after falling down shows a compression fracture of C6 and of the bone plug.

Diagnosis: Failed (unincorporated) fusion with fracture.

Discussion: In this patient, the bone graft was obtained from his iliac crest. Autologous graft are preferred by some patients because of the possibility of hepatitis, HIV, or bacterial infection. There is, however, a small risk of infection at the donor site. Chronic pain at the donor site is reported by up to 15% of patients. Rarely, injury to the lateral femoral cutaneous nerve results in myalgic paresthesias. Osseous complications after anterior approaches include dislodgement of the graft(s), angulation deformity, fracture of the graft, pseudoarthrosis, and aseptic necrosis and diskitis. The rate of nonunion for single level diskectomies is approximately 5% and is 15% for multilevel diskectomies.

Clinical History: You are shown two patients. The first (Figs. A–C) underwent an anterior diskectomy and fusion; he is now asymptomatic. The second (Figs. D and E) underwent multilevel fusions and is now asymptomatic.

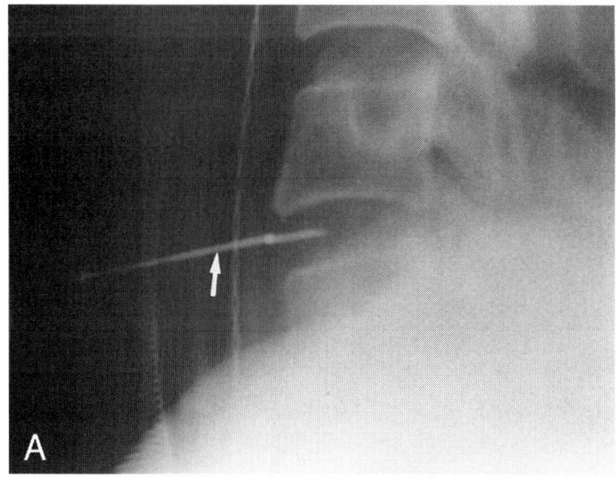

Figure 7.3 A

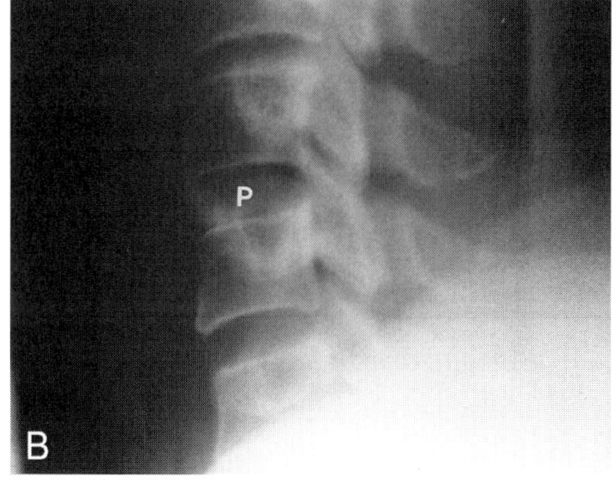

Figure 7.3 B

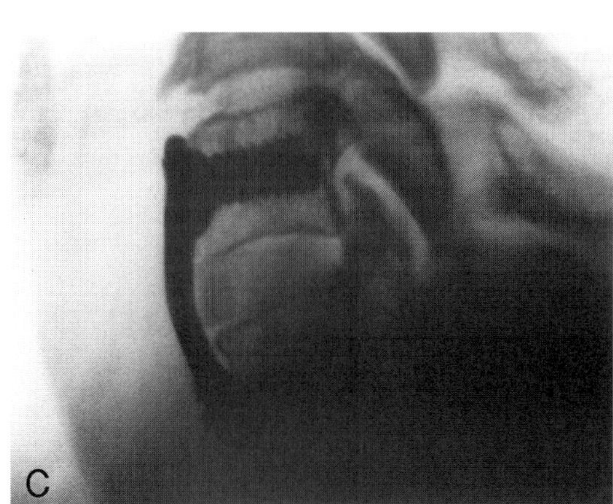

Figure 7.3 C

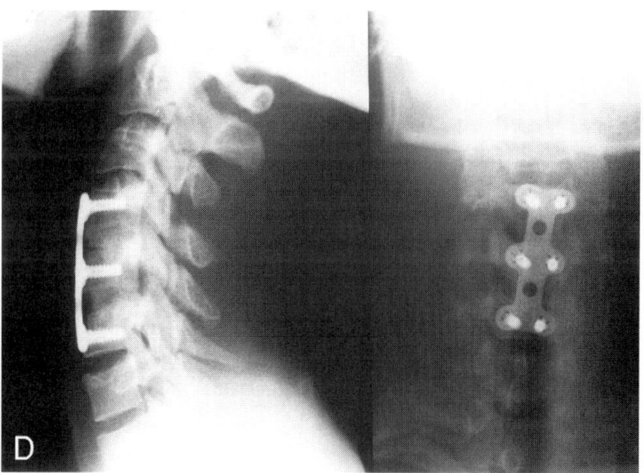

Figure 7.3 D

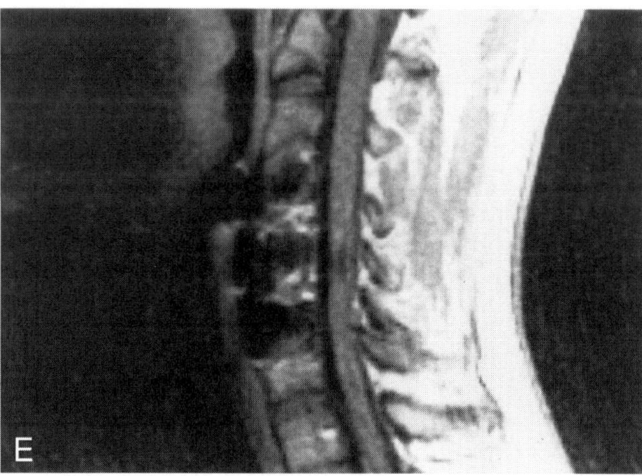

Figure 7.3 E

(continued)

Findings: Lateral intraoperative radiograph (Fig. A) shows probe (arrow) identifying the C5-C6 disk space. Intraoperative lateral radiograph (Fig. B) shows bone plug (P) at C5-C6. Lateral radiograph (Fig. C) shows anterior plate bridging the diskectomy site. The plate is held in place by bicortical screws. In a different patient (Fig. D), lateral and frontal radiographs show a self-locking titanium H-shaped plate extending from C4-C6 where diskectomies were done and bone plugs were placed. The plate is held in place by unicortical screws. In the same patient, midsagittal MR T1-weighted image (Fig. E) shows that the titanium hardware results in little artifact. The spinal cord is well seen and contains an area of low signal intensity at the level of C5.

Diagnosis: Successful anterior diskectomies and fusions. The spinal cord abnormality in the second patient may be related to myelomalacia.

Discussion: Placement of metallic plates and screws are considered when the following situations are found: burst fractures, traumatic disk herniations, tumors, multilevel diskectomies, and grossly unstable injuries. Plates are usually held in place by paired screws above and below the level of the diskectomy. The most commonly used plates are Caspar and Mosher plates. The Caspar plates are slightly curved to accommodate the normal configuration of the cervical spine. Bicortical screws provide better stability than do unicortical screws. Because bicortical screws burrow into the posterior cortex of the vertebral bodies, a greater chance of neurologic injury exists. Unicortical screws traverse only the anterior cortex and their tips lie in the bone marrow cavity of the vertebral bodies. Screws may have spiral fenestrations which are thought to promote the growth of bone into the screws. Hollow screws have a greater incidence of fatigue and failure than do solid ones. Titanium is commonly used because of its increased compatibility with CT and MR imaging.

CASE 4

Clinical History: You are shown two patients. The first (Figs. A–D) suffered bilateral facet dislocations at C6-C7. The reduction was difficult and was done by both a posterior and an anterior approach. The patient was quadriplegic after surgery and was ventilator-dependent. The second (Fig. E) awoke quadriplegic after a posterior open reduction for cervical spine trauma.

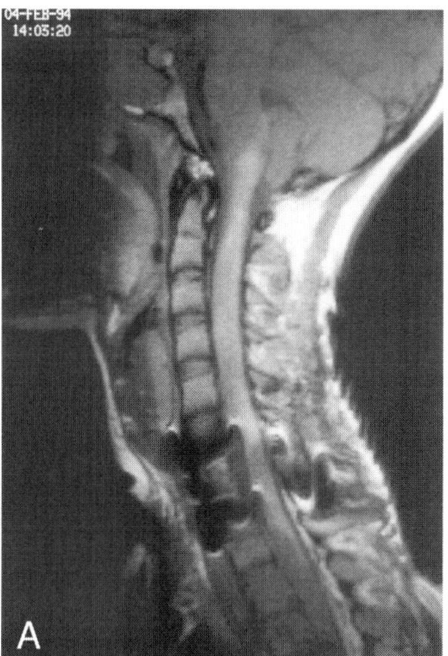

Figure 7.4 A

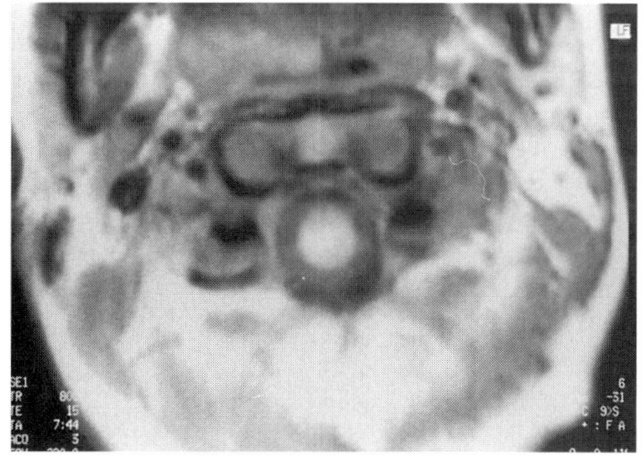

Figure 7.4 B

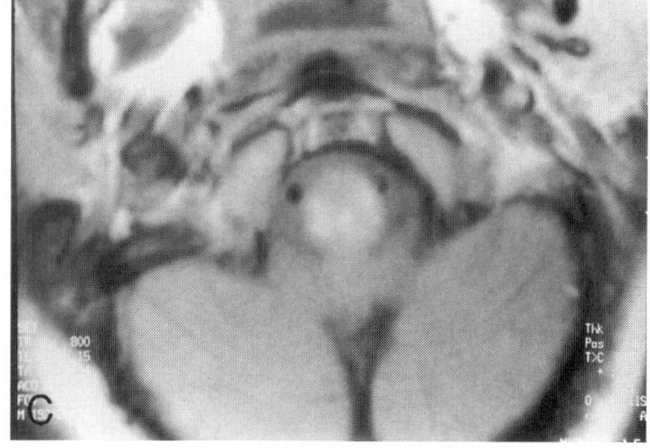

Figure 7.4 C

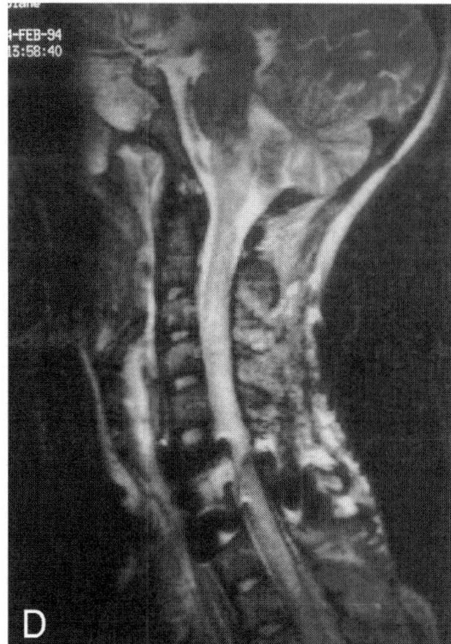

Figure 7.4 D

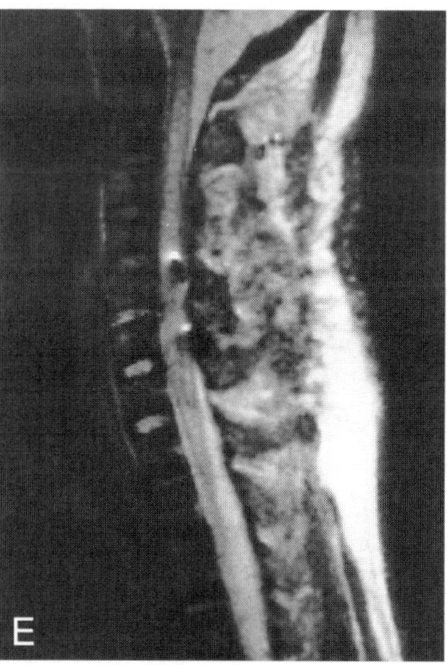

Figure 7.4 E

(continued)

Findings: Midsagittal MR T1-weighted image (Fig. A) shows metal artifact at C5-C7 from an anterior titanium plate as well as posteriorly (at the same level) from cables. The spinal cord has abnormal increased signal intensity from the medulla to the upper thoracic region and is swollen. Axial MR T1-weighted images (Figs. B and C) at the medulla and cervical spinal cord respectively show increased signal intensity. A midsagittal MR T2-weighted image (Fig. D) shows diffusely increased signal intensity in the entire cervical spinal cord. Note artifacts from wires and anterior plating at the C5 and C6 levels. In the second patient (Fig. E), a midsagittal MR T2-weighted image shows abnormal increased signal intensity in the spinal cord extending from C2 to T1. Note artifacts at C5 and C6 from posterior wires.

Diagnosis: Spinal cord infarctions (possibly hemorrhagic in the first patient) as complications of surgical reduction and stabilization.

Discussion: Vascular complications of the anterior approach include injury to the vertebral and carotid arteries and to the jugular veins. The vertebral arteries may also be damaged during the posterior approach. The vertebral arteries are generally injured by direct trauma or wandering instrumentation. The carotid arteries are more commonly injured during retraction. The risk of spinal cord damage secondary to anterior diskectomy and fusion is approximately 0.2%. Contributing factors include neck manipulation during anesthesia, edema, hypertension, and other vascular disorders (such as diabetic vasculopathy). Incomplete neurologic complications of spinal cord injury are the Brown Sequard syndrome, progressive myelopathy, and impaired sphincter control. Removal of the posterior longitudinal ligament has been implicated in injury to the spinal cord presumably by alteration in blood flow through the anterior spinal arterial system. The exact rate of complications between anterior and posterior approaches is not definitely established. Some series report an increased overall rate of complications with anterior approaches, whereas others do not.

CASE 5

Clinical History: You are shown three different patients. The first (Fig. A) is asymptomatic after surgery. The second (Figs. B and C) is experiencing severe neck pain after surgery. The third (Fig. D) has severe pain, fever, and difficultly breathing and swallowing 2 weeks after surgery.

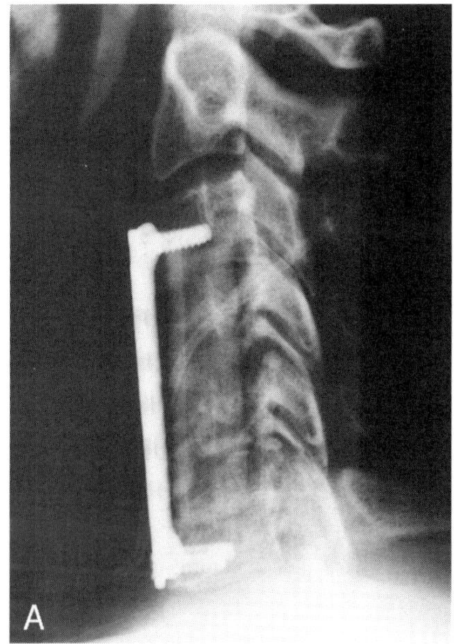

Figure 7.5 A

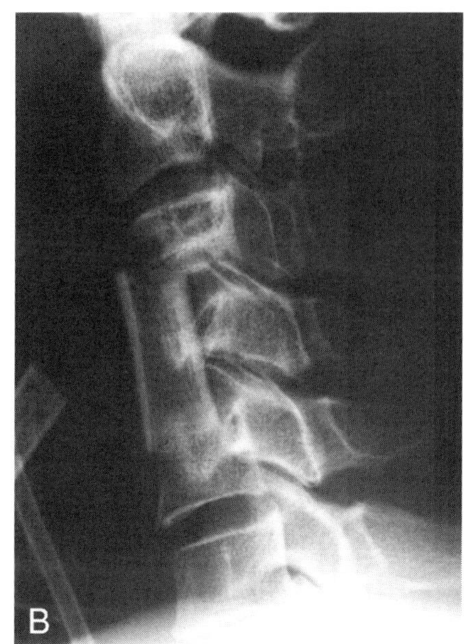

Figure 7.5 B

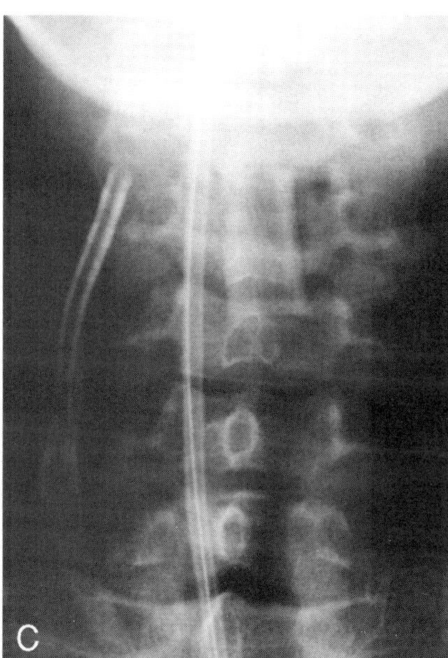

Figure 7.5 C

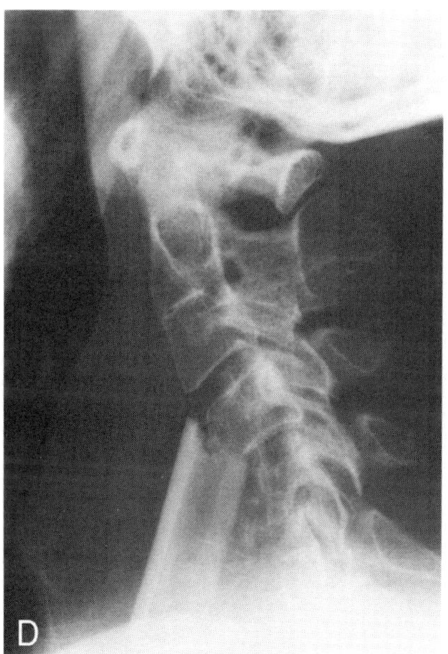

Figure 7.5 D

(continued)

Findings: Lateral radiograph (Fig. A) shows a bone strut graft extending from C3 to C7. The graft is in good position and is held in place by a long plate with unicortical screws. In the second patient, a lateral radiograph (Fig. B) shows slight anterior subluxation of the strut graft. A frontal radiograph (Fig. C) in the same patient shows no lateral dislodgement of the graft. In the last patient, a lateral radiograph (Fig. D) shows complete anterior dislocation of the strut graft. The underlying vertebral bodies are eroded and there is a large, soft tissue mass in the retropharyngeal/precervical space compressing the airway. A large abscess was found at this level.

Diagnosis: Bone strut graft in adequate position (first case), anteriorly subluxated bone strut graft (second case), and dislocated graft with abscess and osteomyelitis (third case).

Discussion: Displacement of bone grafts may occur in up to 13% of patients. Anterior displacements may result in pain or pseudoarthrosis, or it may be asymptomatic. Significant displacement may encroach on other soft tissues of the neck. Posterior displacements are uncommon and may result in compression of the neural structures. Perforation of the upper aerodigestive tract is uncommon because of dislodged grafts and occur most often secondary to forceful intraoperative retraction. Graft displacement may injure the sympathetic chain, resulting in a Horner's syndrome. Fractures of bone strut may also occur. Dissolution in the graft is uncommon with struts and is more commonly seen with dowels of bone. Overall, infections rates vary from 1–3%.

CASE 6

Clinical History: Patient who underwent an anterior fusion and bone grafting now presents with a history of fever and neck pain.

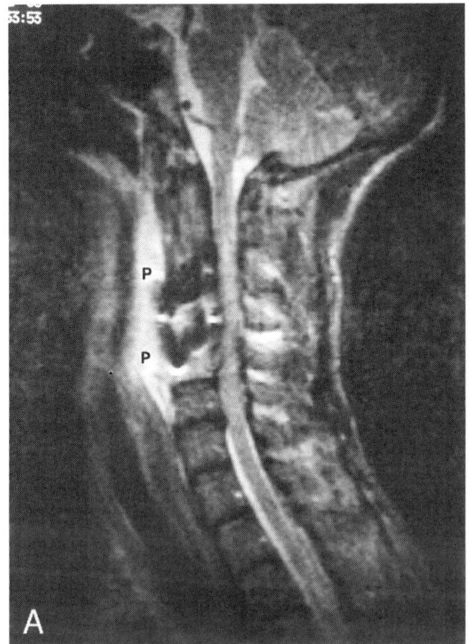

Figure 7.6 A

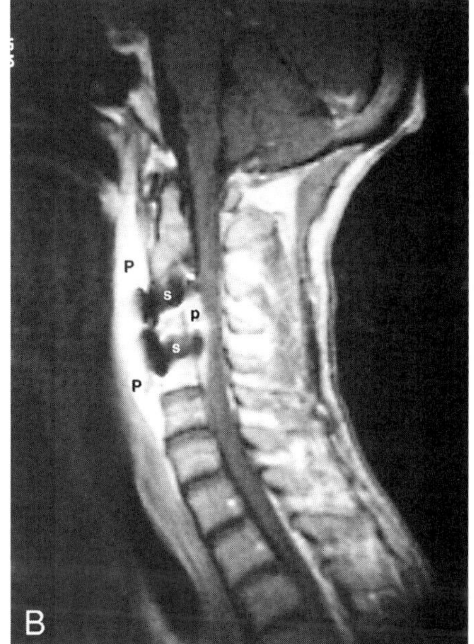

Figure 7.6 B

Findings: Midsagittal MR T2-weighted image (Fig. A) shows abnormal increased signal intensity (P) and thickening of the precervical tissues from the base of the skull to C5. There is questionable high signal intensity in the spinal cord. Corresponding postcontrast T1-weighted image (Fig. B) shows enhancement of the precervical (P) and ventral epidural (p) tissues without evidence of necrosis. The findings suggest the presence of phlegmons. There is compression of the spinal cord at the C3-C4 level. The screws (s) fixating the anterior plate are well seen. The C3-C4 vertebral bodies also enhance. The bone graft is not identified.

Diagnosis: Postsurgical infection with phlegmon formation and compression of the spinal cord.

Discussion: Bone grafts undergo a well-established change in their MR appearance during the first 6 months. Immediately after surgery they are hyperintense on T1-weighted images and mostly isointense to the adjacent vertebrae on T2 sequences. However, the adjacent vertebrae may be bright on T2-weighted images because of edema. At 1 month, T1-weighted images show the grafts to lose some of their brightness and to become minimally hyperintense on T2-weighted images. The edema of the adjacent vertebrae begins to resolve. The graft's appearance remains unchanged at 3 months but the bone marrow of the adjacent vertebrae regains its normal fatty content. At 6 months, the bone grafts are minimally hyperintense with respect to the adjacent vertebrae and isointense on T2-weighted images. Enhancement and thickening of the adjacent paraspinal soft tissues and of the epidural space should be viewed cautiously because they may be related to infection. Infection occurs in 1–3% of all spinal surgeries. Lack of the normal progression just described may be related to infection, pseudoarthrosis, non-union, and dissolution of the graft.

CASE 7

Clinical History: This patient underwent a posterior fusion for instability secondary to trauma. He is asymptomatic.

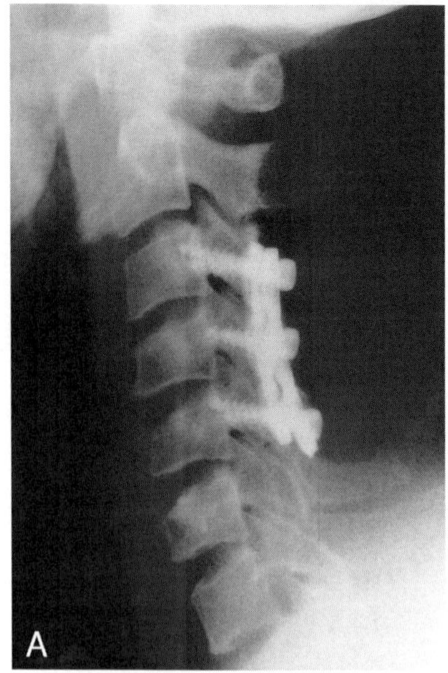

Figure 7.7 A

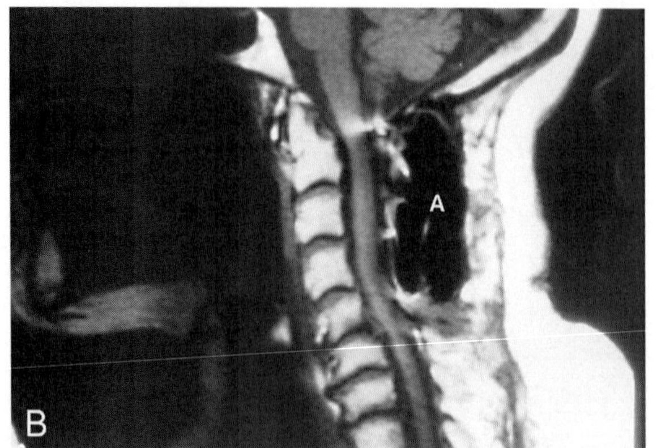

Figure 7.7 B

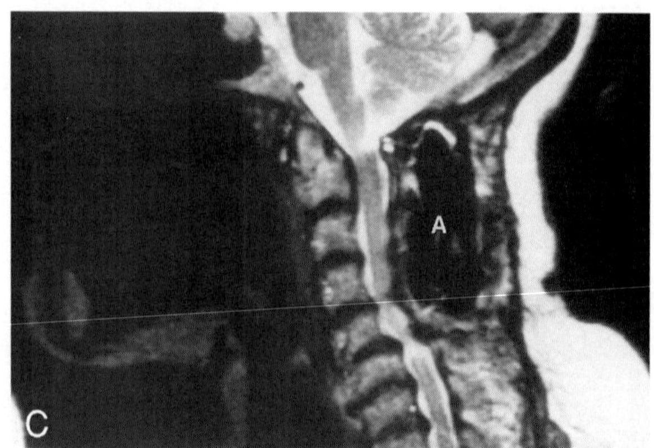

Figure 7.7 C

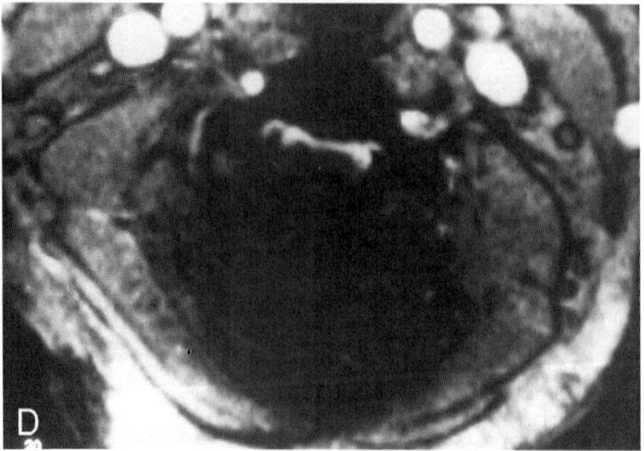

Figure 7.7 D

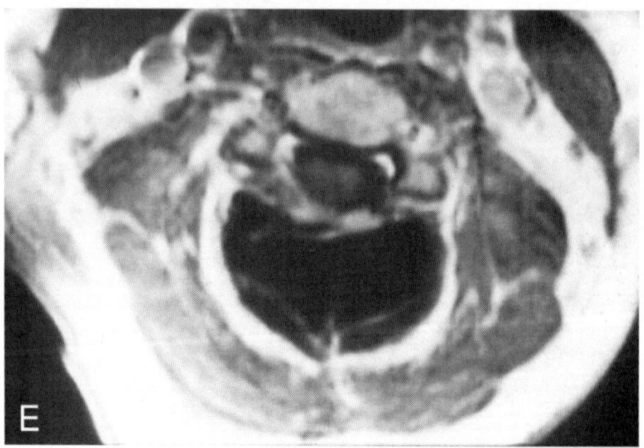

Figure 7.7 E

(continued)

Findings: Lateral radiograph (Fig. A) shows bilateral plates fixed with three pedicular screws each. The bone alignment is normal. Midsagittal MR T1-weighted image (Fig. B) in the same patient shows artifact (A) from the hardware and minimal deformity of the spinal cord. The artifact projects into the posterior spinal canal. Corresponding fast spin echo T2-weighted image (Fig. C) shows mild blooming of the artifact (A) which, however, also obscures the posterior aspect of the spinal canal. Axial T2*-weighted image (Fig. D) shows considerable blooming of the artifact obscuring most of the spinal canal. Corresponding T1-weighted image (Fig. E) shows good visualization of the spinal canal with minimal artifact.

Diagnosis: Adequate posterior fixation with blooming artifact on gradient echo (T2*) images.

Discussion: The increased magnetic susceptibility effects produced by ferromagnetic and paramagnetic materials used in spinal hardware create a potential problem in the imaging of these patients. Although most hardware used nowadays is said to be MR compatible, this does not mean that it will not produce artifacts. This denomination reflects the lack of significant deflection when exposed to the magnetic field. Magnetic susceptibility results in local field inhomogeneities and field distortions leading to increased dephasing of spins, which translates as artifacts (lack of signal intensity). Gradient echo (T2*) sequences are very sensitive to these effects and therefore produce the most artifact. Fast spin echo sequences require multiple, refocusing 180° pulses and result in considerable shortening of the echo time (TE). These factors lead to decreased magnetic susceptibility effects and better images. Conventional spin echo images result in intermediate artifacts (between those produced on T2* and fast spin echo T2-weighted images). Titanium hardware results in less artifacts than those caused by stainless steel materials.

Clinical History: You are shown radiographs of four patients who underwent posterior spinal fixation (one of these patients also had an anterior stabilization procedure).

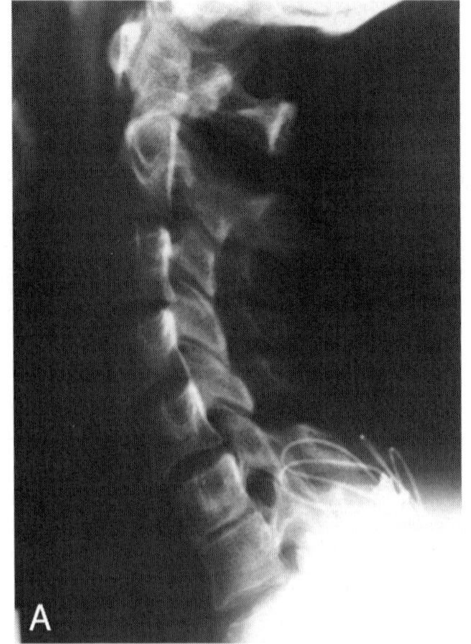

Figure 7.8 A

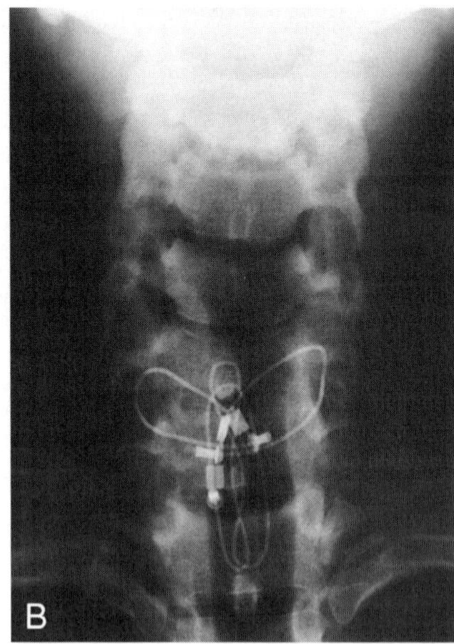

Figure 7.8 B

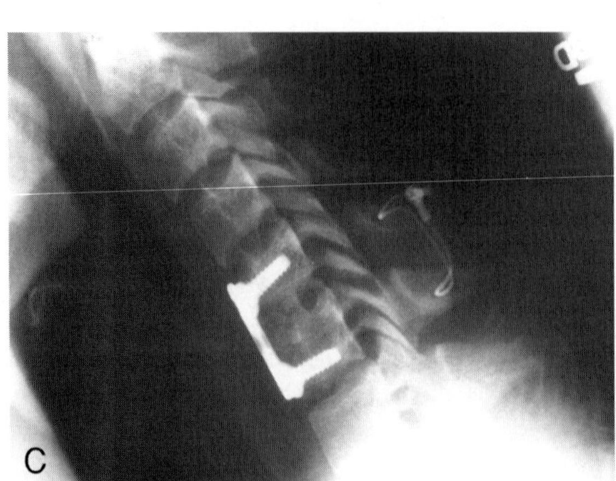

Figure 7.8 C

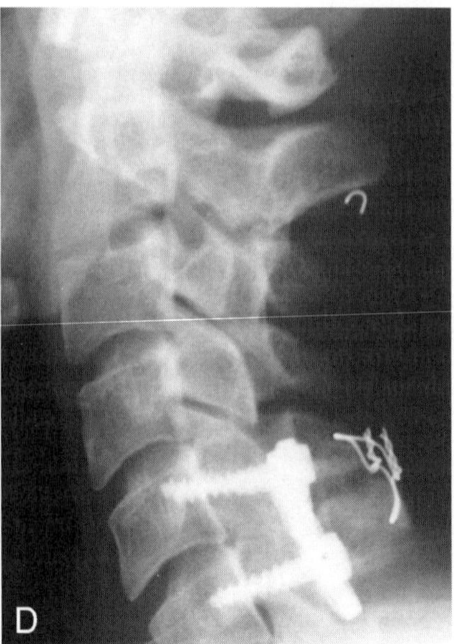

Figure 7.8 D

(continued)

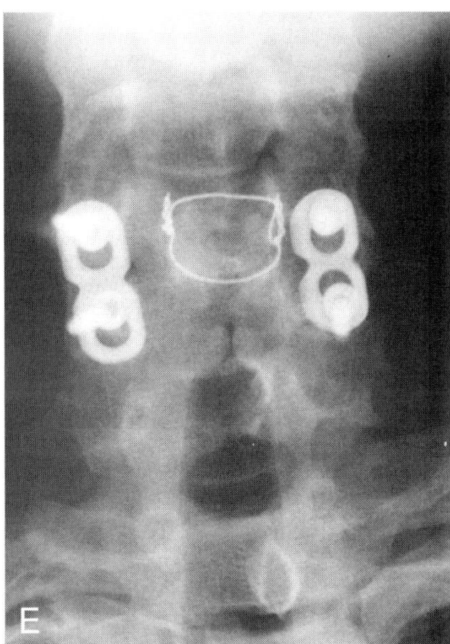

Figure 7.8 E

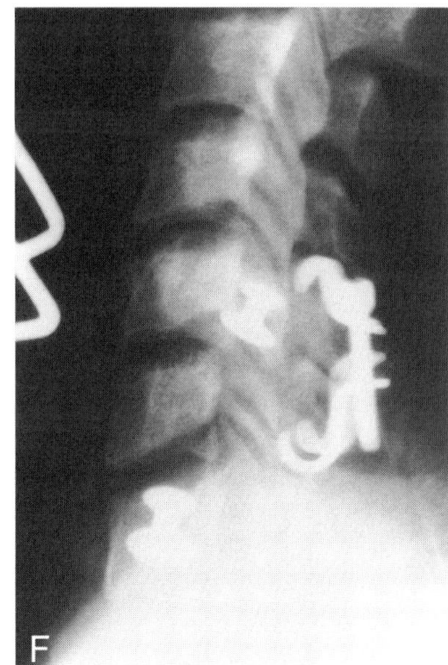

Figure 7.8 F

Findings: In the first patient, lateral and frontal radiographs (Figs. A and B) show Songer steel cables wrapping around the laminae and spinous processes of C6-C7. Note the decreased disk space height as this level. In the second patient, a lateral radiograph (Fig. C) shows anterior plating of C5-C6 held by unicortical screws and a solid appearing bone fusion at this level. Interspinous cable is also present. In the third patient, lateral and frontal radiographs (Figs. D and E) show bilateral plates and screws in the lateral masses of C5-C6. There is interspinous wire at this level and a wire fragment posterior to C2. In the last patient, a lateral radiograph (Fig. F) shows Halifax clamps at the C5-C6 level.

Diagnosis: Adequate appearing posterior fusions (and anterior fusion in the second patient).

Discussion: The posterior surgical approach is the most common procedure for stabilizing the cervical spine. Placement of wires and plates are commonly done in unstable trauma patients. The posterior procedures include: wraparound interspinous wiring or cabling, interfacetal wiring, facet wiring with bone grafting, and interspinous wiring reinforced with methylmethacrylate. These procedures are generally done at the C2-C7 levels. Interspinous and interfacetal wirings are considered safe because the dura does not need to be opened. Wiring of facets does carry the risk of injuring the vertebral arteries. Sublaminar placement of wires or cables is a relatively simple and common procedure. Plating of the lateral masses and facets provides greater strength but carries the risk of the screws injuring the nerve roots, fatigue and fracturing of the devices, dislodgement, pseudoarthrosis formation, and instability. Dural tears may also occur. Songer self-locking cables provide greater tensile strength than do Luque wires. These cables are made of braided steel filaments. Halifax clamps work by attaching the adjoining laminae until no motion is possible. This procedure is commonly used in the upper cervical region (C1-C2) and less often in the lower cervical spine. An H-shaped bone graft is often placed between the spinous processes to promote fusion.

CASE 9

Clinical History: You are shown the images of a patient who underwent a procedure for increasing the diameter of the spinal canal.

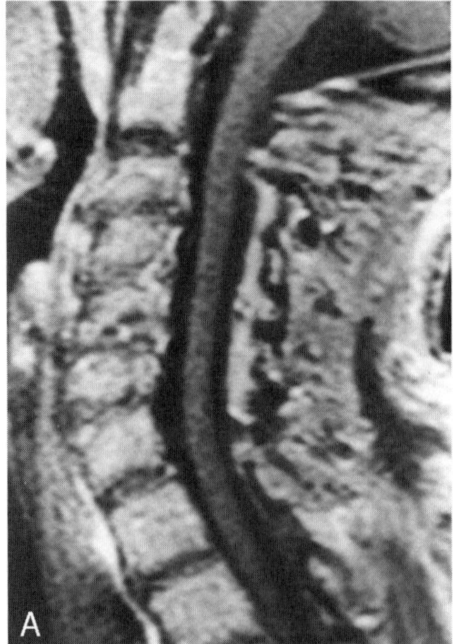

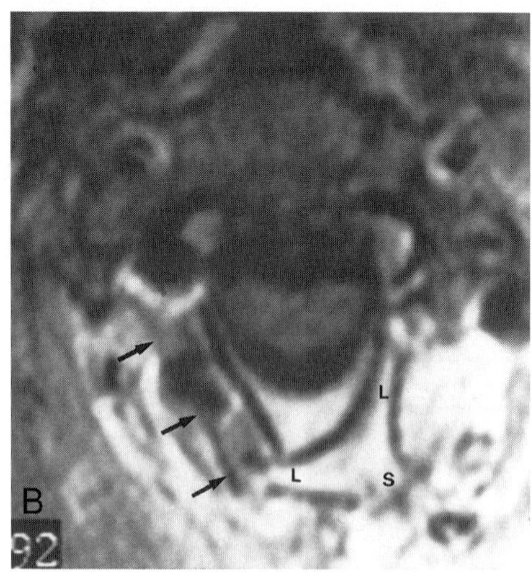

Figure 7.9 A   Figure 7.9 B

Findings: Midsagittal MR T1-weighted image (Fig. A) shows increased anteroposterior diameter of the spinal canal from C3 to C6. At these levels, the configuration of the posterior elements appears unusual. Axial MR T1-weighted image (Fig. B) at C4 shows that the posterior vertebral arch (L = laminae, S = spinous process) has been rotated and hinged by a tubular bone graft (arrows) on the right side, resulting in augmentation of the spinal canal area. (Case courtesy of R. M. Quencer, M.D., Miami, FL.)

Diagnosis: Laminaplasties.

Discussion: A laminaplasty is a procedure used for increasing the diameter of the spinal canal while preserving the protection and stability offered by the posterior elements. This procedure is used in cases of myelopathy secondary to multilevel spondylolysis and ossification of the posterior longitudinal ligament. For this procedure, the laminae are incised bilaterally and one side is sutured with the posterior arch rotated outwardly. The "open door" side is then fixed by inserting a graft in its place. The overall diameter of the spinal canal is increased about 5 mm in its anteroposterior dimension using this procedure, and the stability of the spine is preserved, obviating fixation procedures. Complications of this procedure include recurrence of spinal canal narrowing secondary to misplacement of the bone "open door" and transient paresis of the shoulder girdle muscles secondary to a tethering effect upon the lower cervical nerve roots. This last complication is usually seen in the immediate postsurgical period and resolves spontaneously in the majority of cases.

CASE 10

Clinical History: You are shown images from four patients who underwent different posterior stabilization procedures at the craniocervical junction.

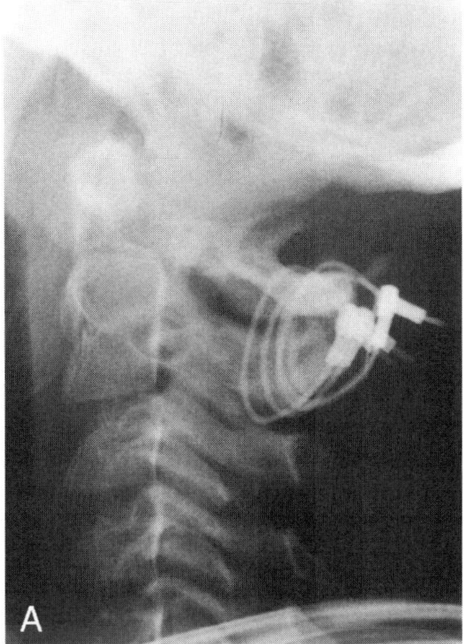

Figure 7.10 A

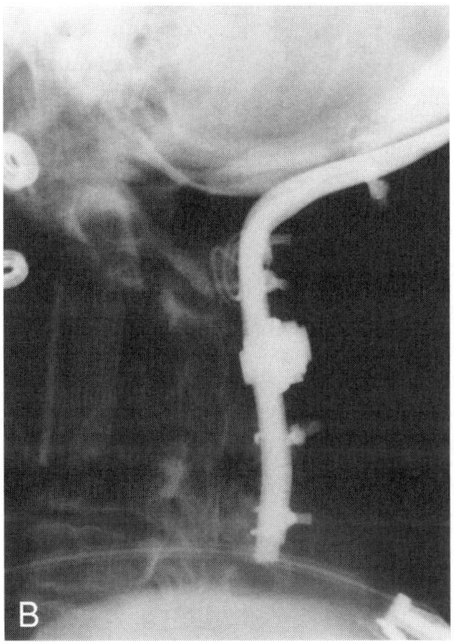

Figure 7.10 B

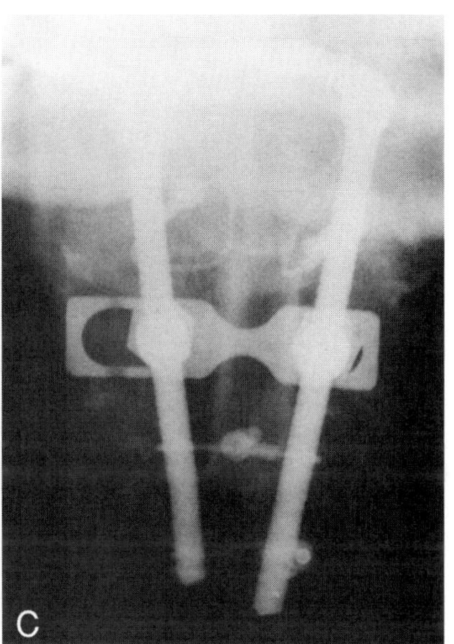

Figure 7.10 C

(continued)

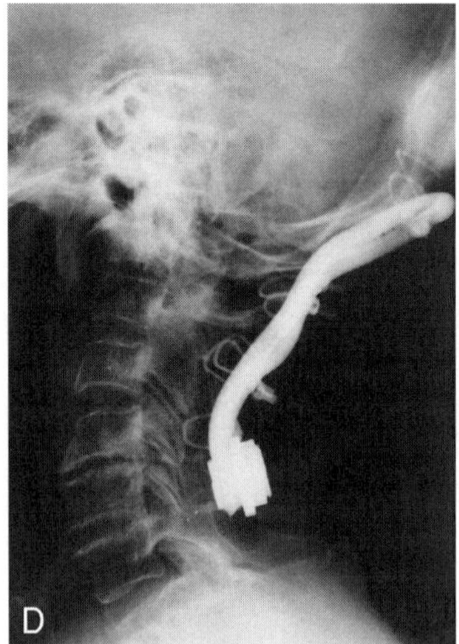

Figure 7.10 D

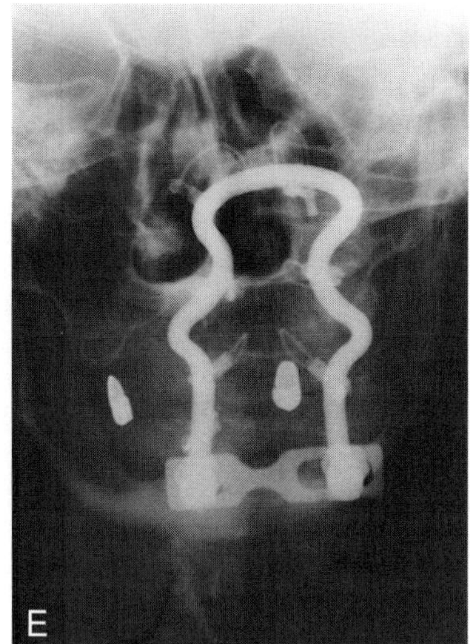

Figure 7.10 E

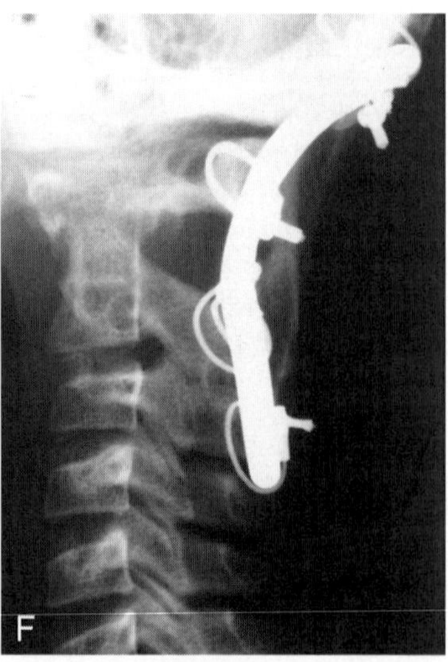

Figure 7.10 F

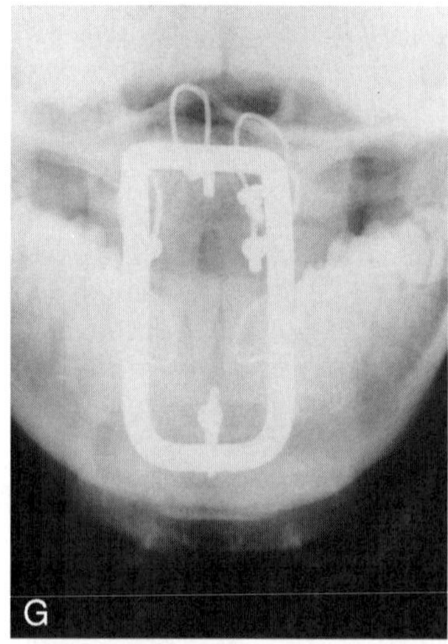

Figure 7.10 G

Findings: In the first patient, a lateral radiograph (Fig. A) shows interspinous cables bridging C1 and C2. Lateral and frontal radiographs (Figs. B and C) in the second patient show a metal loop extending from the occiput to the upper cervical vertebrae. In the third patient, lateral and frontal radiographs (Figs. D and E) show the same procedure, but the metal loop extends further down anchoring the first five cervical vertebrae. In the last patient, lateral and frontal radiographs (Fig. F and G) show a different device extending from the occiput to C1 and C2.

Diagnosis: Brooks fusion (first case), Hartshill-Ransford loop (second and third cases), and Luque rectangle (fourth case).

Discussion: Indications for posterior fusion of the craniocervical junction include instability, intractable pain, cervical osteoporosis with loss of bone substance, severe rheumatoid arthritis, congenital anomalies of the dens, and trauma. In a Brooks fusion, Songer steel braided cables are passed under the spinous processes of C1 and C2. In addition, a bone graft is inserted between the laminae to promote permanent fusion. This technique prevents subluxation because it limits flexion at this level. The Hartshill-Ransford device is a malleable metal loop developed to maintain occipitocervical and atlantoaxial stability and to control progressive vertical migration of the dens. These loops are contoured to fit each patient and are attached to the laminae with wires and to the plates with screws. The Luque rectangles are made of smooth, round, and prebent metal which fits the occipitocervical junction. It is fixed in place with wires in the occipital bone and laminae. The last two procedures may require the placement of interlaminar bone grafts to promote a permanent fusion.

CASE 11

Clinical History: Both of these patients underwent the same procedure for C1-C2 trauma and instability.

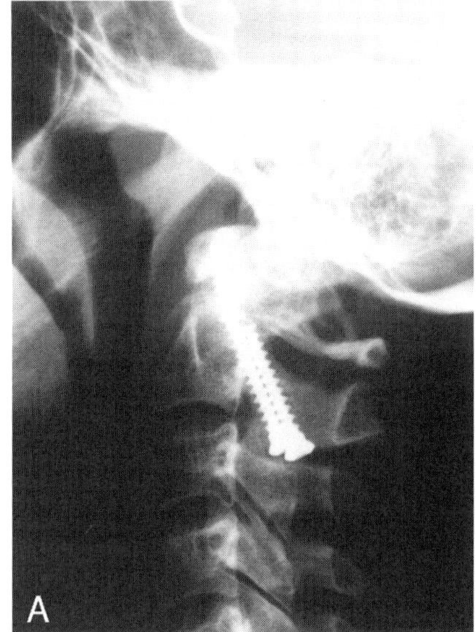

Figure 7.11 A

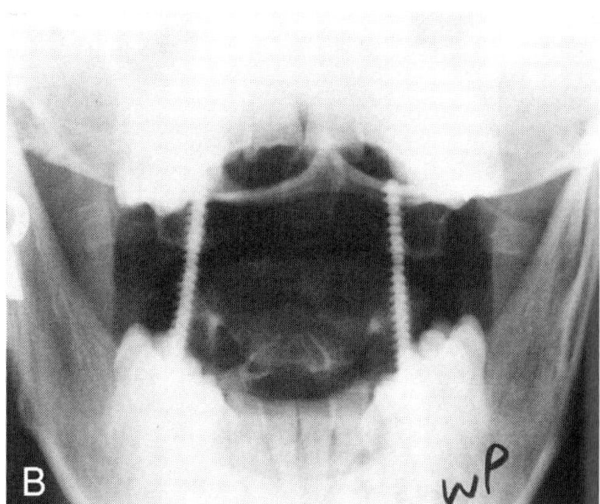

Figure 7.11 B

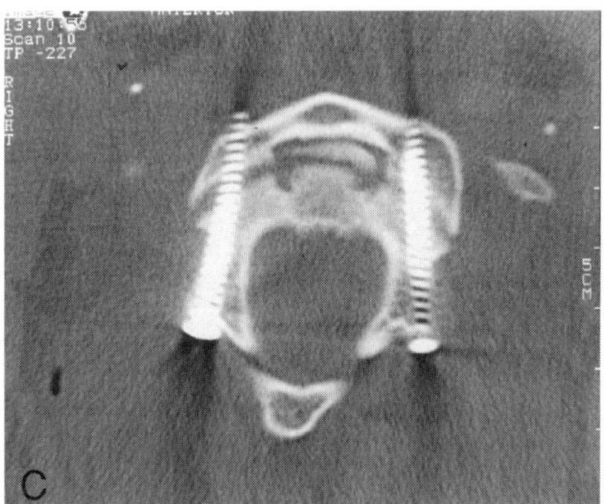

Figure 7.11 C

(continued)

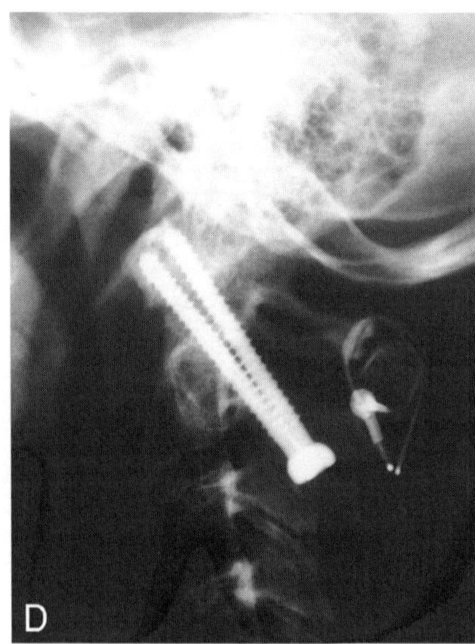

Figure 7.11 D

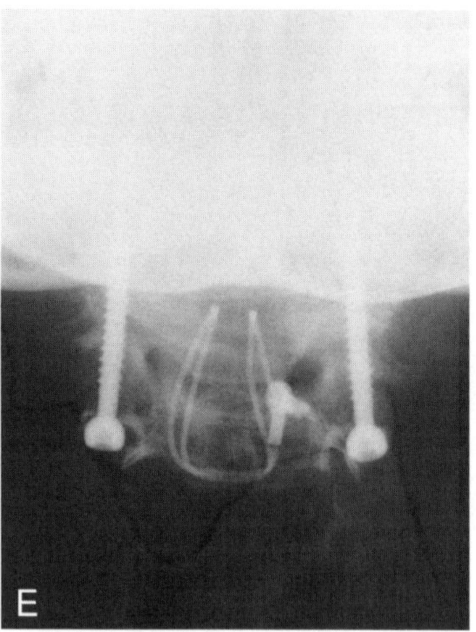

Figure 7.11 E

Findings: In the first patient, lateral and frontal radiographs (Figs. A and B) show bilateral screws fixating C1 and C2. Axial and oblique CT (Fig. C) in the same patient shows the screws crossing the facet joints and a fracture at the base of the dens. In the second patient, lateral and frontal radiographs (Figs. D and E) show transarticular screws and in addition an interspinous cable.

Diagnosis: Posterior transarticular screw fixation of C1 and C2.

Discussion: Posterior transarticular screw fixation was introduced in 1979 and has become a popular alternative to C1-C2 posterior wiring. The screws traverse the articular pillars of C2 and end in the lateral masses of C1 crossing the facet joints. After this procedure, there is no motion of C1 on C2, and instability is reduced. There is a risk of injuring the vertebral arteries, and determining their position before surgery is important. For this purpose, either CT or MR imaging may be used. There is an aberrant and deep course of one or both vertebral arteries through the lateral masses of C2 in approximately 10% of the population. Such a course precludes the insertion of one or both transarticular screws. The planar images need to be obtained in an angle that allows for optimal visualization of the lateral masses of C2 and their relationship to the C1 counterparts. On MR, gradient echo images are optimal as they allow for good definition of bone and flow-related enhancement. CT may be done by angulation of the gantry or by obtaining spiral images through C1-C2 and then reformatting them to the correct angle. Unilateral transarticular screw is said to offer adequate stability when two screws may not be used.

Clinical History: A young male patient suffered a fracture of T11 and underwent treatment. He is now asymptomatic.

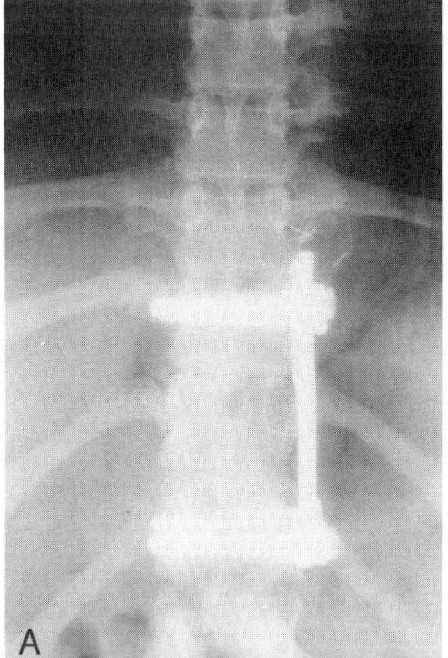

Figure 7.12 A

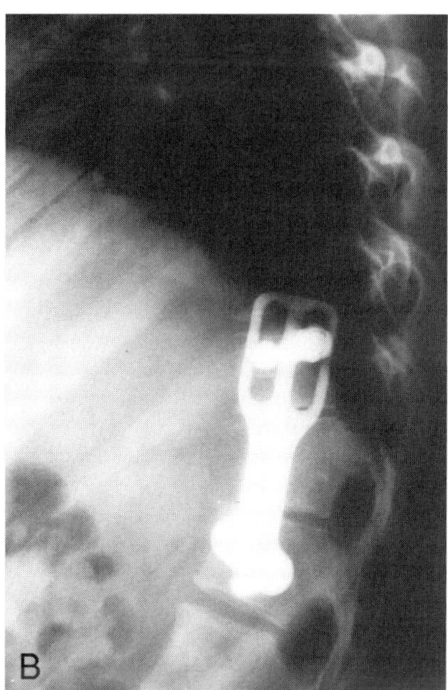

Figure 7.12 B

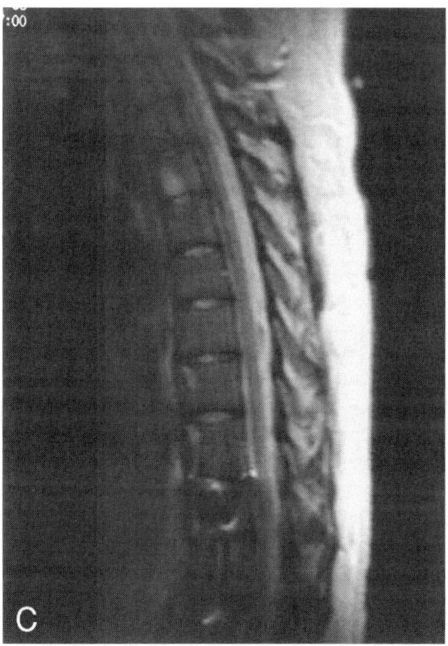

Figure 7.12 C

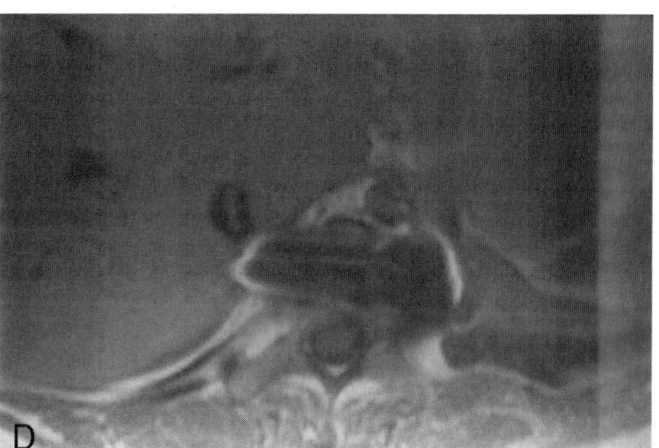

Figure 7.12 D

Findings: Frontal and lateral radiographs (Figs. A and B) show a short lateral vertebral plate bridging T10-T12. There are bicortical titanium screws and a fibular graft. In the same patient, midsagittal MR fast spin echo T2-weighted image (Fig. C) shows artifact from the hardware that does not obscure the spinal canal. Axial MR T1-weighted image (Fig. D) at T10 shows good visualization of the spinal canal and its contents. It was obtained by placing the frequency encoding direction parallel to the long axis of the screws.

(continued)

Diagnosis: Lateral plate and fibular bone graft fusion of the thoracic spine.

Discussion: The anterior thoracic approach is used for placement of hardware either in the frontal or lateral aspects of the spinal column. It was first used for the treatment of tuberculosis and spondylisthesis and is now used for patients with degenerative disease, failed posterior fusions, other infections (including pyogenic), and some tumors that affect the vertebral bodies. In addition, it may be used to treat patients with fractures, particularly when posterior displacement of bone fragment arising in the vertebral bodies is present. The fusion may be further stabilized by the use of methylmethacrylate cement and placement of bone grafts. Anterior plating increases stability but does not alter the deformity. Intraoperative complications of this procedure include vascular, pleural, and pulmonary injuries. Postoperative complications are infection, paralytic ileus, and hematomas. Inaccurate placement of the hardware may lead to compression of the nerve roots and spinal cord.

Clinical History: You are shown two examples of posterior fixation.

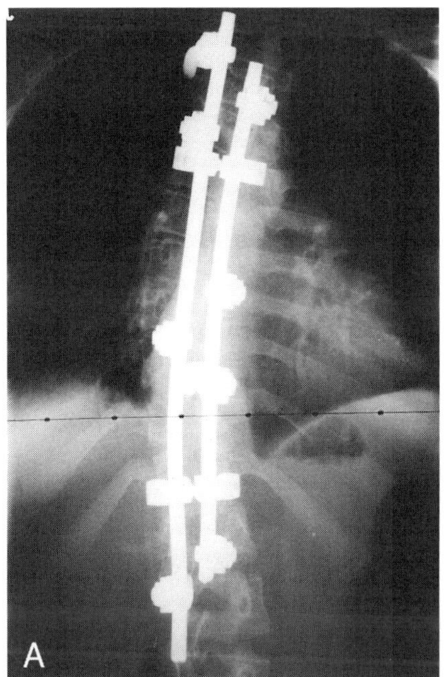
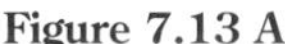

Figure 7.13 A

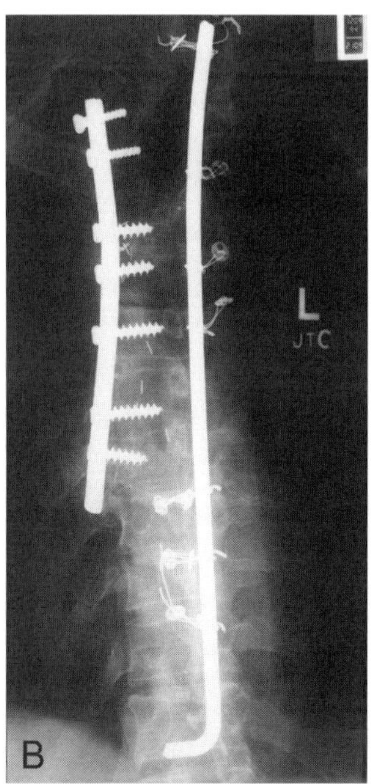

Figure 7.13 B

Findings: In the first patient, a frontal radiograph (Fig. A) shows bilateral Harrington rods attached to the spine with multiple sublaminar hooks. There is mild thoracic dextro-scoliosis. In the second patient, a frontal radiograph (Fig. B) shows a right lateral long plate attached by unicortical screws. There is a left posterior Luque rod attached to the laminae by Luque wires (Drummond buttons prevent the wires from pulling through the bone). This patient had progressive scoliosis after resection and radiation for a costovertebral chondrosarcoma.

Diagnosis: Two methods of posterior fixation.

Discussion: Most stabilization and fixation procedures in the thoracic and lumbar regions are accomplished by a posterior approach. Fixation may be achieved by devices resulting in compression or distraction of the spine. Most of these devices are comprised of rods or plates or a combination of both. They are attached to the spine by sublaminar and interspinous wires or cables, laminar or pedicle hooks, and pedicle screws. Rods are employed where long spans are needed. Harrington rods are some of the most commonly used and are attached to the spine with upgoing (under the laminae) and downgoing (over the laminae) hooks. The use of both types of hooks greatly reduces the risk of dislodgement. Luque rods are also popular and may be recognized because of the smooth, L-shaped appearance. They are attached to the spine by wires, and one of the advantages of these rods are that the wires are able to slide on them freely, allowing for better position during surgery. Luque rods may also be bent to configure to each individual patient. The short limb of the L of these rods is passed through a spinous process to prevent rotation of the device. They are used primarily in patients with scoliosis where they apply lateral flexion in an attempt to correct it.

Clinical History: You are shown the imaging studies of two patients who had prior spinal surgery. The first (Figs. A–C) underwent an occipito-atlantal decompression for a Chiari 1 malformation. The second (Figs. D–F) underwent repair for a myelocele.

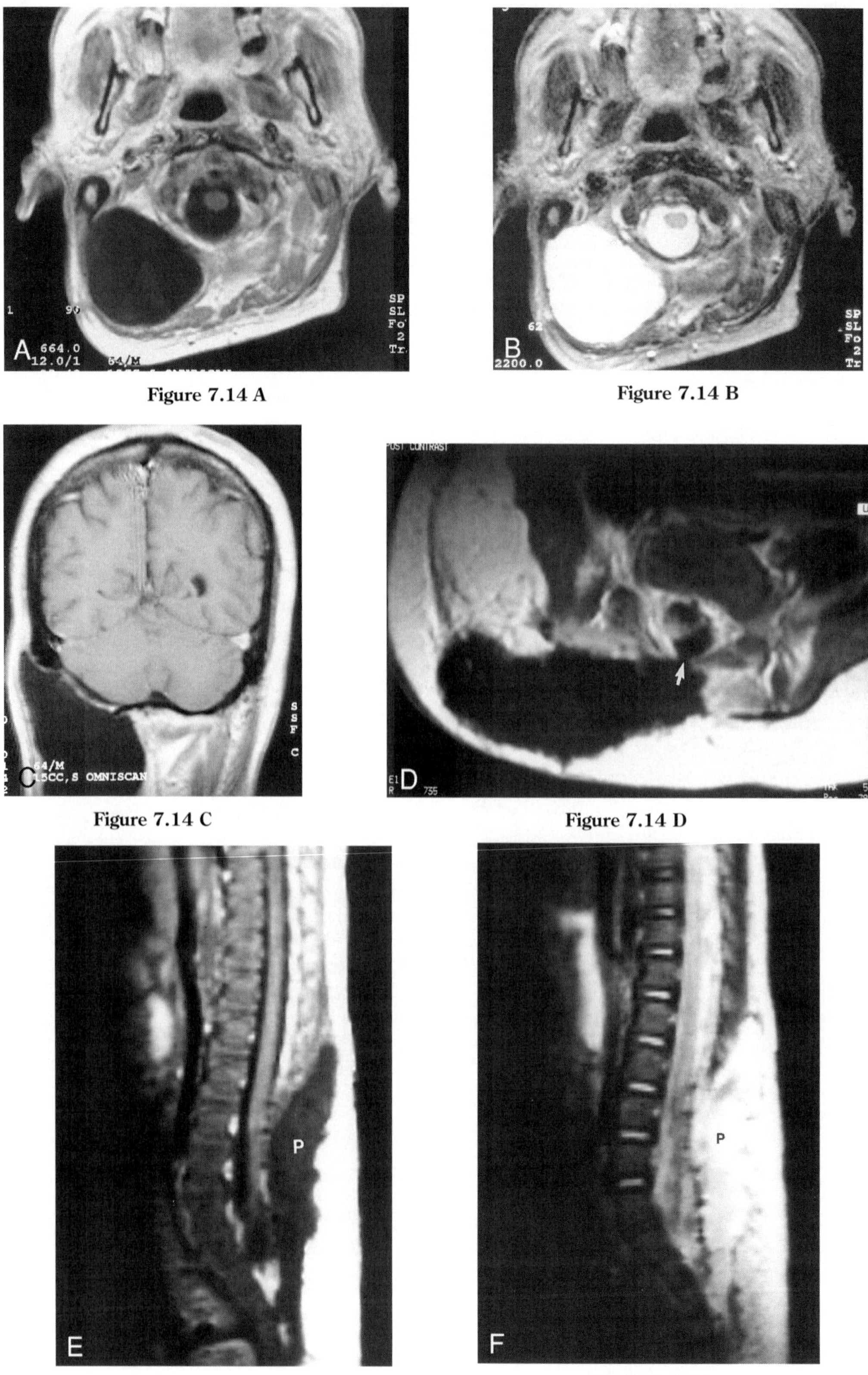

Figure 7.14 A

Figure 7.14 B

Figure 7.14 C

Figure 7.14 D

Figure 7.14 E

Figure 7.14 F

(continued)

Findings: In the first patient, an axial MR postcontrast T1-weighted image (Fig. A) shows a nonenhancing collection of fluidlike signal intensity in the right suboccipital region. On a corresponding T2-weighted image (Fig. B), the abnormality is of high signal intensity (equivalent to cerebrospinal fluid [CSF]). Coronal T1-weighted image (Fig. C) shows the extent of this fluid collection. In the second patient, axial MR T1-weighted image (Fig. D) shows a large right posterior fluid collection communicating (arrow) with the thecal sac. Midsagittal T1-weighted image (Fig. E) shows the full extent of this collection (P) and a low positioned spinal cord ending at L5. Corresponding T2-weighted image (Fig. F) shows that the collection (P) is of high signal intensity.

Diagnosis: Postsurgical pseudomeningoceles.

Discussion: Pseudomeningoceles are collections of CSF adjacent to the cranium or the spine. They are generally the sequelae of surgery or trauma. A tear in the dura and arachnoid leads to escape of CSF and its accumulation in the soft tissues. They have no true capsule. They generally present as a mass and continuous headaches caused by escape of CSF. Patients may also report low back pain in the lumbar region when they arise. Occasionally, these patients may become infected, resulting in meningitis. When pseudomeningoceles are located paraspinally, they are usually posterior but rarely may be anterior and present as masses in the neck, pleural cavities, retroperitoneum, and pelvis. Pseudomeningoceles are generally only filled with CSF but some large ones may contain nerve roots and, rarely, even the spinal cord. Large pseudomeningoceles may also erode bone. In babies, most pseudomeningoceles occur as a complication of the surgery for open spinal dysraphism.

CASE 15

Clinical History: This patient underwent surgery for a congenital anomaly.

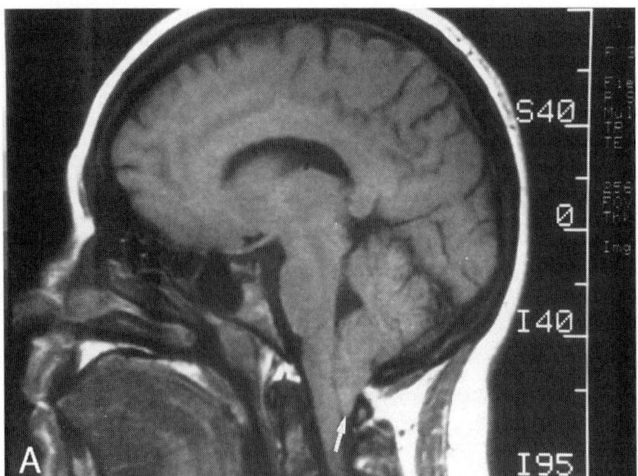

Figure 7.15 A

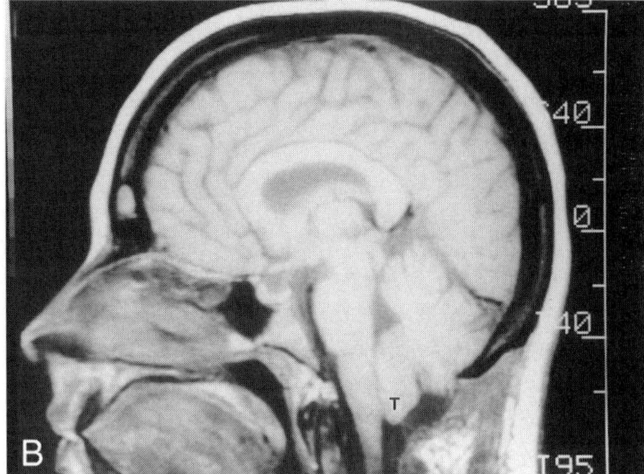

Figure 7.15 B

Findings: Preoperative midsagittal MR T1-weighted image (Fig. A) shows a low position of the cerebellar tonsils (arrow). They are approximately 8 mm below the level of the foramen magnum and are triangular. Postoperative corresponding T1-weighted image (Fig. B) shows that the cerebellar tonsils (T) are now in a more normal position and have a more normal shape. The occipital aspect of the foramen magnum and the posterior arch of C1 have been resected to increase the diameter of this region.

Diagnosis: Occipito-atlantal decompression for a Chiari type 1 malformation.

Discussion: A Chiari 1 malformation (see Case #17, Chapter 4) is a structural abnormality and, as such, its treatment is surgical. There is no medical therapy for this condition. In asymptomatic patients, observation may be an alternative to surgery. Patients with syringohydromyelia have progressive symptoms, and therefore decompression is almost always indicated. The presence of increased intracranial pressure is a requirement before embarking on surgical treatment of a Chiari 1 malformation. In some patients, ventricular shunting relieves all symptoms. After surgery, over 70% of patients show stabilization or improvement in their symptoms.

CASE 16

Clinical History: This patient underwent surgery for a spinal cord abnormality.

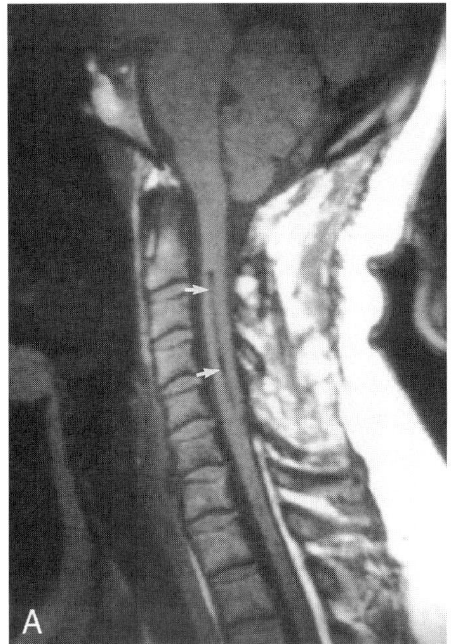

Figure 7.16 A

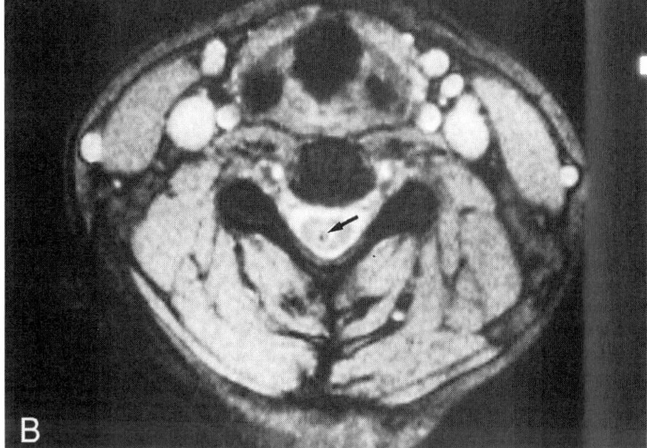

Figure 7.16 B

Findings: Midsagittal MR T1-weighted image (Fig. A) shows a linear hypointensity (arrows) corresponding to a catheter. Axial T2-weighted image (Fig. B) shows the catheter (arrow) inside the spinal cord.

Diagnosis: Decompressed syringohydromyelia. Intramedullary catheter.

Discussion: In some patients with Chiari malformations, decompression of hydrocephalus leads to decompression of syringohydromyelia, whereas in other patients, direct treatment of the spinal cord fluid-filled cysts is required. Successful therapy of a syrinx leads to improvement or stabilization of the patient's symptoms, including scoliosis. Syringohydromyelia secondary to tumors or arteriovenous malformations requires treatment of the primary disorder. Patients with posttraumatic cord cysts do not show dramatic clinical improvement after shunting of cysts. They do, however, experience improvement in pain. When surgery is done, a 1-cm incision is made on the dorsal surface of spinal cord at its thinnest level and in the region of the posterior columns. A silastic wick may be left at this opening to ensure its patency. Treatment may also be accomplished by insertion of a micro-shunt catheter into the cyst. Multicompartmental cysts may be evaluated presurgically by MR imaging or intraoperatively by sonography (see Case #19, Chapter 4). The shunts extend from the cyst to the subarachnoid space and less often to the pleural or peritoneal cavities.

Clinical History: You are shown the CT study (Fig. A) in a patient with known rheumatoid arthritis who underwent a decompression procedure.

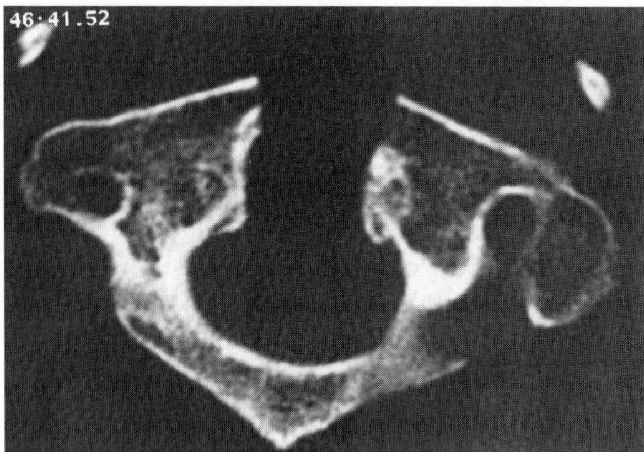

Figure 7.17

Findings: Axial CT section (bone window setting) shows complete absence of the dens.

Diagnosis: Transoral resection of the dens.

Discussion: Transoral resection of the dens provides the most direct route for decompression at this level. The palate needs to split and it is a technically demanding procedure which is not widely performed. It is generally used for patients with rheumatoid arthritis and pannus about the dens, basilar invagination, drainage of C1 and C2 abscesses, and biopsy of tumor at this level. This procedure carries risk of damaging the spinal cord and a postoperative infection risk of up to 50% (due to proximity of the mucosa). Intraoperative fluoroscopy is used to guide the resection. A significant number of patients are at risk of developing instability at the atlanto-axial level and require a posterior cranio-cervical fusion.